LOSE WEIGHT, TARGET BELLY FAT, AND LOWER BLOOD SUGAR WITH THIS TESTED PLAN FROM THE EDITORS OF Prevention

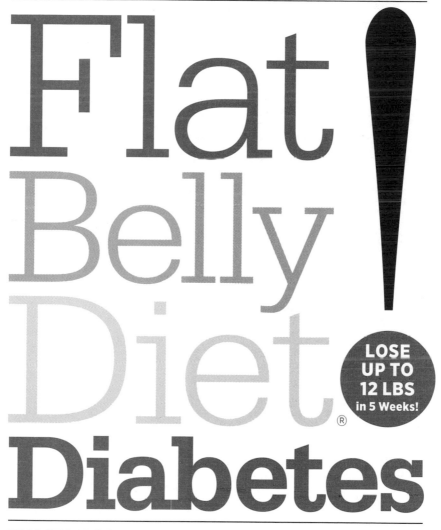

Flat Belly Diet!
Diabetes

LOSE UP TO 12 LBS in 5 Weeks!

BY LIZ VACCARIELLO, Editor-in-Chief, coauthor of the *New York Times* best-selling diet, with Gillian Arathuzik, RD, CDE, and Medical Advisor Steven V. Edelman, MD

RODALE

© 2010 by Rodale Inc.

Printed in the United States of America
Rodale Inc. makes every effort to use acid-free ♾, recycled paper ♻.

Book design by Jill Armus and Maureen O'Brien

Photo credits for insert: Orange Frappe with Strawberries, Grilled Pork Chops with Olives, Oranges and Onion, Roasted Potatoes with Blue Cheese and Walnuts, Chocolate Zucchini Snack Cake, Mexican-Style Stuffed Peppers, Garlic Shrimp with Spanish Smoked Pepper Sauce © Marcus Nilsson; Tortellini Pasta Salad, Salmon with Snow Peas, Chocolate-Almond Macaroons © Con Poulos; Baked Lemon Chicken © Rita Maas; Fusilli with Mushrooms and Chard © David Prince

Before/after/now photos by Jonathan Pozniak; exercise photos by Tom MacDonald/Rodale Images; photo page 54 by Marcus Nilsson, food styling by Anne Disrude, prop styling by Deborah Williams, photo editing by Leah Vinluan

Library of Congress Cataloging-in-Publication Data

Flat belly diet! diabetes : lose weight, target belly fat, and lower blood sugar with this tested plan from the editors of prevention / by Liz Vaccariello, editor-in-chief ; with Gillian Arathuzik and medical advisor Steven V. Edelman.
    p.   cm.
Includes bibliographical references and index.
ISBN-13 978-1-60529-685-2 hardcover
ISBN-10 1-60529-685-6 hardcover
   1. Diabetes—Diet therapy.   2. Reducing diets.   3. Abdomen.   I. Vaccariello, Liz.
II. Arathuzik, Gillian.
RC662.F657 2010
616.4'620654—dc22   2009051069

2   4   6   8   10   9   7   5   3   1   direct hardcover

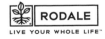

RODALE
LIVE YOUR WHOLE LIFE™

We inspire and enable people to improve their lives and the world around them
For more of our products visit **rodalestore.com** or call 800-848-4735

FOR THE MILLIONS LIVING
WITH DIABETES, SO THEY CAN LEARN
HOW DELICIOUS AND FILLING
HEALTHY FOOD CAN BE!

—Liz and Gillian

contents

acknowle

We dedicate the Flat Belly Diet to the readers of *Prevention*—all 11 million of you—who have told us in no uncertain terms that belly fat is your biggest physical challenge.

OUR GRATITUDE to the Rodale family. For generations, through their magazines, books, and online properties, they have been committed to a special mission, that of giving people the tools and inspiration to live their whole lives. Our most heartfelt thanks to CEO Maria Rodale and former CEO Steve Murphy, whose leadership means Rodale is the kind of company where creativity is nurtured and the highest standards are set—and met—daily.

Like magazines, books are a collaborative effort, and this one is no exception. Very special thanks to Gregg Michaelson, Karen Rinaldi, Beth Lamb, Jenny Sucov, Bill Stump, and Marlea Clark, who were there at the beginning. To Robin Shallow, who never met an idea she didn't improve, and Bethridge Toovell and Lauren Paul, who are tireless in their enthusiasm, support, and belief in this plan.

You would not be holding this book in your hands without editor Andrea Au Levitt. All thanks to her dedicated team, including Marielle Messing, Carol Angstadt, Chris Krogermeier, Sara Cox, JoAnn Brader, Hope Clarke, Brooke Myers, and Liz Krenos. We couldn't have crossed the finish line without Gillian Arathuzik, Sari Harrar, and Steven Edelman, who worked relentlessly to make this plan diabetes-friendly, design all-new

dgments

delicious Flat Belly Diet recipes, and run our test panel. We'd also like to extend our gratitude to the initial test panel members, who bravely sought flat bellies as our guinea pigs during the spring of 2009. Thank you, Donna Branson, Jay Hargis, Anne Harrington, Phil Hernandez, Susan Hoar, Beth Gregory, Steve Lipman, Paula Martin, and all their families for providing us with the essential insights that helped us develop this book beyond daily meal plans.

Big hugs to *Prevention*'s dazzling creative director, Jill Armus, and deputy art director Maureen O'Brien, for their vision of *Flat Belly Diet! Diabetes*. And to *Prevention* fitness director Michele Stanten, whose expertise makes Chapter 11 one of the most authoritative sources of information on banishing belly fat with exercise.

Thanks also to Susan Graves, Courtenay Smith, and Polly Chevalier for their wise counsel and endless and sunny support. And to the smartest photo team in the business, including *Prevention*'s Danielle Planells and Leah Vinluan. Our deep gratitude to original *Flat Belly Diet!* coauthor Cynthia Sass, MPH, RD, and former brand editor Leah McLaughlin, who were critical to developing the original plan upon which this is all based.

Finally, thank you to our husbands, Steve Vaccariello and John Arathuzik, for putting up with all the late—late!—nights and helping us come up with creative recipe ideas, and to our daughters, Olivia and Sophia Vaccariello and Molly Arathuzik—whose birth, conveniently one week late, helped Mommy keep her deadline! We love you all!

WHY

THE FLAT BELLY DIET

DIABETES?

YOUR BELLY FAT and your blood sugar. The two are tightly entwined, linked by a simple cause-and-effect equation—the more belly fat you have, the greater the odds that blood sugar issues will touch your life someday (or already have!). Once upon a time, scientists tell us, the ability to store fat in our torsos was an amazing, life-saving asset. But as you stand in front of your mirror or sit in your kitchen flipping through the pages of this book, I suspect that the belly behind your waistband is a source of frustration and worry. Same goes, I'm thinking, for your blood sugar: If you've been diagnosed with type 2 diabetes or with prediabetes or are concerned about your risk for developing diabetes, I bet you'd like to feel that *you* control your blood sugar rather than having it control your life. And, of course, who wouldn't like a flatter belly?

I'm here to tell you that you can accomplish both.

You *can* lose your belly fat. You *can* erase stubborn pounds. You *can* protect yourself from developing type 2 diabetes. And if you already have diabetes, you can gain tighter control over your blood sugar—and lower your risk for serious complications such as high blood pressure, heart disease, vision problems, kidney failure, and nerve damage. The great news: You can accomplish all of these important goals without feeling hungry or deprived or signing up for a lifetime of bland and tasteless food. Yes, my friends, you can have pasta! You can get there *because* you're eating four delicious meals a day, each one packed with real food that just happens to be research-proven to take aim at diabetes and belly fat—including *nuts, peanut butter, chocolate, olive oil, avocados, and olives.*

You read that correctly! On the Flat Belly Diet Diabetes, these belly-flattening, blood-sugar friendly, super-satisfying treats are in the mix of healthy foods you'll eat *at every meal*. This isn't just a nice theory. Rigorous scientific research *and* the real-life experiences of our own Flat Belly Diet Diabetes test panelists prove that this plan works, at every level, to fight fat and pamper your blood sugar.

Grounded in Science

PREVENTION MAGAZINE PUBLISHED THE original Flat Belly Diet! in 2008—and as editor-in-chief, I was amazed by the outpouring of enthusiasm for this innovative, belly-blasting plan and by the response from people with one specific issue: blood sugar. Time and again, women and men who had diabetes, or were at risk for it, asked me: Will this plan work for me? Some readers didn't wait for an answer. One, Lisa Stevens, an Illinois woman with type 2 diabetes, really got my attention when she shared that she'd lost 17 pounds in 4 months, whittled 5.5 inches from her waist, and improved her blood sugar levels dramatically. Wow! At *Prevention*, we've been talking for a decade about the growing diabetes crisis in America and around the world. Not only do more than 24 million Americans already have diabetes,[1] but more than 100 million more are at risk—and most don't even know it. It's a health crisis tied directly to the obesity epidemic—and experts say the link is . . . you guessed it . . . deep belly fat.[2]

Could we formulate a version of the Flat Belly Diet that meets the specific health needs of people with—or at risk for—type 2 diabetes? Could it help with blood sugar control and with lowering diabetes risk for those worried about this important health threat? And, could it target the belly fat that makes us buy oversized shirts and elastic-waist pants, too?

In early 2009, a study conducted by preventive medicine expert David Katz, MD, an associate professor adjunct at the Yale University School of Public Health, gave us an important piece of the answer. Dr. Katz put the Flat Belly Diet to the test. He tracked nine extremely overweight women as they followed this eating plan for 4 weeks, and the results were nothing short of amazing. The study volunteers lost an average of 8.4 pounds and trimmed as much as 3.9 inches from their waistlines—but that wasn't all.

Their visceral fat—the deep and dangerous abdominal fat that wraps around internal organs and pumps harmful, diabetes-related chemicals into the bloo stream—shrank significantly. Measured via high-tech magnetic resonance imaging equipment at the beginning and end of the study, visceral fat shrank by an average of 20 percent and in some women, by as much as 40 percent.

And signs of insulin resistance—a body-chemistry "glitch" you'll be hearing more about in this book because it triggers type 2 diabetes, prediabetes, and an even earlier and very common health condition called metabolic syndrome—were reduced, too. In other words, the foods and portions you'll eat on the Flat Belly Diet Diabetes take aim at two major diabetes triggers: visceral fat and insulin resistance.

Diabetes-Friendly!

As EXCITING AS THESE results were, the Yale study of the Flat Belly Diet looked only at the eating portion of the plan. And it didn't address the plan's effects on women and men who already have diabetes. Before we could bring you this book, I needed confirmation that the full Flat Belly Diet Diabetes plan—our unique eating plan plus an easy exercise routine and stress reduction—would be safe, healthy, and effective for people coping with type 2 diabetes.

Why type 2? Ninety to 95 percent of people with diabetes in the United States have type 2. While it has some genetic origins, type 2 is considered a "lifestyle disease"—meaning that your weight, your activity level, your food choices, and, yes, the amount of belly fat you have all powerfully determine whether and when you'll develop this serious blood sugar problem. In contrast, type 1 diabetes develops when your body simply stops making insulin. If you have type 1, controlling blood sugar involves daily insulin injections. The Flat Belly Diet Diabetes won't necessarily help you with blood sugar control, but it can help you reap plenty of other benefits, including weight loss and a sleeker midsection. Check with your doctor first to be sure the plan is right for you.

I enlisted two compassionate and respected diabetes specialists. Steve Edelman, MD, a professor of medicine in the division of endocrinology and metabolism at the University of California, San Diego, School of Medicine, is the founder and director of the dynamic diabetes self-help organization Taking Control of Your Diabetes (he also wrote a book by the same name) and has had type 1 diabetes himself since the age of 15. Dr. Edelman knows the ins and outs of daily blood sugar management on a very personal level. Then I called registered dietitian Gillian Arathuzik, RD, LDN, CDE, a certified diabetes educator at the world-renowned, Harvard Medical School–affiliated Joslin Diabetes Center in Boston, where every day she helps people with diabetes make healthy diet and lifestyle changes that work for them.

With Dr. Edelman and Gillian, we reviewed hundreds of studies analyzing the effects of food, exercise, and stress reduction on belly fat, blood sugar, and weight. Together, we also reviewed the original Flat Belly Diet plan. Dr. Edelman and Gillian weighed in on issues like blood sugar testing, cholesterol, and blood pressure testing; on the importance of exercise in maintaining healthy blood sugar levels; the effect of nutrients such as carbohydrates, protein, fat, and fiber on blood sugar in people with diabetes; and emerging research on the role of stress reduction in blood sugar control.

Their conclusion: The healthy eating plan at the core of the original Flat Belly Diet, combined with our exercise and stress reduction components, offered some unique advantages for people with blood sugar concerns.

The mix of vegetables, fruit, lean protein, good fats, and whole grains you'll find here is proven to lower diabetes risk. In the landmark Diabetes Prevention Program study sponsored by the National Institutes of Health, it helped people with prediabetes cut their odds for progressing to full-blown, type 2 diabetes by an impressive 58 percent!

But our plan doesn't stop there—and here's where we're unique! Every meal features a delicious, belly-flattening monounsaturated fatty acid—as we like to say, a "MUFA" (pronounced MOO-fah) at every meal. As delicious as they are satisfying, MUFAs are key to the success of the Flat Belly Diet Diabetes—and you won't find them featured like this in any other healthy blood sugar plan! Emerging research points to MUFAs as a potentially powerful strategy for controlling blood sugar and for reducing insulin resistance.

Because controlling blood sugar requires a comprehensive mind-body approach, we knew that exercise and stress relief belonged in the plan, too. Physical activity, Dr. Edelman and Gillian told me, is powerfully effective for lowering blood sugar and sensitizing cells throughout your body to insulin, the hormone that persuades cells to absorb blood sugar. That's why exercise is an integral part of this plan. We also include a 10-minute, progressive muscle relaxation program. We knew it could help melt away tensions that can lead to emotional eating, and we were impressed by studies showing that people who de-stress every day see important blood sugar benefits, too.

BINGO! We had a winner—and this groundbreaking plan is the result!

Real-World Success

OUR PLAN HAD TO pass one more hurdle: the "real world" test. Could the Flat Belly Diet Diabetes help real people with type 2 diabetes and prediabetes lose pounds, shed belly fat, and improve their blood sugar levels?

I'm here to tell you that it does all of those things and more. Our *Prevention*-sponsored test of the plan confirms it: In just 5 weeks, our nine test panelists—all diagnosed with type 2 diabetes or prediabetes—lost a total of 27.5 inches from their waists and hips, dropped more than 58 pounds, and were thrilled by their consistently lower, steadier blood sugar levels. Many also saw improvements in LDL and HDL cholesterol and in levels of a heart-threatening blood fat called triglycerides. (That's important, because diabetes quadruples heart attack risk!)

Cooking and Eating— For the Whole Family

When Donna Branson, 51, a registered nurse, began cooking the Flat Belly Diet Diabetes meals, her husband jumped right in. "He absolutely loves it," she says. "He doesn't have diabetes like I do, and sometimes he ate larger portions, but he lost 14 pounds in 5 weeks, his total cholesterol dropped from 200 to 144, and he lost a couple of inches from his waistline. His pants were getting too loose!" Donna never had to prepare two meals—the couple both loved everything from the almond and pork meatballs to the broiled fish to the chicken piccata paired with a spinach and pear salad. "The test panel is over, but we're still eating this way because it tastes so good," she raves.

The filling, tasty, and quick-to-prepare meals in this plan are intended to work for the whole family—no need to make two different meals! Proof that it works: Many of

It's no wonder, then, that our test panelists raved about their results:

■ "My blood sugars were absolutely amazing on this diet—that's really, really inspiring," Anne Harrington told us.

■ "I love nuts, I love avocado, and I love olives, so I loved this diet," said panelist Steve Lipman. "And when I heard I could also eat chocolate, I was excited! The results were great—I lost 11 pounds. My blood sugar was already very healthy, but it got even better."

■ "I was never hungry. And my morning blood sugars were the healthiest they've ever been," noted Beth Gregory, who lost 3 inches from her waist and 1½ inches from her hips.

■ "I've lost weight before, but this time everybody's telling me how great I look—it's as if my whole body has changed shape," said Susan Hoar.

■ "I've been battling prediabetes for 15 years now," said Joe Sicurella. "Diabetes runs in my family, and I've seen what it can do to your health and to your life. I lost nearly 13 pounds in 5 weeks, lost an inch and a half from my waist, and saw my A1c drop a little. It's all good news."

our test panelists told us that their spouses and their children enjoyed the food as much as they did. And while your spouse may also opt to follow the plan along with you as a way to lose weight, we want to emphasize that this is not a weight-loss plan for kids. "Even if you and your pediatrician think your child is overweight, the best approach is a healthy diet and getting enough physical activity—such as about an hour a day—so that they can grow into their weight, rather than losing pounds," says Gillian. "Children need plenty of nutrients and sufficient calories for growth and development. Cutting calories is not recommended for them." (You'll find more details about adjusting the plan for kids, preteens, and teens in Chapter 8.) Looking for even more delicious recipes? Watch for the *Flat Belly Diet! Family Cookbook*!

The Flat Belly Diet Diabetes Is for You If . . .

PREVENTION ESTIMATES THAT AT least 100 million American adults have metabolic syndrome, prediabetes, or undiagnosed type 2 diabetes right now—and don't even know it. That's almost half of all adults in the United States. In November of 2008, the Centers for Disease Control and Prevention released a survey showing that *just 4 percent* of people with prediabetes have been told by their doctors that they have it.[3] Experts note that doctors sometimes downplay the importance of prediabetes—shrugging it off as a "borderline" or "mild" problem. Same goes for another prediabetic condition called metabolic syndrome.

This book is for you if you meet any *one* of the following criteria:

1: YOU HAVE TYPE 2 DIABETES. The most common form of diabetes, type 2 is usually associated with insulin resistance—when cells throughout your body stop obeying insulin's commands to let in blood sugar. (In contrast, type 1 diabetes happens when your body stops producing insulin.)

2: YOU'VE BEEN DIAGNOSED WITH PREDIABETES. You have prediabetes if your blood sugar is between 100 and 125 mg/dl on a fasting blood sugar test (measured first thing in the morning before breakfast) or 140 to 200 mg/dl on an oral glucose tolerance test. One in four people with prediabetes develops full-blown, type 2 diabetes within 3 to 5 years, and 8 out of 10 develop it over the course of their lifetimes—*if they don't take steps to prevent it*, says the Centers for Disease Control and Prevention.[4]

3: YOUR WAIST MEASURES 40 INCHES OR MORE FOR MEN, 35 INCHES OR MORE FOR WOMEN. A wide waistline is an indicator of dangerous fat accumulating deep in your abdomen. In one study, it raised risk for prediabetes and diabetes 5 to 10 times higher than for people whose waists were below 40 inches for men and 35 for women.[5]

4: YOU'RE OVER AGE 45. Aging increases diabetes risk: If you have no other risk factors, your odds for developing diabetes rise from 1 in 100 at age

50 to 11 in 100 at age 70. According to the American Diabetes Association, risk begins to rise at age 45—especially if you're overweight, have a large waistline, are inactive, or have any of the other diabetes risk factors listed here.[6]

▪ **5: YOU HAVE THE "LITTLE" WARNING SIGNS OF INSULIN RESISTANCE AND/OR METABOLIC SYNDROME.** You have metabolic syndrome if you have any three of the following: A waist measurement of 40 inches or more for men and 35 inches or more for women; triglyceride levels of 150 milligrams per deciliter (mg/dL) or above, or taking medication for elevated triglyceride levels; HDL, or "good," cholesterol level below 40 mg/dL for men and below 50 mg/dL for women, or taking medication for low HDL levels; blood pressure levels of 130/85 or above, or taking medication for elevated blood pressure levels; fasting blood sugar levels of 100 mg/dL or above, or taking medication for elevated blood glucose levels.[7] Even if your blood sugar is still in the normal range, metabolic syndrome boosts your risk for eventually developing diabetes five times higher than the risk for people without it.[8]

▪ **6: YOU HAD GESTATIONAL DIABETES DURING PREGNANCY OR DELIVERED A BABY THAT WEIGHED 9 POUNDS OR MORE.** About 7 percent of pregnant women develop gestational diabetes, a form of diabetes that resolves after labor and delivery—but that raises risk for type 2 diabetes significantly. Up to 50 percent of women who've had gestational diabetes develop full-blown diabetes in the next 10 years.[9]

▪ **7: YOU HAVE A FAMILY HISTORY OF DIABETES.** Having one parent with type 2 diabetes raises your risk two to three times higher than average; if both parents have type 2 diabetes, your risk is up to 5.6 times higher than average, studies show.[10]

▪ **8: YOU BELONG TO A HIGH-RISK RACIAL OR ETHNIC GROUP.** Compared with Caucasians, African Americans are twice as likely to be diagnosed with—and die from—diabetes. Latino/Hispanic Americans, Native Americans, Asian Americans, and Pacific Islanders are also at increased risk.[11]

9: YOU'RE OVERWEIGHT AND/OR INACTIVE. For women, being overweight doubles diabetes risk; being obese triples it. For men, overweight increases diabetes risk by about 50 percent, and being obese nearly triples it.[12] Skipping physical activity also raises your risk—even if you're not overweight. In one study, inactivity doubled diabetes risk for lean women and increased it sixteenfold for obese women, compared to active women who maintained a healthy weight.[13]

The Flat Belly Diet Diabetes Plan

THE FLAT BELLY DIET Diabetes is made up of two phases. Together, they take 35 days, which is just enough time to turn any dietary or exercise change into a habit for life. After you've mastered the plan and have seen your weight, your waist, and your blood sugar change for the better, you'll find tools at the end of this book for following the diet long-term.

Phase 1 is the 7-Day Start-Up Plan—in these first 7 days, we walk you through every aspect of the diet. You'll see exactly what to eat, when to exercise, and how to use your "me time" for stress reduction. You'll begin tracking your food intake and exercise. And you'll have the experience of fitting all the pieces into your busy week. You'll have the chance to try a variety of Flat Belly Diet Diabetes

Flat Bellies Are for Men, Too

Guys, this plan's for you. We've even included a provision for an extra 200-calorie snack that can help bigger, taller, more active men feel satisfied. You may be surprised, however, by just how satisfying this four-meals-a-day plan really is. The men who participated in our test panel all said that they rarely added the extra snack, even though most thought beforehand that they were going to need it. "The peanut butter, the nuts, and the avocado really helped me stay satisfied," says Steve Lipman, 63, who lost 10.4 pounds and 1.5 inches from his waist in 5 weeks. "I even took the plan on vacation with me. It was meals and foods and experience the flavors, the satisfaction, and the energy boost you get from following this healthiest of eating styles. Some test panelists began losing weight and inches and seeing blood sugar changes immediately, during Phase 1!

"I started seeing better blood sugars within the first week," said Donna Branson. "I use insulin, and by the end of the first week, I had to adjust my dose because my blood sugars were lower."

That's not all. Phase 1 will also introduce you to the attitude shift we believe is essential for making the plan so successful. Every day, I'll give you a quick and easy mind trick to remind you that you've embarked on a new way of living with and caring for your body.

In Phase 2, you'll let freedom ring. For the next 28 days, you can choose your own breakfasts, lunches, dinners, and snacks from our lists of easy-to-assemble favorites. If you have time, there are options that make use of our scrumptious Flat Belly Diet Diabetes recipes—two test panelists found them so delicious that they serve them when company's coming! No time? No problem. Turn to our grab-and-go meals and our list of convenience foods and even restaurant and fast-food choices that keep you on the plan and on schedule no matter how busy your day is. Any way you do it, you'll enjoy three super-satisfying 400-calorie meals and one 400-calorie snack each day. Each meal

easy with the grab-and-go meal options."

We've also kept it simple and straightforward, so that you can sit down to breakfast or get together meals and snacks for the day in seconds flat. "When you're busy and rushed, keeping it simple is vitally important," says Phil Hernandez, 47, a child psychiatrist who lost 11.4 pounds in 5 weeks and trimmed 2.75 inches from his waist. "You can put a meal together with three or four ingredients. Most of the foods are staple items you can keep on hand at home. Shopping is easy, too. That makes it so much easier to stick with."

and 400-calorie snack contains just the right amount of MUFA to help melt belly fat. It's so simple that you never have to count a single calorie. We've even worked treats like dark chocolate and nuts into healthy meals, so that you can enjoy them without feeling guilty!

We've chosen 1,600 calories as our calorie target each day because that's the amount most adult women and many adult men need to achieve an ideal body weight while maintaining a high energy level, healthy immune system, and strong muscles. It also ensures that you won't feel tired, cranky, irritable, moody, or hungry. That said, we've built in some flexibility. Taller men and women, as well as men or women who are more active, can add an optional 200-calorie snack. (We'll show you how to assess whether this extra snack is right for you.)

Like Phase 1, Phase 2 isn't just about what you eat. It's about how you move. You'll continue to walk for 15 to 30 minutes, 6 days a week. We'll ask you to try a "Calorie Torch" walk that incorporates faster-paced brisk walking, a proven

If You Have Diabetes

If you have already been diagnosed with type 2 diabetes and are under treatment, please be sure to discuss this plan with your doctor before you start! The plan has been formulated to work for people who have diabetes who control their blood sugar with diet and exercise and for those who use oral or injected medications for blood sugar control. Throughout the book, you'll find special information tailored to the needs of people with diabetes. These include blood sugar testing, avoiding episodes of low blood sugar during exercise, and ways that stress reduction—another key component of the Flat Belly Diet Diabetes—can improve your blood sugar.

fat-burner. You'll be introduced to our Metabolism Boost moves, which use light dumbbells to build more calorie-burning, body-toning muscle, and to our Belly Routine, a set of easy moves to tone and tighten your midsection. *No crunches required!*

We'll also ask you to keep a journal—studies show tracking what you eat can double your weight-loss success. (Our test panelists agree wholeheartedly on that one!) Every day, we'll prompt you to reflect for a few minutes on your relationship to food, exercise, your health, your body, or your goals. We call these reflections Core Confidences—not just because your belly is at the physical center of your body, but because your attitude is at the core of your ability to succeed . . . at anything you choose to do in life!

Flat Belly Diet!
Diabetes
At a Glance

> Phase 1:
The 7-Day Start-Up Plan

Seven days is all it takes to fall in love with the Flat Belly Diet Diabetes—and to begin seeing results. On Phase 1, you will:

■ EAT FOUR 400-CALORIE MEALS A DAY. Just follow the fast and easy directions for a quick introduction to delicious eating. Each meal features a MUFA, such as nuts, olive oil, avocado, and even olives and chocolate.

■ DO A MIND TRICK EVERY DAY. These fast mental tune-ups help get your head into the Flat Belly Diet Diabetes game.

■ WALK 15 TO 30 MINUTES A DAY. Exercise is crucial for lowering your blood sugar and improving insulin sensitivity—a key to cutting your risk for diabetes and keeping blood sugar in better control if you have diabetes.

■ RELAX FOR 10 MINUTES A DAY. De-stressing with a progressive relaxation exercise not only feels great, it can help you sidestep emotional eating and, as a growing stack of studies demonstrates, can help control your blood sugar.

> Phase 2:
The 28-Day Flat Belly Diet Diabetes

Four weeks of delicious, MUFA-rich meals—with recipes you can mix and match plus options for healthy grab-and-go meals and even guilt-free, nutritious restaurant and fast-food fare. On Phase 2, you will:

EAT FOUR 400-CALORIE MEALS A DAY, plus an optional 200-calorie snack for larger or more active people.

HAVE A MUFA AT EVERY MEAL. These superhealthy fats keep you feeling full and make every meal a taste sensation.

WALK AT LEAST 15 TO 30 MINUTES A DAY. In addition, each week we'll introduce a new element to your exercise routine, including a 10-minute strength training and 10-minute tummy-toning workout.

SET ASIDE 10 MINUTES OF "ME" TIME. Making a commitment to stress reduction with the progressive relaxation exercise can help you stay on track for success.

In addition, we encourage you to keep a daily journal to track your meals and your activity. Your journal will also include your Core Confidences. Spending a few minutes a day exploring your relationship to food and keeping track of what you eat (plus blood sugar readings if you use a blood sugar monitor) can give you powerful new insights that help you reach your goals.

READ A FLAT BELLY
SUCCESS
STORY

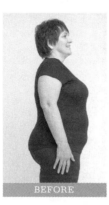

BEFORE

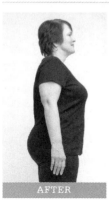

AFTER

Paula Martin

AGE: 54

POUNDS LOST:

13

IN 35 DAYS

ALL-OVER INCHES LOST:

4.5

✳ **BLOOD SUGAR: A1C FELL FROM 7.7 TO**

7.0

PERCENT

* The A1c is a test of long-term blood sugar control; levels below 7 percent are considered ideal for most people with diabetes.

"I TELL EVERYONE TO EAT MUFAS NOW! NO MATTER what diet I tried before, I was always so hungry," reports Paula, 54. "Even if I ate healthy foods, I didn't feel full. Eating 400 calories every 4 hours means I don't get the real 'hungry horrors' anymore. MUFAs—the olives and peanut butter and dark chocolate— make a huge difference. They're delicious. I don't even feel like I'm dieting. And I don't feel a need to overeat. The portions are perfect."

For the past 14 years, Paula's blood sugar readings "have been all over the place." But on the Flat Belly Diet Diabetes, her numbers "don't get as high and don't drop as low, and that's a good thing! I feel my blood sugar is under better control." Seeing her A1c level—a sign of long-term blood sugar control— drop to 7 percent was a cause for celebration. "For a person with diabetes, an A1c of 7 is very healthy," she says. "It's a sign of good blood sugar control and a lower risk for complications in the years ahead."

Paula confesses that she was never a breakfast eater—"I only had coffee"— and that she was always tempted by

the candy, cookies, and bagels coworkers brought to work at the hospital
where she's a psychiatric nurse. That's
all changed for the better. "Every day
on this program, I had oatmeal with
walnuts and a banana," she says.
"I felt like I had a lot more energy
all morning. And I was so satisfied
that I didn't even look at the treats!
In fact, my coworkers are asking
me for Flat Belly Diet recipes
because the meals look so good!"
Among her favorites: salad with
cranberries and walnuts and pork with
sweet potatoes.

Taking a minute to relax at the
start of each meal helped Paula release
daily stresses and focus on enjoying
the food on her plate. "If I have other
things on my mind when I sit down to
eat, I can eat anything without even
noticing," she says. "Being mindful
made a big difference." At the end of
each day, she recorded her meals on
her Flat Belly Diet Diabetes journal
pages—a strategy she credits with
helping her stay on track.

Paula was thrilled to discover that
she'd dropped a dress size—and slid
easily into a flattering, form-fitting
outfit for her photo shoot for this book.
"I was totally surprised—it fit perfectly
and was really cute! I might just go out
and buy it for myself now!"

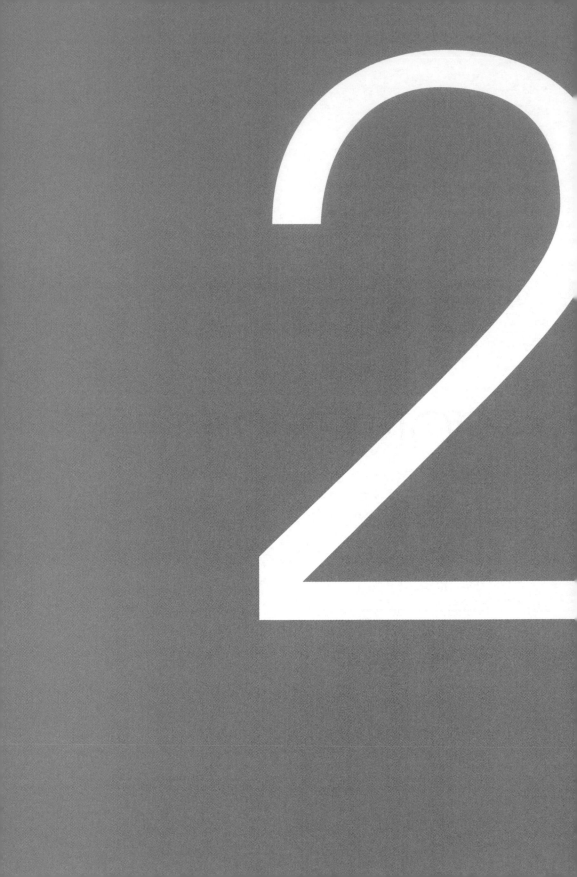

THE BELLY FAT–
BLOOD
SUGAR
CONNECTION

VISCERAL FAT DOESN'T jiggle when you dance. It won't spill over the waistband of your skinny jeans. And it's not the stuff of love handles, little belly pooches, muffin tops, or "pinching an inch" at your waistline.

No, the most dangerous fat in your body lies deep within your abdomen, beneath your skin, behind puffy subcutaneous fat (the fat you can notice on your waist, hips, thighs, etc.), and under your abdominal muscles. I consider visceral fat to be "deep" belly fat, so throughout the book I use the terms *visceral fat, deep belly fat,* and *deep abdominal fat* interchangeably (as opposed to subcutaneous, or "surface," belly fat). Doctors catch glimpses of it only during major surgical procedures (they report that it's butter-yellow and firm, whereas subcutaneous fat is white and squishy). Researchers who use high-tech magnetic resonance machines and computed tomography scanning equipment to measure visceral fat say that while everyone has a little bit (it protects organs and may even play a role in immunity), if you're overweight, you may have several pounds of it.

It's not benign. The "v" in visceral fat truly stands for "vicious." Medical experts now say this deep belly fat is strongly associated with diabetes and pre-diabetes, as well as with metabolic syndrome, a common and often overlooked condition that leads to both. It also contributes to high blood pressure, heart disease, strokes, and even dementia and some forms of cancer.

It's no wonder, then, that when it comes to health, researchers say we should worry about hidden *visceral* fat, not the subcutaneous fat padding your waist, hips, thighs, arms, and butt. Of course, if you're hoping to fit back into your skinny jeans, you're going to worry about both. The good news? On the Flat Belly Diet Diabetes, you'll lose 'em both. What could be sweeter?

Location, Location, Location

WHY IS VISCERAL FAT so deadly? In part, because it occupies some prime real estate within your abdomen.

It's no coincidence that the word "visceral" comes from *viscera*, the Latin word for internal organs. Visceral fat cozies right up against the organs that keep you alive and well—and that keep your blood sugar on an even keel. Connected by tiny blood vessels to your portal vein, the "superhighway" that delivers blood to your heart, liver, and other internal organs, visceral fat affects the important functions of these organs in ways that subcutaneous fat does not.

We're not talking about a little dab of fat. When researchers in Hong Kong measured visceral fat with magnetic resonance imaging (MRI) machines, they discovered layers $\frac{1}{2}$ to 1 inch thick in people who were about 5 to 20 pounds overweight.[1] Less is better; researchers have found that risk for metabolic syndrome—which raises diabetes risk—begins to rise when visceral fat is just

$^4/_{10}$ inch thick.[2] Your age, your gender, and your genes all play roles in how much fat you store deep in your abdomen, but body weight plays a big role. The more you weigh, the more visceral fat you're likely to have.

The Toxic Chemical Factory in Your Torso

THE SECOND REASON VISCERAL fat is so dangerous is that it's *active* fat. Scientists used to think that the human body's 40 billion to 120 billion fat cells were like the plastic containers in your refrigerator—they just held stuff (in this case, extra calories) until needed. Today, we know that fat is more like the leaky faucet on your kitchen sink—it drips constantly. Sometimes, the "drip" benefits our health: I'm intrigued by a recent announcement from Harvard Medical School that subcutaneous fat—such as hip fat, thigh fat, butt fat, and the fat just below the skin on your belly—may produce substances that protect against diabetes.

But visceral fat's drip is oh-so-deadly. It churns out dozens of chemicals and hormones that interfere with the healthy functioning of your liver, your heart, and your pancreas, as well as with your blood vessels, your muscle cells, and even your brain and the tissue in a woman's breasts and in a man's prostate gland. Among the worst:

Inflammatory compounds. Visceral fat produces chemicals such as tumor necrosis factor[3] and interleukin-6.[4] These compounds raise levels of chronic inflammation in your body, wreaking havoc. Chronic inflammation is intimately connected with insulin resistance—the glitch that leads to metabolic syndrome, prediabetes, and diabetes. When cells are insulin resistant, they don't obey signals from the hormone insulin to absorb blood sugar.

Inflammation also raises risk for heart disease, the number one killer of people with diabetes, prediabetes, and metabolic syndrome. It does this by triggering the growth of heart-threatening plaque in artery walls, by boosting blood pressure, and by making blood stickier—and more likely to form the clots that cause heart attacks (and strokes).[5, 6]

Free fatty acids. These blood fats stream out of visceral fat like gravy pouring from a pitcher. Their first stop: your liver. That's trouble, because a fatty liver pumps out extra blood sugar and makes cells throughout your body more resistant to insulin. It also raises your risk for heart disease by churning out more harmful LDL cholesterol and triglycerides (another blood fat) and less of the helpful HDL cholesterol that protects your heart. A fatty liver is shockingly common: Researchers at St. Mary's Hospital in London who used MRIs, ultrasound, and computerized tomography scans to look for liver fat estimate that 20 to 30 percent of adults have dangerous levels of it.[7]

Hormones. New research suggests that a hunger-triggering hormone called neuropeptide Y—NPY for short—is produced by visceral fat. If theories about NPY are correct, this could mean that extra visceral fat makes you hungrier. This sets up a nasty cycle: hunger, overeating, more visceral fat, more hunger, more overeating . . .

In the rest of this chapter, we'll delve into the health effects of visceral fat. But for now, I wanted to describe a dramatic study that illustrates its power. In a controver-

Yes, There IS Good Body Fat!

Your body needs a little padding in order to function—without it, you'd freeze in a winter wind, have trouble healing from the smallest cut or scrape, run out of energy between meals, and run the risk of damaging your internal organs just by bumping into a kitchen counter. An estimated 2 to 5 percent of a man's body weight comes from "essential" fat; for women, it's 10 to 15 percent. Body fat's metabolic benefits include:

- Providing energy
- Maintaining proper hormone levels
- Regulating body temperature
- Protecting vital organs
- Aiding fertility
- Stimulating bone growth
- Boosting immunity and healing
- Releasing hormones that regulate appetite

The latest? Harvard Medical School researchers, in a study published in the journal *Cell Metabolism*, recently found that a mysterious factor in the fat just below the skin (subcutaneous fat) *may* protect against diabetes![8,9]

sial Swedish experiment involving 50 weight-loss surgery patients, those who had visceral fat surgically removed saw blood sugar improve two to three times more than those who only had subcutaneous fat removed.[10] While this surgery is still strictly experimental—it's currently in the early stages of study in the United States as a potential fix for type 2 diabetes—it shows just how strongly this fat affects the way your body functions. Lucky for you, you don't need surgery to remove this fat!

Insulin, Blood Sugar, and Belly Fat

WHAT DOES ALL THIS mean for you? To understand deep belly fat's implications for diabetes, I want you to understand how your body handles blood sugar when everything's operating properly.

The story begins when you eat a meal, such as a quick lunch consisting of a tuna fish sandwich, an apple, a cookie, and a glass of milk. Your digestive system converts the carbohydrates from the bread, the fruit, the cookie, and even from the milk into blood sugar. This is your body's primary source of fuel—without it, you wouldn't have the physical energy to run after your kids, the mental energy to balance your checkbook, or the internal energy to maintain the thousands of functions your body performs every day.

Getting that fuel into cells is insulin's job. Normally, your pancreas—a cone-shaped, spongy, 6-inch-long organ located just behind your liver—produces this hormone and releases a squirt when blood sugar levels begin to rise after you eat. Insulin tells cells to open up and let the sugar in. And normally, your cells obey. But if your body stops obeying insulin's commands—or if your pancreas can't produce enough insulin—you wind up with one of these blood sugar problems:

Type 1 diabetes. About 5 percent of people with diabetes have type 1 diabetes, in which your pancreas stops producing insulin entirely. Type 1 usually strikes in infancy or childhood, but can occur later in life. It happens when your body's immune system attacks and destroys beta cells. Treatment always includes insulin injections.

Visceral fat doesn't play a direct role in type 1 diabetes. But thanks to the obesity epidemic, more and more people with type 1 are also becoming overweight—and are developing insulin resistance (described below) as a result. That means your cells may not respond readily to the insulin you take, requiring you to use more and making daily blood sugar control more challenging. (Daily blood sugar control, of course, is important for ensuring your cells get the blood sugar they need and for avoiding diabetes-related complications.) It makes sense, then, that an eating and exercise plan that fights deep visceral fat, like the Flat Belly Diet Diabetes, could help you fight insulin resistance and remain sensitive to the insulin you use to keep your blood sugar in control.

Type 2 diabetes. In contrast to type 1, type 2 diabetes is the result of insulin resistance. Your pancreas continues to make insulin. But your cells don't obey its signals readily. Your body must then force blood sugar into cells by pumping out extra insulin. If your body can't keep up with the demand for extra insulin,

Can you be thin on the outside, fat on the inside?

Absolutely. When Jimmy Bell, PhD, a professor of molecular imaging at Imperial College London, used magnetic resonance imaging (MRI) to make "fat maps" of nearly 800 people, he discovered that 45 percent of the thin to normal-weight women and 65 percent of the thin to normal-weight men he checked were carting around excess visceral fat.[11] While their body mass indexes (BMI—a measure that compares your weight to your height) were within the slender to normal range of 20 to 25, they harbored hidden belly fat. Dr. Bell coined the acronym TOFI (thin outside, fat inside) to describe the phenomenon, which raises risk for diabetes and other health problems regardless of the number on your bathroom scale. Dr. Bell says TOFIs are on the threshold of becoming overweight—they're eating too many foods high in saturated fat and exercising too little. Consider that a wake-up call and a good reason to eat the Flat Belly Diet Diabetes way, even if your waistline isn't in the danger zone (generally, over 35 inches for a woman and 40 inches for most men)!

blood sugar eventually rises—ultimately leading to type 2 diabetes.

Reversing insulin resistance is an important goal of treatment for type 2 diabetes. Sometimes, diet and exercise are enough. For many people, however, adding medications that further increase insulin sensitivity, boost insulin production, or enhance blood-sugar absorption is also necessary.[12]

The visceral fat connection: Carrying fat in your torso boosts your odds for developing type 2 diabetes significantly—*even if you're not overweight.* Plenty of studies have found a strong connection between this deep belly fat and type 2 diabetes. One, published in the *Archives of Internal Medicine,* looked at waist sizes and health of 14,924 Americans. Researchers found that a big waistline— over 35 inches for women, 40 for men—raised the risk for developing diabetes 10 times higher than normal for people who were not overweight and five times higher than normal for those who were. If you already have type 2 diabetes, visceral fat makes controlling it more difficult.[13] In an Italian study of 63 people with type 2 diabetes, those with the most visceral fat were five times more insulin resistant than those with the least visceral fat. As a result, their blood sugar was two to three times higher.[14]

The good news: *Losing* even a little of this dangerous belly fat can make your blood sugar easier to control. In one study of 114 people with type 2 diabetes who used oral medications to control their blood sugar, those who lost just 15 percent of their weight needed less medication because their cells became three times more sensitive to insulin.[15]

Gestational diabetes. Between 3 and 8 of every 100 pregnant women develop this form of diabetes. Not a visceral fat problem, gestational diabetes happens when hormonal shifts and the weight you gain while carrying a baby conspire to temporarily boost insulin resistance so high that your blood sugar rises into the danger zone.

It's perilous for moms and babies. Excess sugar in your bloodstream pads a developing baby with extra fat, raising the risk for a longer, more difficult delivery. Gestational diabetes can also contribute to breathing problems and low blood sugar for a newborn; low blood sugar can lead to everything from lethargy and feeding problems to seizures and brain injuries in babies.

While gestational diabetes usually clears up soon after you give birth, it raises your lifetime risk for type 2 diabetes to nearly 70 percent. If you're pregnant, follow your doctor's advice for controlling diabetes—the Flat Belly Diet Diabetes is not intended for women who are pregnant or nursing a baby (you may need more calories). But if you've had gestational diabetes in the past, the Flat Belly Diet Diabetes could help you lower your risk for developing type 2 diabetes later in your life.[16]

Metabolic syndrome. Long before prediabetes or full-blown type 2 diabetes develops, many people have metabolic syndrome—a "silent" condition that raises your odds for diabetes, as well as for heart attacks, strokes, some forms of cancer, and even dementia. You have metabolic syndrome if you have any three of these five warning signs:

- A waist measurement of 40 inches or more for men and 35 inches or more for women
- Triglyceride levels of 150 milligrams per deciliter (mg/dL) or above, or taking medication for elevated triglyceride levels
- HDL, or "good," cholesterol level below 40 mg/dL for men and below 50 mg/dL for women, or taking medication for low HDL levels
- Blood pressure levels of 130/85 or above, or taking medication for elevated blood pressure levels
- Fasting blood sugar levels of 100 mg/dL or above, or taking medication for elevated blood glucose levels, which is also a sign of prediabetes[17]

The visceral fat connection: In one French study, risk for metabolic syndrome increased fivefold for women and eightfold for men whose waistlines grew by 3 inches in 9 years.[18] The toxic chemicals released by visceral fat cause metabolic syndrome long before they trigger full-blown type 2 diabetes.

Prediabetes. You have prediabetes if your blood sugar is higher than normal but hasn't yet reached the "tipping point" for type 2 diabetes. While a normal reading on a fasting blood sugar test is below 100 mg/dL, a reading of 100 to 125 mg/dL means prediabetes—and levels of 126 mg/dL or higher usually mean type 2 diabetes.

Don't shrug prediabetes off as "just a touch of sugar" or "high-normal" blood sugar. It's serious: One in four people with prediabetes develop full-blown, type 2 diabetes within 3 to 5 years; 8 in 10 develop it over the course of their lifetimes—*if they don't take steps to prevent it*, says the Centers for Disease Control and Prevention.[19] Your risk may be even higher if you're of African American, Latino, Pacific Islander, or Native American descent. But the risk doesn't end there. Prediabetes ratchets up heart disease risk, doubling your odds for a fatal heart attack.[20]

The visceral fat connection: Living for years with excess visceral fat means ever-worsening insulin resistance and a weakening of your body's ability to release insulin. Eventually, blood sugar levels begin to rise into the prediabetic range. The more visceral fat you have, the more likely it is that you'll go on to develop full-blown type 2 diabetes, say researchers from the University of Texas Health Science Center in Austin.[21]

Belly Fat and Other Big Health Risks

Blood sugar problems are just part of the story. These serious health problems have also been associated with higher levels of visceral fat:

Heart attack and stroke. If you have diabetes, prediabetes, or metabolic syndrome, the health of your heart should be one of your top priorities. Blood sugar and insulin problems go hand-in-hand with cardiovascular problems—and visceral fat is involved. A wide waist (more than 35 inches in this case)—an indicator of visceral fat deep inside your torso—tripled risk for fatal heart disease in a Harvard Medical School study of 44,636 women.[22] The same connection has been found in men. Visceral fat threatens your cardiovascular system in several ways. Researchers have found that it quadruples your risk for high blood pressure and raises your risk for high levels of "lousy" LDLs and low levels of "helpful" HDLs by 30 percent to 100 percent.[23]

In a study of 382 people with type 2 diabetes, researchers at Chicago's Rush University Medical Center found that those with the most visceral fat had a more lethal cholesterol profile—they had more small LDL particles and more particles called very low density lipoproteins (VLDLs), factors that raise risk for heart attacks and strokes.[24]

Cancer. Visceral fat increases risk for cancers of the breast, prostate, and colon.[25-27] The connection? Experts suspect it's excess insulin, which acts like a growth factor and encourages cells to grow and divide. A big waistline also makes it more likely you would not survive cancer treatment, Harvard researchers have found.

Dementia. Visceral fat also increases your odds for dementia. When researchers at the Kaiser Permanente Division of Research in Oakland, California, tracked more than 6,000 people, they found that those with big bellies were 65 percent more likely to develop fuzzy thinking and memory lapses later in life than those with the slimmest midlines.[28] The link in this case? The researchers suspect it may be inflammation.

Exercise, Belly Fat, and Blood Sugar?

HAVE YOU MOVED AROUND much today? If you haven't weeded the garden, walked the dog, gone to the gym, or gotten some other type of physical activity, put this book down immediately and treat yourself to a 5-minute stroll.

There. You've just taken an important step in vanquishing visceral fat.

The fact is, leading a sedentary life is a big contributor to the worldwide widening of waistlines. We know you're busy, and we know it's tough to find a half hour for exercise. But the fact is, any kind of activity helps fight this fat, even if you're fitting in a couple of 10-minute walks per day or making a point of finding time to dance along to the radio or spending a sweaty 20 minutes planting green beans in your vegetable garden.

Does it count? You bet. University of South Carolina researchers who questioned nearly 1,500 people about their activity levels and then checked their insulin resistance levels found that out. People who moved 5 days a week—whether it was formal exercise, an active job, or keeping up with the yard work—were 70 percent more insulin-sensitive than those who were the least active.[29]

And while everyone deserves time to unwind in front of the TV, be sure screen time is balanced with activity: Harvard School of Public Health researchers have found that every 2 hours a day in front of the tube boosts risk for insulin resistance by 23 percent![30] (Of course, exercising while you watch TV, as you'll be able to do on the Flat Belly Diet Diabetes plan, solves that problem neatly!)

Stress, Belly Fat, and Your Blood Sugar

YOU'RE LATE FOR WORK. Fuming after a spat with your spouse. Worried about finances . . . your kids . . . or your aging parents. Stress, whatever its cause and whenever it strikes, unleashes "fight-or-flight" hormones intended to help you escape from danger. But in today's world, the human stress response is more likely to fuel belly fat and high blood sugar, research shows.

When levels of the stress hormone cortisol rise, your liver converts stored carbohydrates and protein into sugar (glucose) and releases it into the blood. At the same time, the hormones epinephrine and norepinephrine reduce your pancreas's production and release of insulin—the hormone that tells cells to absorb blood sugar. The result: Your body gets a rush of extra blood sugar so you can run faster and think more clearly. It came in handy in prehistoric times, when our ancestors needed fuel to outrun attacking saber-toothed tigers. But today, when stress has become a 24/7 way of life, it can lead to trouble.

Duke University researchers have found that stresses, large and small, can raise blood sugar. And cortisol also contributes to belly fat accumulation. Surprising research from the University of California, San Francisco, suggests that cortisol also triggers cravings for high-calorie food—and directs your body to store excess calories as belly fat. In one study, women exposed to high-stress situations in a lab experiment chose high-sugar, high-fat foods afterward.[31] Again, this made sense a millennium ago when our bodies needed every single calorie available for survival—refueling after a saber-toothed tiger attack prepared you to fight again. And storing the extra calories as belly fat meant they could be released quickly when needed. But today, it may be fueling a worldwide growth in belly fat. Fortunately, there's hope! Research also shows that soothing stress can break these cycles—helping to lower blood sugar in people with diabetes and making weight loss easier. For details, see Chapter 5.

The Number You *Must* Know

WONDERING WHETHER THERE'S BAD fat lurking in your midsection? Some day soon, your doctor may be able to scan your torso or even check your blood to find out. Researchers at Beth Israel Deaconess Medical Center in Boston have discovered elevated levels of a telltale protein called RBP4 in people with excess visceral fat, a finding that could lead to a "belly fat test" someday. For now, we've got a simpler method. Put down this book for a moment and go grab a soft, flexible tape measure—the kind used for sewing.

Your waist size isn't just easy to measure. Studies show that it's a very accurate picture of your visceral fat status. When Brazilian researchers used high-tech computed tomography scanners to measure visceral fat in 100 women, then checked their weight, waist size, and skin-fold thickness with calipers (like those used in many gyms to check body fat), they discovered that waist size really did accurately reflect the amount of visceral fat inside a woman's torso.[32]

The first thing to remember about checking your visceral fat status is that it's not the same as measuring to see if you're ready for a bathing suit or to check what size pants to buy. Honesty and accuracy really count—no cinching, sucking in your breath, or knocking off a half-inch because you're feeling a little bloated! And you won't necessarily measure your waist at its narrowest point or use your belly button as a landmark for lining up the tape.

For the most accurate belly-fat reading, the National Institutes of Health recommends using the top of your hip bones instead. This ensures that you'll measure across the section of your abdomen that hides significant amounts of visceral fat.

What to do:

1. MEASURE ON BARE SKIN. So strip to your birthday suit or take off your shirt and unfasten your pants. Push pants and underwear down past your hips. (Squeezing tight pants down onto your hips while you measure isn't a good idea—you could get a "muffin top" bulge that makes your waist seem bigger than it really is!)

2. STAND IN FRONT OF A MIRROR WITH YOUR FEET SHOULDER WIDTH APART. Be sure you can see your waist and hips in the mirror.

3. USE YOUR HANDS TO FIND THE UPPERMOST POINT ON YOUR HIP BONES. Wrap the measuring tape around your middle so that the bottom edge rests *just above* these bones. Be sure the tape is snug and straight, not twisted or tight.

4. RELAX AND TAKE TWO TO THREE NORMAL BREATHS. Take your measurement at the end of the third exhale. (Remember, don't suck your belly in!)[33]

5. WRITE THE NUMBER HERE: _____ inches (to the nearest ¼ inch).

6. RECHECK WHEN YOU'VE FINISHED YOUR FIRST 35 DAYS ON THE FLAT BELLY DIET DIABETES AND MONTHLY THEREAFTER. Write your new number here _____.

How does your waist rate? Check our chart to find out.

	HEALTHY RANGE	AT RISK FOR DIABETES AND HEART DISEASE	HIGH RISK
MEN	Below 37 inches	37–39 inches	40 inches and above
WOMEN	Below 32 inches	32–34 inches	35 inches and above [34, 35]
ASIAN MEN	Below 30 inches	30–35 inches	35½ and above
ASIAN WOMEN	Below 28 inches	28–31 inches	31½ and above

Note: Experts recommend lower waist sizes for people of Asian descent, due to a higher genetic risk for diabetes and cardiovascular disease.[36] Studies show that risk rises even at lower body weights and smaller waist sizes for Asians due to an inherited pattern of abdominal fat storage.[37]

The Five Factors Behind Visceral Fat

LEVELS OF VISCERAL FAT have skyrocketed in the past 5 decades. The average American woman's waist size increased 7 inches between the 1960s and the start of the 21st century; the average man's, 4 inches. Today, an estimated 60 percent of women and 39 percent of men have too much fat packed into their midsections. Why the increase? Blame the obesity epidemic—and a curious quirk of the human body. At a healthy weight, 10 percent of your total body fat is visceral fat. But if you're overweight, it's more like 25 percent.

But why do some people store more dangerous fat deep in their bellies—the "apples" of this world—while the "pears" among us pack more of it on hips and thighs? Extra calories and a low-exercise lifestyle are just part of the equation. These five factors play key roles:

■ **1. YOUR GENES.** Your genetic makeup is about 30 to 60 percent responsible for *where* your body stores fat. (But diet and exercise play big roles in *how much* you store there!)

■ **2. YOUR AGE.** Not only do most of us gain fat all over as we age, visceral fat seems to accelerate over the years. In one Canadian study of 174 women, those approaching age 50 had twice as much visceral fat as those in their twenties, even though the older women weighed only about 12 to 15 pounds more. Similar results have been found in men.

3. YOUR GENDER. In general, human beings store 10 to 15 percent of our total body fat as visceral fat.[38] But men store twice as much of their fat deep in their abdomens as premenopausal women do.

4. MENOPAUSE. Thanks to changing hormones, a woman's body burns 30 percent less fat[39] and stores more fat deep in her abdomen after menopause. One Syracuse University study of 54 postmenopausal women found that 20 to 30 percent of their total body fat was visceral fat.[40]

5. FOOD CHOICES. Diets packed with saturated fat—in fatty meats, cheeses, and full-fat milk, yogurt, and ice cream—have been linked with higher levels of visceral fat. Brazilian researchers have found that trans fats—processed fats found in fast food and many packaged foods—seem to concentrate in visceral fat. In contrast, diets rich in monounsaturated fats discourage the formation of this deep belly fat!

Does my dress or pants size say anything about my level of visceral fat?

Surprisingly, yes. Clothing sizes correlate very closely with deep abdominal fat levels. When British researchers compared the clothes sizes, weight, and body mass index (a measure of weight that takes height into account) of 262 women and men, they discovered that an American woman's dress size of 16 or larger and a man's trouser waist size larger than 38 tripled risk for diabetes and heart disease in men and raised risk sevenfold for women, compared to people who wore smaller sizes. Most of the time, height differences didn't affect the outcome. The researchers suggest that you stay aware of changes in abdominal fat by keeping tabs on clothing size and fit. If your clothes become too tight, if you go up a size, or if you find yourself regularly reaching for elastic-waist pants, you may be packing on extra visceral fat.[41]

And Now for the *Good* News

VISCERAL FAT, IT TURNS out, is easier to lose than the fat on our hips, thighs, and bottoms. Research shows that just a little bit of weight loss adds up to big losses of deep abdominal fat—and big health benefits, including better insulin sensitivity, less need for diabetes medications, lower blood pressure, healthy cholesterol levels, and a lower risk for developing diabetes.

This book is one of the first places you'll read this exciting news! In study after study, women and men who've taken smart, belly fat–banishing steps— exercise and healthy eating, the same basic foundation we used for building the Flat Belly Diet Diabetes—saw dramatic reductions in their waist sizes and even bigger drops in the amount of visceral fat lurking below their waistbands. Remember the Yale University study of the Flat Belly Diet that I mentioned in Chapter 1? The participants—who ate marvelous MUFAs (monounsaturated fats) at every meal—lost 8.4 pounds, 3.9 inches from their waists, and 20 percent of their visceral fat! And in case you're wondering, losing belly fat really does improve your health:

DID YOU KNOW ?

Heart-threatening blood fats called triglycerides may hold a clue to hidden belly fat. In a study published in the journal *Diabetes Care*, researchers at Canada's Laval University measured visceral fat levels in volunteers in a study of 249 women.[42] They found that those with the highest triglyceride levels were more likely to have higher levels of this dangerous fat. The connection: Your liver pumps out more triglycerides in response to high levels of free fatty acids in your bloodstream. And those free fatty acids come from visceral fat. If your triglycerides are over 150 mg/dL, the level recommended by the American Heart Association, it's time to eat less saturated fat and fewer sugar-laden goodies, take in fewer calories, and take your risk from visceral fat very seriously.

■ LESS INSULIN RESISTANCE: In a study from Finland, losing visceral fat improved insulin sensitivity by 17 percent. A change like that could mean you'd need a lower dose of blood sugar–lowering medication if you now have diabetes or you would have a significantly lower risk of ever developing diabetes if you don't.

■ REDUCED RISK FOR PROGRESSING TO DIABETES IF YOU NOW HAVE PREDIABETES: Losing abdominal fat was the secret to the success of the landmark Diabetes Prevention Program study, which followed 3,234 people with prediabetes. Researchers recently found that study participants who made healthy lifestyle changes—they ate less saturated fat and more fiber, cut calories, and exercised—reduced their visceral fat by 18 to 22 percent and cut their risk for developing full-blown diabetes by 58 percent.[43]

■ PROTECTION FROM HEART ATTACKS AND STROKES: In a Canadian study, women who lost visceral fat also saw two important signs of cardiovascular health improve: Levels of "helpful" HDLs rose by 50 to 65 percent. And blood pressure fell by 5 to 11 percent.[44]

Dropping visceral fat pampers your heart in other ways, too. In an Australian study of 18 people—9 with diabetes and 9 with normal blood sugar—those who lost weight and trimmed their waistlines saw levels of heart-threatening triglycerides fall about 18 percent.[45]

■ LESS INFLAMMATION: Chronic, low-level inflammation is a culprit behind major health conditions ranging from diabetes and heart attacks to strokes and cancer. Losing belly fat reduces signs of inflammation significantly, studies show. In one from the University of Vermont, women who lost visceral fat saw levels of C-reactive protein (CRP), an important marker of chronic, low-level inflammation, fall by 33 percent.[46] And it doesn't take much weight loss or belly fat loss to get these results. In the Diabetes Prevention Program, women and men who lost just 7 percent of their body weight—a little more than 12 pounds if you now weigh 175—saw CRP levels drop 29 to 33 percent.[47]

On the Flat Belly Diet Diabetes, you'll find out how easy and delicious it can be to make the small, everyday changes that reap big rewards.

READ A FLAT BELLY
SUCCESS
STORY

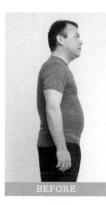

BEFORE

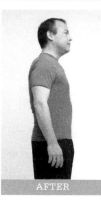

AFTER

Phil Hernandez

AGE: 47

POUNDS LOST:

11.4

IN 35 DAYS

ALL-OVER
INCHES LOST:

3.75

✳ **BLOOD SUGAR: A1C FELL FROM 6 TO**

5.9

PERCENT

* The A1c is a test of long-term blood sugar control; levels below 7 percent are considered ideal for most people with diabetes.

"I HAVE MORE ENERGY AND STAMINA! I'M DOWN TO MY lowest weight ever—206 pounds!" says Phil, a child psychiatrist. "When I test my blood sugar in the morning or 2 hours after a meal, I notice that it's lower *and* steadier. It's down in the ranges that would be normal for someone who doesn't have diabetes."

Making a commitment to the Flat Belly Diet Diabetes rules taught Phil that he can make the kind of healthy eating changes he once considered an impossible dream. "I've gotten some hands-on skills I never had before," he says. "I have three sons to help get ready for school in the morning while I get myself ready for work. But I discovered I can make time for an egg with avocado and cheese on an English muffin—and it's really satisfying. *And* I have time to pack lunch and snacks."

Phil confessed that he felt worried that carrying lunch to work might make him look geeky. "I used my son's old lunch box, and I was a little self-conscious at first," he says. "I did it anyway, and the feedback was really positive. There were doughnuts one day at work, and someone said, 'Don't even offer any to Dr. Hernandez—he eats healthy!' I was happy to realize my colleagues see my new routine as some-thing so positive.

"I only have time to make foods with three or four ingredients. With this, I can remember what I need when I go to the grocery store. When you're busy and rushed, keeping it simple is vitally important. Everything I need for a Flat Belly Diet meal or snack is ready to go."

Eating meals on time was another revelation. "I used to get busy and skip meals. Now, I eat every 4 hours. I never thought I could make time for it, but I did it and learned another new skill—and my work day didn't fall apart! On the contrary, it went better because my blood sugar wasn't swinging between highs and lows. I even keep a can of soup in my car now as an emergency meal."

He feels good that his sons are watch-ing him follow such a healthy eating plan. "Some diets depend on highly processed food and food substitutes. But this one is all about real food. My sons see me doing everything to take care of my diabetes and even help me get out my medications," he says. "As I eat this way, they see something healthy happening that's good for me. That sends a strong message that could help them stay healthier in the future, too."

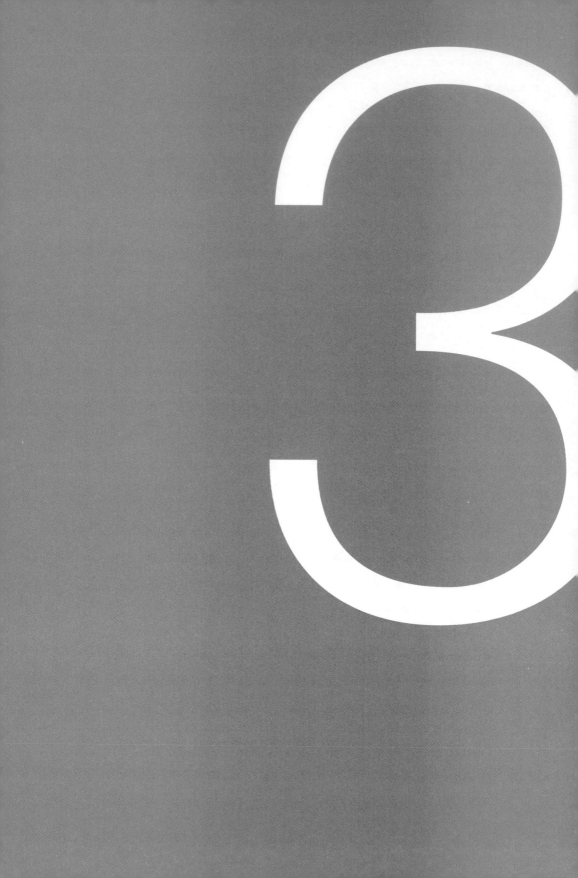

ON YOUR PLATE: THE AMAZING FLAT BELLY DIET DIABETES FOODS

I LOVE—NO, MAKE that adore—good food. Sharing a delicious meal with my family and friends is one of life's greatest pleasures. So you can imagine how thrilled I was to hear from our test panelists that not only did they love their Flat Belly Diet Diabetes meals—their families and friends fell head over heels in love with all of the goodies in this eating plan, too!

Test panelist Phil Hernandez came home a little late for dinner on Valentine's Day to discover that his 9-year-old son had prepared a meal he'd seen his Dad cook on the plan: cod, red potatoes, and snap peas. "He decided he wanted to cook it for the whole family," Hernandez recalled. "I was able to eat it when I came home, too." The family liked the meal so much that, he says, "they ate most of the fish!"

Donna Branson told us that she couldn't decide which Flat Belly

Diet Diabetes meal she and her husband liked best: Was it the turkey sliders, the chicken piccata, the spinach-and-pear salad . . . or the pork and almond meatballs? "It's all delicious. We've definitely continued to eat this way," she said a few weeks after the test panel ended. "My husband says this is definitely a way of eating he can stick with for the long term!"

Susan Hoar brought Chocolate-Zucchini Snack Cake to a family party—and it was such a hit that her brother-in-law now requests it. "It's his favorite dessert!" she notes. "With food like this, it's hard to believe this is a weight-loss diet!"

I hope you're noticing the pattern here. The Flat Belly Diet Diabetes is all about hearty, tasty *real* food including our signature "MUFA at every meal"— and by that I mean treats rich in monounsaturated fats such as nuts and seeds, olive oil, avocados, olives—*and chocolate!* If you were to analyze the menu, as Gillian has, you'd find that each meal is packed with vegetables, fruit, whole grains, lean protein, and a MUFA. If you were to simply savor the food on your plate, you'd find that it's great cuisine that you can feel good about eating.

With every tasty bite, the foods on this plan work hard to fight belly fat, help you lose extra pounds, keep your blood sugar healthier, and more. This chapter outlines how this breakthrough plan came to be, and why it has such a uniquely powerful effect on your health. As you savor Flat Belly Diet Diabetes meals, we hope you get a little extra enjoyment knowing that there's solid science behind it!

The Rise and Fall of the Low-Fat Diet

IF EATING (AND *enjoying*) fat in moderation feels forbidden—or downright dangerous—to you, you're not alone. We've all become a bit too fat-phobic thanks to the "fat is bad" message drummed into us over the years—something that's frustrated Gillian and Dr. Edelman as they worked with people with diabetes and prediabetes on weight loss and maintaining healthy blood sugar levels.

"All fat is bad" is simply a myth. It implies that there are no good fats and that less fat is always better—theories now proven to be false and even unhealthy. But until *very* recently, some of the world's foremost health organizations—including the American Diabetes Association, the American Heart Association, the National Institutes of Health, and the World Health Organization—advocated low-fat diets as *the* healthy way to reduce risk for diabetes, heart disease, stroke, high blood pressure, and overweight.

The thinking behind this dates back to the 1950s, when Ancel Keys, PhD, a University of Minnesota researcher, noticed that well-fed Americans had rising heart disease rates, while Europeans living with post–World War II food shortages had declining rates. After studying the diets and heart disease rates of men in seven countries—the United States, Japan, Italy, Greece, the Netherlands, Finland, and Yugoslavia—Dr. Keys concluded there was a "strong association" between saturated fat, high cholesterol, and heart trouble. That became the foundation for America's first heart-healthy "prudent diet," recommended by the American Heart Association in 1957.

The "fat is bad" myth gathered momentum through the years. By the 1980s, we were munching fat-free cookies, crackers, and frozen treats with abandon. The trouble was, we weren't really becoming any healthier or any slimmer. We were just eating more refined carbohydrates and more calories in general. Between 1970 and 2000, Americans cut their fat consumption as a percent of total calories by more than 10 percent. But a look behind the statistics shows that thanks to bigger and bigger portion sizes, the average American woman increased her calorie intake from 1,542 to 1,877 between 1970 and 2000; men's calorie intakes rose from 2,450 to 2,618! And women increased their actual fat consumption by 6.5 grams a day (men's fell somewhat).

Meanwhile, a fat backlash happened. Some diet gurus began recommending diets packed with meat, cheese, butter, and other fats and low in carbohydrates—found in breads, noodles, rice, fruit, and even vegetables. The most severe drastically slashed intake of some of the healthiest foods you can eat, including veggies, fruits, and whole grains—foods important for maintaining a healthy weight and protecting yourself from heart disease and diabetes.

Remember I mentioned bigger portions? While everyone debated the merits of low-fat versus low-carb, we were busy piling our plates higher than ever before. Between the 1950s and the year 2000, the size of a fast-food hamburger has tripled; fries and muffins and pasta entrées have at least doubled; a glass of soda has gone from 7 ounces to between 16 and 64 ounces![1] Without realizing it, Americans were eating more and more calories at every meal.

There's one more piece to this puzzle. We were, and are, burning far fewer calories going about our daily lives compared to levels in the 1950s. Thanks to dishwashers, electric car windows, TV remote controls, riding lawn mowers, 500-channel TVs, video games, and the Internet, some experts estimate the average adult burns 700 fewer calories per day now than she or he would have 60 years ago!

Bottom line? More calories. Less activity. The stage was set for the twin epidemics of overweight and diabetes that are gripping our nation—and the world. Rates of overweight have increased from 14.5 percent in 1971 to 68 percent today.[2] Diabetes rates in the United States doubled between 1990 and 2005, according to the Centers for Disease Control and Prevention (CDC) in Atlanta, and continue to rise.[3, 4] This "diabesity" epidemic is now affecting our children, too. Experts have stopped referring to type 2 diabetes as "adult-onset diabetes." The CDC now estimates that one-third of the 10-year-olds in the United States will develop diabetes in their adult years.

Clearly, low-fat and low-carb diets weren't the answer. But a newer, healthier picture was emerging, about a way of eating, a way of living, and a type of fat that might hold the key.

Good Fats: The Way to Eat!

BY 2006, RESEARCHERS HAD solid proof that low-fat living didn't work, for weight loss or for better health. Many studies showed this, but one of the largest and most convincing is the landmark, federally funded Women's Health Initiative. It tracked nearly 49,000 women for 8 years as they followed their regular diets or stuck with a low-fat diet. In the end, the low-fat group had rates of heart attacks and strokes *nearly equal to that of women who ate higher-fat diets.* Both groups also gained *similar amounts of weight.*[5]

If low-fat wasn't the long-term solution, what was? Thousands of miles away, people on the beautiful Greek island of Crete had the answer. Researchers had noticed decades earlier that people there ate large amounts of fat, yet had extremely low heart disease rates. Why? It turns out that instead of saturated fats from fatty meats, creamy salad dressings, full-fat dairy products, and baked goods, most of the fat in classic Crete home cooking was *monounsaturated*—primarily from extra-virgin olive oil. The Cretan people consumed a whopping 100 cups of it per person, per year. That's more than a quarter-cup a day! And these monounsaturated fats—MUFAs (MOO-fahs) for short—were part of a super-healthy diet that also included lots of fruit and vegetables and moderate amounts of whole grains, beans, fish, nuts, olives, wine, cheese, and grass-fed meat.

Why are MUFAs so healthy? It's all in the chemistry. All dietary fats are chains of carbon, oxygen, and hydrogen atoms. If a fat is *saturated,* all of the carbon atoms are bound to hydrogen atoms; it's *unsaturated* if some of the carbon is free. At room temperature, saturated fats are sticky and hard (like a stick of butter) while MUFAs and other unsaturated fats are liquids (like a bottle of golden olive oil).

The difference between MUFAs and saturated fats is like the difference between pouring high-octane gasoline and molasses into your car. MUFAs make the human body purr (we'll show you how later in this chapter). Saturated fat makes it run amok—producing more heart-threatening blood fats, damaging insulin-producing cells, and making cells throughout your body insulin-resistant.

Of course, you can't simply add a MUFA to an unhealthy diet and expect great results. MUFAs are effective when eaten in the right quantities, as part of a healthy diet that features vegetables and fruit, whole grains, lean protein, fish, and low-fat dairy products—and few refined carbohydrates or foods high in saturated fat.

You won't find this comprehensive, forward-looking strategy anywhere else, but the experts are catching up to its wisdom. The US Department of Agriculture, in its 2005 Dietary Guidelines for Americans, advocated a moderate-fat—not low-fat—diet and came out in favor of MUFAs (along with polyunsaturated fats, such as the good fats found in fish). *Most of the fats you eat should be polyunsaturated and monounsaturated fats*, the guidelines say. *Keep total fat intake between 20 percent and 35 percent of calories.*[6] Wow! That's a seismic shift! It means there's now enough research to convince the government's careful,

Isn't chocolate candy unhealthy for people with diabetes or prediabetes?

Dark chocolate is packed with antioxidants called flavonols that keep arteries flexible, lower blood pressure, and—when eaten in small quantities—even improve the way your cells absorb blood sugar. In an Italian study of 19 people who had high blood pressure and insulin resistance (their cells didn't absorb blood sugar readily), those who ate a small piece of dark chocolate (about the size of a Hershey's Kiss) every day for 18 weeks saw blood pressure and insulin resistance improve.[7] A cup of hot cocoa works, too—just be sure to make your own using unsweetened cocoa powder, skim milk, and a pinch of sugar or a sugar substitute. In a recent Yale University study, blood vessels relaxed twice as much in people who drank cocoa without sugar compared to those who drank it with added sugar.[8]

We're here to tell you that when you follow two important rules, enjoying chocolate in moderation is not only healthy, it's a cornerstone of the Flat Belly Diet Diabetes. Things to remember:

1. Eat this decadent treat *only* in small quantities—and have it once a day at most.
2. Make sure it's *dark* chocolate—aim for a cocoa content of 70 percent or higher.[9]

thoughtful health experts that the healthiest fat *isn't* no fat . . . it's the *right* fats, in the *right* quantities.

MUFAs Aid Weight Loss

MARVELOUS MUFAS CAN HELP you lose weight more easily, keep it off more effectively—and fall in love with healthy eating for life. (What's not to love about chocolate, nuts, and olives?)

If you're like most people, you've lost and regained the same pounds time after time. Now, you won't have to see the numbers on the scale creep back up. Like the finely tuned engineering behind a gorgeous sports car or the well-planned, perfect fit that makes a beautiful dress look great when you slip it on, our MUFAs do more than please your taste buds. They work hard to help you lose weight in three important ways:

■ THEY'RE SUPER-SATISFYING. MUFAs like nuts and olive oil are automatic insurance against between-meal cravings. In the hours after you eat a few nuts, for example, satisfaction levels soar—so you won't have that "I've gotta eat, eat, eat" urge at your next meal. Weight loss researchers from Purdue University report that we automatically compensate for 55 percent of the calories in walnuts, for example, by eating fewer calories later on![10]

■ THEY HELP YOU STICK WITH A HEALTHY EATING PLAN. Three times more people stayed on a MUFA-rich diet than a conventional low-fat diet in one study from Brigham and Women's Hospital in Boston and the Harvard School of Public Health.[11] The reason? Fat provides instant gratification while you're eating and keeps you feeling satisfied for hours afterward.

■ THEY HELP YOU KEEP WEIGHT OFF. When an international research team assigned 322 moderately obese people to one of three weight-loss diets—a low-carb diet, a low-fat plan, or a Mediterranean-style diet rich in MUFAs—everyone lost 10 to 15 pounds in the first 5 months. But after 2 years on their respective eating plans, the low-carb and low-fat groups regained 2 to 3 pounds while the MUFA group barely regained an ounce—maintaining an average 11-pound weight loss. Why? Again, because this fat tastes good and keeps you feeling fuller and more satisfied than does a drastic low-fat or low-carb diet. How did they do it? Their eating plan featured lots of fruit, vegetables, and whole grains; lean protein from fish and chicken; and MUFAs at almost every meal. Every day, they used 2 to 3 tablespoons of olive oil and munched a small handful of nuts.

MUFAs Target Visceral Fat

WHEN YOU SPRINKLE OLIVE oil instead of a creamy dressing on your salad, snack on a handful of nuts instead of chips, or slide a slice of avocado into your sandwich instead of Swiss cheese, you set in motion beneficial body-chemistry changes that usher dangerous visceral fat *out:*

■ LOSE MORE VISCERAL FAT. **When researchers at Pennsylvania State University assigned 53 overweight women and men to a low-fat diet packed with carbs or a higher-fat diet with plenty of MUFAs, the MUFA group saw a 20 percent greater reduction in visceral fat.[12] And when 16 overweight Australians with type 2 diabetes followed either a high-carb diet or a moderately high-MUFA diet for 3 months, researchers made an amazing discovery. Everyone lost a few pounds, but the MUFA group lost fat mostly from their midsections while the carb eaters lost it mostly from their legs and hips.[13]**

■ DISCOURAGE THE STORAGE OF NEW BELLY FAT, EVEN WHEN YOU'RE NOT DIETING. **In a groundbreaking Spanish study that tracked 59 people who followed a high-carbohydrate eating plan or one that was high in saturated or monounsaturated fats for 4 weeks, nobody lost or gained weight. But their body fat redistributed itself. The carb group lost lower body fat and gained belly fat, while the MUFA group's belly fat shrank.[14]**

MUFAs Reverse Insulin Resistance

IF YOU TAKE AWAY just a few health concepts from this book, we hope one of them is *insulin resistance*—when cells throughout your body stop responding to insulin's commands to take in sugar from the bloodstream. Insulin resistance can exist for decades before you notice anything, but all the while it's raising your risk for metabolic syndrome, prediabetes, type 2 diabetes, heart disease, high blood pressure, even dementia and cancer. The more visceral fat you have, the more insulin resistant you are, report researchers from Laval University in Canada.[15]

Weight loss and exercise help overcome insulin resistance. And by adding MUFAs to the equation as part of a healthy diet, you can reverse it.

■ MUFAS LOWER INSULIN RESISTANCE; SATURATED FAT RAISES IT. In one international study that followed the health of 162 people on diets high in either saturated fat (the kind found in cheese, ice cream, and fatty meats) or monounsaturated fats, Swedish researchers found that the MUFA diet increased insulin sensitivity 9 percent, while the saturated fat group saw insulin sensitivity decrease by 12 percent.[16]

■ MUFAS WORK QUICKLY. When 11 people with insulin resistance and a high risk for developing type 2 diabetes (all had at least one parent with diabetes) ate diets packed with carbs, saturated fat, or MUFAs for 4 weeks,

DID YOU KNOW ?

Half of the heart-protecting, disease-fighting antioxidants in nuts are lost when you remove their fragile, papery skins. Some nuts, like walnuts and hickory nuts, are almost always sold with skins intact—no worries there. But peanuts and almonds come both ways—so when possible, choose those with skins intact.[17]

Spanish researchers learned an important lesson. The MUFA eaters saw the biggest improvements in insulin sensitivity. After a single breakfast, the MUFA group had lower insulin and blood sugar levels than the high-carb group—a sign that their bodies were more responsive or sensitive to insulin, thus requiring less of it to control blood sugar levels.[18]

MUFAs Fight Metabolic Syndrome

AS YOU MAY REMEMBER from chapter 2, metabolic syndrome is one step before prediabetes. You've got it when you have any three of these five signs:

- A big belly
- Slightly high blood pressure
- Elevated triglycerides
- Low levels of "helpful" HDL cholesterol
- Above-normal blood sugar

Salted Peanuts and Briny Olives: The Sodium Question

Modern food processing has turned two MUFA-rich superfoods, nuts and olives, into blood-pressure-raising traps—thanks to gobs of salt sprinkled on the outside, in the case of many packages of nuts, or infused throughout, in the case of most olives. Since many people with diabetes, prediabetes, and metabolic syndrome also have high blood pressure—and in fact, 90 percent of us are at risk for developing this heart risk at some point in our lives—it's important to enjoy these foods without getting unwanted sodium.

- Avoid salted nuts. Instead of buying your nuts in the party-foods aisle of the grocery store, check out the natural foods aisle and the produce department for bags and packages of unsalted nuts. While you're at it, avoid nuts roasted in oil—no one needs the extra calories.
- Enjoy olives once a day, period. Limiting olives in this way will help you keep the lid on blood-pressure-boosting sodium—and still let you enjoy this Mediterranean treat.

DID YOU KNOW

It raises your risk for diabetes, heart disease, stroke, and other serious medical conditions—and there's no drug that fights it. What does? Physical activity—and the right diet. That means eating plenty of fruit, vegetables, whole grains, lean meats, fish, and poultry—and getting some MUFAs every day.

In one recent Spanish study, a team of researchers put diets remarkably similar to the Flat Belly Diet Diabetes to the test in 1,224 women and men. They followed one of three plans: a low-fat diet, a Mediterranean diet with an extra serving of virgin olive oil, or a Mediterranean diet with extra nuts. When the study began, 61 percent had metabolic syndrome. After a year, metabolic syndrome was reduced in both Mediterranean diet groups—by 14 percent among nut eaters and 7 percent among olive oil users; it fell just 2 percent in the low-fat group.[20]

The results suggest why including just a small handful of nuts in many Flat Belly Diet Diabetes meals and snacks is so important. The study's authors say antioxidants in nuts may help lower your risk for metabolic syndrome by protecting against oxygen-related cell damage and chronic inflammation. How many nuts did it take? About seven walnuts, five or six almonds, and five or six hazelnuts a day. Of course, as you can see, olive oil also helps reverse this condition, so why choose? On the Flat Belly Diet Diabetes, you get nuts, olive oil, and more!

MUFAs: Are Part of the "Ideal" Diabetes Diet

IF YOU HAVE TYPE 2 diabetes, you may be thinking at this point: All that's fine for people who don't have diabetes . . . but my needs are a little different. I have to keep my blood sugar under control all day, every day. Can this kind of eating plan give me any help there?

We're happy to report that the answer is *yes:*

■ MUFAS CAN LOWER FASTING BLOOD SUGAR LEVELS. In one large, international weight-loss study that included 36 people with type 2 diabetes, those who followed a Mediterranean-style diet enriched with MUFAs got a big blood sugar benefit. Their fasting blood sugar levels fell by 30 mg/dL—a drop that can mean you'd need lower doses of diabetes medications or might even, in some cases, be able to eliminate some diabetes drugs entirely.

■ MUFAS HELP WITH LONG-TERM BLOOD SUGAR CONTROL, TOO! Even better: In the same study, MUFA eaters saw their scores on an A1c test—a blood test that measures long-term blood sugar control over 2 to 3 months—fall by 0.5 percent. That may sound small, but it's enough to reduce risk for diabetes complications like heart disease, blindness, and kidney problems by 20 percent. And compared to those on a low-fat diet, the MUFA group saw insulin sensitivity improve sevenfold.[21]

How do MUFAs exert such a powerful effect on blood sugar? Experts are still trying to answer that question, but so far, they have some fascinating clues:

■ MUFAS INCREASE ADIPONECTIN. This crucial hormone helps control blood sugar, and levels are usually low in people with diabetes. Boosting it improves insulin sensitivity and lowers levels of inflammation.

■ MUFAS SLOW THE ABSORPTION OF GLUCOSE—BLOOD SUGAR— FROM THE CARBOHYDRATES YOU EAT. The sugar in your bloodstream all comes from carbs—from grains, fruit, even vegetables and dairy products.

They're converted to glucose during digestion. When a meal also includes MUFAs (or any fat or protein), this sugar is released into the bloodstream at a slower pace than in a meal without fat—the reason that you feel hungrier sooner if you have a piece of dry toast than if you have toast with margarine or peanut butter. The result: lower, steadier blood sugar, instead of roller-coaster highs and lows. Any fat has this effect, but by choosing a MUFA, you get this benefit plus all of the others mentioned in this chapter. MUFAs are amazing multitaskers!

■ MUFAS STIMULATE YOUR INTESTINES TO RELEASE MORE GLP-1.[22] This antidiabetic hormone "tells" your body to pump just the right amount of insulin into your bloodstream, at the right time, after you eat. Levels drop in people with diabetes—and in fact, several pharmaceutical companies are trying to turn GLP-1 into a diabetes drug right now.

■ MUFAS BUILD HEALTHIER CELL WALLS. The walls of every cell in your body contain fatty acids. Scientists suspect that when these membranes contain more oleic acid, a type of MUFA found in olives, olive oil, and nuts, they work better. British researchers have found that blood sugar is transported more quickly and easily through cell walls rich in oleic acid—and transport is less efficient when membranes contain more saturated fatty acids.[23]

MUFAs Protect Your Heart

THE RESEARCH ON MUFAs and heart disease is so compelling that the National Heart, Lung, and Blood Institute (part of the National Institutes of Health) has set a daily MUFA target as part of its recommendations for preventing and managing cardiovascular risk. It recommends a total fat intake of 25 to 35 percent of daily calories, with saturated fat no more than 7 percent of calories and MUFAs up to 20 percent. That's especially important if you have diabetes, prediabetes, or metabolic syndrome because these conditions raise your odds for heart disease two to four times higher than normal. High blood pressure, low levels of "helpful" HDLs, and high levels of heart-threatening fats called triglycerides often accompany these blood sugar–related problems.

Here's why the world's leading heart experts are over the moon about these good fats:

■ MUFAS PROTECT AGAINST HEART DISEASE; LOW-FAT DIETS DON'T. When researchers in Israel, Germany, and the United States tracked 322 people who followed three different weight-loss diets, they discovered that a MUFA-rich plan was better for heart health than a low-carbohydrate diet and even better than the American Heart Association's recommended low-fat, restricted-calorie diet.

All three diets contained healthy foods and healthy calorie ranges—1,500 for women, 1,800 for men. But after 2 years, the MUFA group saw the most improvement in their cholesterol and triglyceride balance. "Bad" LDL cholesterol fell 5.6 points, and heart-threatening triglycerides dropped 22 points, while "helpful" HDLs increased by 6.4 points. The drop in triglycerides is especially significant, because this blood fat is often too high in people with metabolic syndrome, prediabetes, and diabetes.

■ MUFAS BOLSTER "HELPFUL" HDL CHOLESTEROL. For too long, cardiologists and family doctors only paid close attention to LDL cholesterol—a blood fat that, at high levels, triggers growth of plaque in artery walls and raises heart attack risk. But experts at Johns Hopkins University now say that slashing nasty LDLs is just half the equation. It's also important to raise your heart-friendly HDLs—the long-overlooked cleanup crew that helps get LDLs out of your bloodstream. MUFAs have a unique ability to reduce LDLs without also shrinking levels of heart-friendly HDLs. In some studies, MUFAs have even helped raise HDL levels. Every 1-point increase in HDLs lowers your risk for a fatal heart attack 3 percent, and MUFAs are on the short list of strategies that work—along with exercise, quitting smoking, and losing weight.[24]

■ MUFAS LOWER BLOOD PRESSURE. In one study of European men, those who consumed 4 teaspoons of olive oil a day for 9 weeks saw systolic blood pressure—the top number in a blood pressure reading, when a heart beat is exerting maximum pressure on artery walls—drop 3 points.[25] What made the men's blood vessels more flexible? Spanish researchers suspect that oleic acid, found in high concentrations in olive oil and in some nuts, is responsible. This fat is used to build healthy cell membranes—the walls that surround cells and play important roles in sending chemical signals in and out.[26]

MUFAs Cool Inflammation

ONE REASON A MUFA-RICH diet is so good for your heart and blood vessels is that it reduces levels of chronic inflammation in your body. Inflammation is our immune system's response to stress, injury, illness, aging, and (you guessed it) too much belly fat. Short-term inflammation aids in healing, such as after you cut yourself. But when inflammation doesn't get turned off—due to low-grade infections, advancing years, or, yes, too much visceral fat—it alters body chemistry and triggers diabetes, heart attacks, strokes, and other illnesses.

But MUFAs, as part of a healthy diet, are tops at quelling inflamation's "flames." Italian researchers measured levels of inflammatory compounds in the blood of nearly 200 women and men before and after they followed a Mediterranean-style diet rich in MUFAs versus a "prudent" diet that was higher in carbs and lower in fat. After 2 years, the MUFA group had significantly lower levels of C-reactive protein and interleukin-6, two compounds in the bloodstream associated with chronic inflammation throughout the body.[27] The blood vessels of the MUFA group were more flexible and less likely to trigger the formation of heart-threatening blood clots. The researchers say that every food group in the MUFA-rich diet (good fats plus fruit, vegetables, and whole grains) fights inflammation, while the typical Western diet, packed with refined carbohydrates (such as white bread and sweets), saturated fat, and red meat actually fuels it.

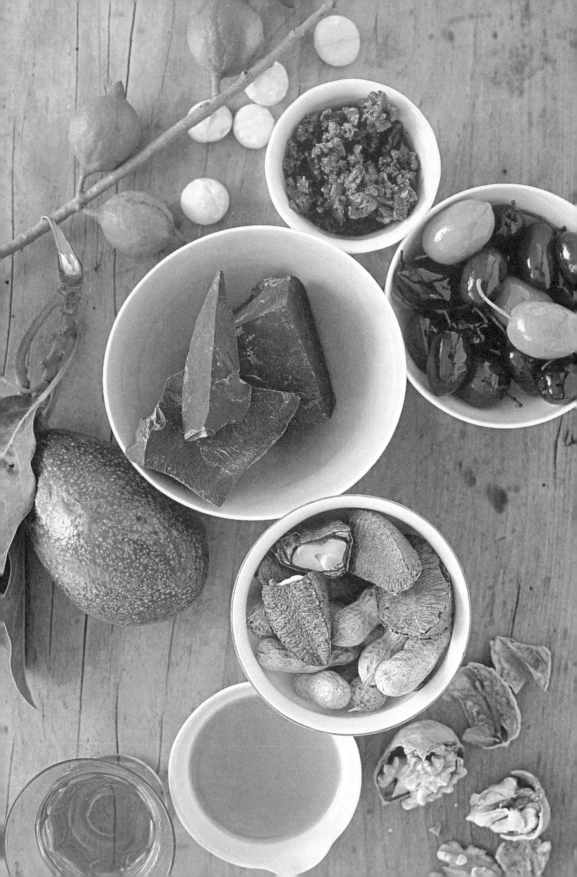

CHOOSE YOUR MUFA

The near-magical health benefits of monounsaturated fat–rich foods begin with less belly fat and better blood sugar, but they don't stop there. Our favorite MUFAs pack an astonishing variety of important nutrients that deliver plenty of surprising health benefits.

1. Oils: The MUFA-rich oils we recommend on the Flat Belly Diet Diabetes pack many different health bonuses. Extra-virgin olive oil contains antioxidants that short-circuit the growth of heart-threatening plaque in artery walls. Using olive oil frequently may reduce risk for asthma, bone fractures, colon cancer, and even rheumatoid arthritis. MUFA-rich oils such as canola, safflower, sesame, soybean, and sunflower are also rich in vitamin E.

2. Olives: Surprisingly rich in copper and iron—which protect your nerves, thyroid gland, and connective tissue throughout your body—these Mediterranean treats are also a super source of vitamin E, which destroys free radicals, and protects LDL cholesterol from the damage that leads to atherosclerosis and shields colon cells from changes that lead to cancer.

3. Nuts and Seeds: Fiber-rich almonds not only guard your heart and keep you feeling satisfied, they're also full of the nutrients manganese, copper, and riboflavin. Eating ground flaxseeds or walnuts is a great way to get inflammation-soothing omega-3 fatty acids, in the form of alpha-linolenic acid. These plant-based good fats worked just as well as fish for lowering blood pressure in one study.[28] The magnesium in sunflower seeds may reduce asthma attacks, migraine headaches, and high blood pressure. In general, nuts and seeds are little nutritional powerhouses, full of fiber, protein, iron, zinc, B vitamins, and more.

4. Avocados: The creamy, pale-green flesh of this luscious fruit is full of folate, a heart-healthy B vitamin that lowered heart attack risk 55 percent in one study of more than 80,000 women.[29] Avocado also contains the antioxidants lutein, zeaxanthin, and beta-carotene. They help fight prostate cancer, promote eye health, and battle oral cancers. Adding avocado to a salad doubles absorption of carotenoids from greens and other vegetables, giving your body further protection from heart disease and macular degeneration, a leading cause of blindness.[30]

5. Dark Chocolate: Packed with flavonols and proanthocyanidins, dark chocolate can help raise levels of "good" HDL cholesterol and lower blood pressure. In one German study, people who ate 30 calories' worth of dark chocolate a day—one good-size bite of a chocolate bar or the amount in one Hershey's Kiss—lowered their blood pressure—enough to cut the risk of a deadly stroke by 8 percent and of a fatal heart attack by 5 percent.[31]

The Flat Belly Diet Diabetes All-Stars

How ABOUT WAKING UP to a hearty breakfast sandwich made with a whole wheat English muffin, an egg cooked as you like it, avocado, and reduced-fat cheese? A weeknight supper of whole grain pasta topped with tomato sauce, mushrooms, and ground turkey sautéed in olive oil? A lunch salad packed with walnuts, cranberries, and orange slices, drizzled with a generous amount of olive oil vinaigrette? Or a special snack that includes an exquisitely flavorful piece of dark chocolate?

Getting hungry? Good! These yummy choices illustrate what the Flat Belly Diet Diabetes is all about—MUFAs *plus* a winning combination of fruit, vegetables, whole grains, beans, lean protein, fish, and low-fat dairy products. A cornucopia of research studies, and the experiences of our happy test panelists, show that this combination of healthy, delicious foods works together to help you lose weight, improve your blood sugar, and lower your risk for diabetes-related complications at the same time. Simply tossing a few nuts and a chocolate bar into a junk-food diet won't work. You need all of these healthy foods to get the benefits. In fact, this way of eating has stood the test of time. How? It's actually the classic Mediterranean-style diet we described earlier in this chapter. Lucky for you, the Flat Belly Diet Diabetes has updated this super-healthy cuisine to fit modern tastes and our real-world, crazy-busy lives. You'll get all the benefits even on hectic days when you're eating out or need a grab-and-go meal.

And the benefits are huge. When researchers from the Harvard School of Public Health looked at the diets and health histories of 74,886 women, ages 38 to 63, they found that those whose diets contained the most monounsaturated fats, produce, beans, whole grains, and fish were 29 percent less likely to have heart disease, 13 percent less likely to have a stroke, and 39 percent less likely to die from either one, compared to women whose diets contained very little of these superfoods.[32] In contrast, women with the highest risk ate the most red meat, butter, margarine, fried foods, and highly processed foods.

Here, then, is a brief summary of the rest of the Flat Belly Diet Diabetes building block foods:

FAT-FIGHTING FRUIT AND VEGETABLES

The Flat Belly Diet Diabetes's five to eight servings of fruit and vegetables a day aren't just tasty and super-filling (without bogging you down with excess calories!). Fresh fruits and veggies are crucial for flattening your belly, losing weight, and controlling your blood sugar for these reasons:

■ THEY'RE PACKED WITH FIBER. Fiber fills you up, slows digestion, and slows the release of glucose into your bloodstream. Fruits and vegetables, for the most part, have a low "glycemic load"—a hot-button concept in nutrition that refers to how fast and how high carbs boost blood sugar. Including produce at every meal helps slow the rise in your blood sugar afterward. (So do fiber-rich whole grains, the fats you eat, and protein.)

■ THEY PUT THE CHILL ON INFLAMMATION. Low-level inflammation interferes with absorption of blood sugar by scrambling signals meant to tell cells to carry sugar molecules inside. But produce cools off inflammation. In a recent Harvard School of Public Health study of 486 women, those who ate the most fruits and vegetables had the lowest levels of C-reactive protein, a marker of chronic inflammation. Those who ate the most fruit were 34 percent less likely to have metabolic syndrome; those who had the most vegetables cut risk 30 percent.[33]

■ THEY'RE FULL OF VITAMINS, MINERALS, AND ANTIOXIDANTS. You'll get healthy levels of blood pressure–pampering potassium from bananas, spinach, lima beans, sweet potatoes, and avocados. (Some people with diabetes need to be careful not to get too much potassium, though, if they have kidney problems. But if you follow the Flat Belly Diet Diabetes guidelines, you're in no danger of getting too much.) Carotenoids—which the body turns into cell-protecting vitamin A—from tomatoes, leafy greens, broccoli, melons, sweet potatoes, and others, seem to help protect against cancers of the lungs, mouth, prostate, and stomach.[34] And so much more!

■ THEY PROTECT YOUR HEART. A diet full of fruit and veggies cuts the risk of heart disease by 28 percent and of stroke by 20 percent.[35, 36] One reason: Many fruits and vegetables are also rich in pectin, a type of water-soluble fiber that helps lower levels of "bad" LDLs.

HEARTY WHOLE GRAINS

Here's why whole grain bread, whole wheat pasta, oatmeal, and other whole grains are the grains of choice on the Flat Belly Diet Diabetes—and why they belong on your plate:

■ THEY CUT DIABETES RISK. Swapping just two pieces of white bread for whole grain bread could lower your risk for type 2 diabetes by 20 percent, says one study that followed over 150,000 women for more than 15 years.[37] The fiber and bran in whole grains resist easy digestion, so it takes longer to convert a whole grain's starches into sugars. Some grains, like oatmeal and barley, have a special talent for slowing the rise in blood sugar after a meal and holding it steady for hours on end. Their secret: "resistant starches," a type of starch that acts like fiber and breaks down very, very slowly in the body.

■ THEY FIGHT INFLAMMATION. Eating at least two whole grain servings a day reduced deaths from inflammation-related diseases by 30 percent over 17 years in the Iowa Women's Health Study.[38]

■ THEY REDUCE LDLS. Soluble fiber—the stuff found in oatmeal, barley, and rye—helps lower cholesterol. It forms a gel in your intestinal tract that traps cholesterol-rich digestive substances called bile acids. The result: You eliminate the bile acids, instead of reabsorbing them, and your body has to use more cholesterol to make new ones. That leaves less cholesterol to roam your bloodstream as heart-threatening LDLs!

SATISFYING LEAN PROTEIN

Since one of the goals of the Flat Belly Diet Diabetes is to rein in the amount of saturated fat you eat, we recommend *lean* protein, such as skinless poultry, beans, and lean and well-trimmed cuts of beef and pork instead of fatty cuts of meat. And eat fish, including fattier types like salmon, for reasons you'll discover in the subsequent pages of this chapter. Here's what protein has to offer:

▇ IT SUPPORTS HEALTHIER BLOOD SUGAR LEVELS. Researchers at the University of Minnesota tested two diets, one high in protein and one with only half as much. The fat content was the same in both diets. In the group that followed the high-protein diet (which was also lower in carbs) for 5 weeks, A1c levels—a test of long-term blood sugar control—fell by nearly 1 full point, a significant improvement.[39]

▇ IT PROTECTS AGAINST METABOLIC SYNDROME. In another University of Minnesota study, people who ate red meat, fatty pork, breakfast meats, and other processed meats twice a day raised their risk for metabolic syndrome 25 percent higher than those who indulged just a few times each week.[40] Those who ate little red meat weren't skipping protein, however. They were filling up on chicken, turkey, beans, and other low-fat proteins.

▇ A WEIGHT-LOSS ADVANTAGE. Protein contains an amino acid called leucine that helps preserve more muscle while you diet. In a recent study of 48 overweight women dieters, ages 40 to 56, those who ate more protein lost 20 percent more weight than those on an equal-calorie, higher-carb plan—and most of their loss was body fat, not muscle.[41] The more muscle you have, the more calories your body burns round the clock. Losing muscle, in contrast, slows your metabolism. It's smart to hold onto as much as you can (something our metabolism-boosting exercise routine will also help you do!).

▇ FIBER—IF YOUR PROTEIN IS MEATLESS. You'll enjoy beans several times a week on our plan. Why? Beans are a good source of soluble fiber, the type that helps control blood sugar. And some, like navy beans and lentils, are also packed with an up-and-coming form of fiber called resistant starch, which breaks down extremely slowly in your digestive system—slowing the absorption of sugar into your bloodstream.

MORE GOOD FATS: THE OMEGA-3S AND OMEGA-6S

When you eat certain MUFA-rich foods—such as walnuts, flaxseed, and olive and canola oils—you also get a healthy dose of two other good fats: omega-3 and omega-6 fatty acids. You've no doubt heard about the heart-protecting powers of omega-3s, the good fats that are also found in fatty, cold-water fish like salmon and mackerel (as well as in fish oil capsules).

Worried about toxins in fish? It's true that fatty fish like salmon can accu-

Good Fats versus Bad Fats

Dietary fat is an important energy source. Used in the production of cell membranes and certain hormones, it's critical to the regulation of blood pressure, heart rate, blood vessel constriction, blood clotting, and the nervous system. Dietary fat aids the body in absorbing vitamins such as A, D, E, and K. But not all fats are created equal. Eating large amounts of the wrong fat is very hazardous to your health. But telling good fats from bad fats isn't so easy, unless you know what to look for:

THE HEALTHY
MONOUNSATURATED FAT (MUFA) remains liquid at room temperature but may start to solidify in the refrigerator.

POLYUNSATURATED FAT (PUFA) remains in liquid form both at room temperature and in the refrigerator. Foods high in polyunsaturated fats include vegetable oils, such as safflower, corn, sunflower, soy, and cottonseed oils.

OMEGA-3 FATTY ACIDS are an exceptionally healthy type of polyunsaturated fat (PUFA) found mostly in fat-rich fish. If you'd rather do your taxes than eat two fish meals a week (the number recommended by the American Heart Association), then eat other foods rich in omega-3 fatty acids, including walnuts, flaxseeds, flaxseed oil, and, to a lesser degree, canola oil.

mulate chemical pollutants such as PCBs in their fat and skin, while leaner fish such as tuna can accumulate mercury in their flesh. But don't shy away from fin food—you need the good fats! Minimize your risks by eating two fish meals a week and by eating a variety of fish, the Environmental Protection Agency recommends. Choose types with lower levels of toxins, such as wild salmon (available in cans at the grocery store as well as in pricier fillets at the fish counter), mackerel, and herring. Tuna has some omega-3s, too, and *light* varieties have two-thirds less mercury than white or albacore tuna.[42] In addition, getting some of your omega-3 fatty acids from walnuts, ground flaxseed, and flaxseed oil may help. These contain alpha-linolenic acid, which your body converts into the more potent omega-3 called DHA, the type found in fish and fish oil capsules.

OMEGA-6 FATTY ACIDS, another type of PUFA, are found in many types of vegetable oils, including safflower, sunflower, walnut, soybean, and corn oils. Since this fat is in abundance in most diets, there's no need to go out of your way to add it in, experts say. Until recently, many nutrition experts thought these fats raised levels of inflammation in the body, but in early 2009 the American Heart Association set the record straight—saying that omega-6s help battle inflammation.

THE UNHEALTHY

SATURATED FATS become solid or semi-solid at room temperature. The marbling in red meat is one example, as is a stick of butter. Saturated fat is found mostly in animal foods, but three vegetable sources are also high in saturated fat: coconut oil, palm (or palm kernel) oil, and cocoa butter. Keep in mind that it's almost impossible to get your saturated fat intake down to zero. Even olive oil contains 2 grams of saturated fat per tablespoon—a tiny amount that's okay.

TRANS FATS raise LDL cholesterol and lower HDL cholesterol, increasing the risk of heart disease. They're quite possibly the most hated fats in all of fat-dom. Created when manufacturers alter the chemical structure of liquid oils to increase their shelf life, they're found mostly in packaged products and many commercially fried foods, including French fries and doughnuts from some restaurants and chains.

Among the benefits of good fats:

■ THEY REDUCE RISK FOR HEART DISEASE. **A study at the Harvard School of Public Health found that women with diabetes who ate fish just once a week had a 40 percent lower risk of dying from heart disease than did women with diabetes who rarely had fish.**

■ THEY FIGHT INFLAMMATION. **Omega-3s cool chronic inflammation in the body, a major contributor to numerous chronic diseases of aging, including insulin resistance and diabetes. So do omega-6s, which, according to the American Heart Association, suppress production of inflammation-related compounds including adhesion molecules, chemokines, and interleukins, all of which are involved in the growth of plaque in artery walls.[43] (The heart association recently came out in favor of including some omega-6s in our diets. These fats have been demonized as a cause of inflammation, but in reality, if you eat omega-3s and omega-6s in balance, both are beneficial.)**

I know I should avoid trans fats, but how do I find them on a food label?

You're not alone in wondering. In a recent American Heart Association survey, 92 percent of adults knew trans fats were dangerous, but only 21 percent could name three foods that usually contain them. While the Nutrition Facts label on a food package now lists trans fats, there's a catch: Foods with less than 0.5 gram per serving can say they contain zero trans fats. The problem? Eat several servings and you're getting more trans fats than is healthy (experts recommend getting as close to none as possible). A better plan: Check the ingredients list for "partially hydrogenated" oils and avoid products that contain them. Another strategy: Pass up commercial baked goods, snack foods, and, when possible, fast food, unless you can verify that they're truly trans-fat free. While some cities, including New York City, have banned trans fats, they're still on the menu in many locales.

READ A FLAT BELLY
SUCCESS
STORY

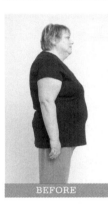

BEFORE

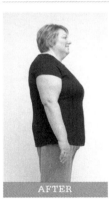

AFTER

Donna Branson

AGE: 51

POUNDS LOST:

7.2

IN 35 DAYS

ALL-OVER
INCHES LOST:

4

✳ **BLOOD SUGAR: A1C FELL FROM 8.2 TO**

7.1

PERCENT

* The A1c is a test of long-term blood sugar control; levels below 7 percent are considered ideal for most people with diabetes.

"I LOVED THE FOOD! I WAS DIAGNOSED WITH TYPE 2 DIABETES 14 years ago, and I've tried lots of weight loss and healthy eating programs—but I've never seen the kind of dramatic improvement in blood sugar that I got with the Flat Belly Diet Diabetes," says Donna, 51. "My blood sugar levels are so much better now that I've been able to reduce the amount of long-acting insulin I take on a daily basis by about 30 percent.** Improvements began in the first week of the plan, and things just kept getting better. I really think having a MUFA at every meal made the difference. I can't say enough about how good my blood sugar numbers are!"

A registered nurse who takes care of mothers and newborns in a busy hospital maternity department, Donna loved Flat Belly Diet Diabetes grab-and-go meals—such as healthy, frozen entrees or a meal-replacement bar paired with a MUFA and a piece of fruit or a vegetable. "There are times when you're waiting, in gown and gloves, for a baby to be delivered, and you just don't know how long you'll be there. So you have to eat when you can. In the past it would have been pizza or Chinese food or something from a vending machine.

Now it's something that's good for me that's also satisfying and energizing. I've absolutely fallen in love with the S'Mores Luna Bar and some peanut butter—it reminds me of a Reese's Peanut Butter Cup, only better!"

A "basic meat-and-potatoes" person, Donna discovered avocados and enjoyed experimenting with new types of nut butters. "My husband made cashew butter, and I went gaga for it," she says. "In fact, my husband followed the diet with me, and he lost 14 pounds in 5 weeks, his total cholesterol dropped 66 points, and he needed a smaller pants size. We both loved the marinara sauce with ground turkey and mushrooms over pasta. I was afraid the portion would be too small, but we were both filled up."

As Donna's waistline shrunk, her pants began "just falling off me—to the point where I had to go out and buy new ones. I bought jeans for the first time in 10 years, and they actually fit my body! I'm definitely wearing more form-fitting clothes, and I love it. We're continuing to eat the Flat Belly Diet Diabetes way, and we've warned our 21-year-old son that when he gets home from college, he'll be eating that way, too!"

** Never adjust your medication on your own—consult your doctor first.

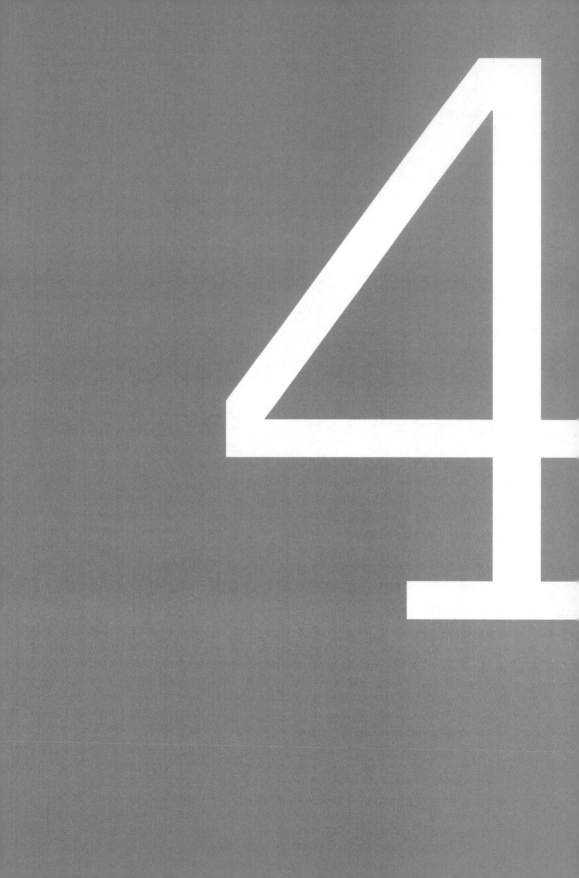

KNOW YOUR NUMBERS

SUCCESS ON THE Flat Belly Diet Diabetes begins with flattening your belly, but it doesn't end there. For you, real success means healthy blood sugar levels—today, tomorrow, and always. As you'll discover in this chapter, it also means taking your cholesterol, triglyceride, and blood pressure levels seriously. And it means working with your doctor to ensure that you're cleared to follow the Flat Belly Diet Diabetes Workout. If you have diabetes, it also means working with your doctor to be sure you know how to protect yourself from blood sugar "lows" and from foot problems during exercise.

Knowing your numbers is crucial for everyone. If you have diabetes, maintaining healthy blood sugar levels is *the* way to lower your risk for serious and even life-threatening complications such as heart attacks, strokes, high blood pressure, kidney failure, nerve damage, vision loss, and amputation. If you're at risk for diabetes, a blood sugar check is the only way to find out whether or not you have prediabetes or have already developed full-blown type 2 diabetes—or (and I hope this is the case!) if your blood sugar is still at a healthy level.

Remember, diabetes often has no symptoms—you may not feel a thing as blood sugar levels rise. This is the reason nearly 6 million people in the United States have type 2 diabetes but don't know it—and why tens of millions more have prediabetes, the step before full-blown diabetes, yet are unaware of it.

Working with Your Doctor

OUR TEST PANELISTS TOLD us over and over about the importance of tracking these numbers. One, Joe Sicurella, has prediabetes—and thanks to regular blood sugar checks and a healthy lifestyle has been able to avoid full-blown diabetes for 15 years. "I see my doctor twice a year for blood sugar tests, and I test my blood sugar at home, too, with a meter," he says. "It's the only way to know how I'm doing. My doctor jokes that if I get diabetes, it won't be until I'm in my nineties!"

One of the most stunning facts I've learned about diabetes, prediabetes, and metabolic syndrome (a step before prediabetes) is how these conditions also raise your risk for heart attacks and strokes. That's why the American Diabetes Association says it's vital for people with diabetes to know their blood pressure, cholesterol, and triglyceride levels—and keep them in a healthy range. It's equally important if you're at risk for diabetes. And in fact, as you'll discover on the following pages, knowing these numbers can even tip you off to early body chemistry changes that can lead to diabetes.

"Knowing your blood sugar, cholesterol, and blood pressure levels is empowering," Dr. Edelman told me. "You feel more in control. You and your doctor have the information you need to take the next steps. You don't have to worry any longer—you know where you stand and you're ready to take action."

You've probably had your cholesterol, triglycerides, and blood pressure checked, but do you know the whole story about your blood sugar status? After discussing the growing diabetes epidemic with Gillian and Dr. Edelman, I believe knowing your blood sugar levels is as basic and important as knowing your telephone number and your e-mail address!

Why am I on my soapbox here? Consider this: The American Diabetes Association recommends diabetes screening start at age 45—earlier if you're at risk. But thanks to the rise in obesity and the drop in physical activity in the United States, "earlier" now applies to most of us! Get checked *now* if you're carrying a few extra pounds and have even one of the diabetes risk factors we mentioned in Chapter 1: an inactive lifestyle; a family history of diabetes; a personal history of high blood pressure, low HDLs, high triglycerides, diabetes during pregnancy, and/or polycystic ovary syndrome; African American, Asian American, Hispanic, Native American, or Pacific Islander ancestry.

How early should you begin? The American College of Endocrinology, an association of physicians who specialize in hormonal disorders including diabetes, recommends starting in your thirties.[1] If type 2 diabetes runs strongly in your family, then testing beginning in your twenties makes sense, too.

If you have diabetes and haven't had an A1c check—an important check of long-term blood sugar control—in the past 3 to 6 months, it's time for an A1c test. And if you have diabetes, this is the perfect time to take a look at your home blood sugar monitoring routine and perhaps brush up your skills and check your equipment.

In this chapter, you'll find everything you need to ask your doctor to be successful on the Flat Belly Diet Diabetes. Let's get started!

For Everyone

"How are my blood pressure, cholesterol levels, and triglycerides?"

YOUR DOCTOR OR HEALTH-CARE practitioner will most likely check these along with a fasting blood sugar test. If not, ask her to do so. These numbers are important because they assess your risk for heart attacks and strokes—major health risks for people with diabetes, prediabetes, and metabolic syndrome. And there's emerging evidence that for people with diabetes, they're not just important indicators of the health of your cardiovascular system. They may also indicate your risk for nerve damage, a complication experienced by three out of five people with diabetes. If you do not have diabetes, they also help determine whether you have metabolic syndrome, a condition that begins raising your risk

Am I Cleared for Exercise?

For most people, the Flat Belly Diet Diabetes exercise program is perfectly safe. But we recommend that you talk with your doctor first if you've had a heart attack, asthma, heart disease, liver or kidney disease, chest pain, joint pain, arthritis, osteoporosis, dizziness or balance problems, persistent pain or other problems from a joint or muscle injury, or if you take medication for a chronic medical condition.

According to the American College of Sports Medicine, you should also discuss your exercise plans with your doctor if two or more of the following describe you:

- You're a man older than age 45 or a woman older than age 55.
- You have a family history of heart disease before age 55.
- You have high blood pressure or high cholesterol.
- You smoke or you quit smoking in the past 6 months.
- You're overweight or obese.

If you have diabetes and have foot problems such as nerve damage or poor circulation, it's also important to discuss exercise with your doctor before you begin. If foot problems mean that walking's not right for you, you can follow our optional program that uses an inexpensive "pedaler"—a small piece of exercise equipment, like the pedals on a bike, that you use while seated in a chair.

for diabetes even if your blood sugar levels look normal.

If any of these numbers are high, your doctor may suggest starting with healthy lifestyle changes—weight loss, exercise, healthy eating (all of which you can achieve via the Flat Belly Diet Diabetes, by the way!)—and may or may not add medication to help you reach healthy targets. You may be rechecked in 3 to 6 months. How often should you be retested after that? Your doctor will probably check your blood pressure at every visit—and at the very least, once a year. Experts recommend that people who do not have diabetes get their cholesterol and triglycerides checked at least once every 5 years, more often if they've ever been high. If you have diabetes, they should be checked annually.

BLOOD PRESSURE Hypertension, or high blood pressure, damages arteries and raises your risk for heart attack and stroke. It also contributes to kidney failure if you have diabetes. The top number, called systolic pressure, measures pressure during a heart beat; the bottom measures diastolic pressure, the force of blood through your arteries between beats. All measurements are in millimeters of mercury.

WHAT THE RESULTS MEAN:

BLOOD PRESSURE	
LOW BLOOD PRESSURE	Below 90/60 mm Hg
HEALTHY	119/79 mm Hg to 90/60 mm Hg (115/75 mm Hg is ideal)
PREHYPERTENSION	120/80 mm Hg to 139/89 mm Hg
HYPERTENSION	140/90 mm Hg and above

NOTE: Your blood pressure is considered low if the top number falls below 90 or the second falls below 60. It's a problem if you're getting dizzy or faint; low blood pressure can also be caused by infections or severe allergic reactions.

WHEN TO RETEST: At least once a year; recheck after 3 to 6 months if you're trying to lower your blood pressure with healthy lifestyle changes.

LDL CHOLESTEROL "Bad" LDL cholesterol packs heart-threatening plaque into artery walls, raising your odds for a heart attack or stroke. It also contributes to circulation problems, already a concern for people with diabetes, especially in the legs and feet.

WHAT THE RESULTS MEAN:

LDL CHOLESTEROL	
IDEAL	Less than 100 mg/dL
HEALTHY	100 to 129 mg/dL
BORDERLINE HIGH	130 to 159 mg/dL
HIGH	160 to 189 mg/dL
VERY HIGH	190 mg/dL and above

WHEN TO RETEST: Repeat every 5 years if normal; after 3 to 6 months if you're using healthy lifestyle changes to lower high LDLs.

HDL CHOLESTEROL This "good" cholesterol protects against heart attack and stroke by ferrying "bad" LDLs to the liver for elimination. When HDLs are low, your body can't eliminate LDLs effectively. This raises risk for heart attacks and strokes.

WHAT THE RESULTS MEAN:

HDL CHOLESTEROL	
LOW	Below 50 mg/dL for women, below 40 mg/dL for men
HEALTHY	50 mg/dL and over for women, 40 mg/dL and over for men
IDEAL	60 mg/dL and above

WHEN TO RETEST: Repeat every 5 years if normal; after 3 to 6 months if you're using healthy lifestyle changes to improve HDL levels.

TRIGLYCERIDES Normally, this blood fat carries extra fat from the food you eat to fat cells for storage. But if you eat too much fat or too many calories, your liver converts the excess into an overabundance of triglycerides—then uses them as raw material for making small, dense LDLs, an extra-lethal type of LDL that accelerates growth of plaque in artery walls. At high levels, these blood fats raise heart attack and stroke risk. If you have diabetes, high triglycerides are troublesome for another reason: They seem to go hand in hand with extra risk for nerve damage, University of Michigan researchers report in a new study. In fact, the researchers say people with diabetes should be as careful with their triglycerides as they are with their blood sugar![2]

WHAT THE RESULTS MEAN:

TRIGLYCERIDES	
NORMAL	Less than 150 mg/dL
BORDERLINE HIGH	150–199 mg/dL
HIGH	200–499 mg/dL
VERY HIGH	500 mg/dL and above

WHEN TO RETEST: Repeat every 5 years if normal; after 3 to 6 months if you're using healthy life-style changes to lower high levels of triglycerides.

If You Do NOT Have Diabetes

What's My Blood Sugar Level?

DOCTORS MOST OFTEN USE the results of a fasting blood sugar test to determine whether you have diabetes or prediabetes (a potent risk factor for diabetes). Some health-care practitioners prefer the oral glucose tolerance test, which takes longer to administer. Which test is right for you? That's a decision your doctor will make. The details:

FASTING BLOOD SUGAR Long the gold standard for diagnosing diabetes and prediabetes, the fasting blood sugar test (also called a fasting plasma glucose test) is quick and only a *little* inconvenient: You can't eat for

8 to 12 hours before your blood is drawn. Studies show that morning tests are twice as likely to catch blood-sugar problems as afternoon tests. The reason is that waiting until afternoon usually means fasting for *more* than 12 hours, and blood sugar often drops precipitously after 14 or more hours without food. So while a morning test might turn up prediabetes or even full-blown diabetes, the evidence could disappear by midafternoon because your body has used up the excess blood sugar for energy. Bottom line: Make sure your appointment is first thing in the morning for best results.

HOW IT WORKS: After an 8- to 12-hour overnight fast, you report to the doctor's office or to a commercial lab (with a lab test order from your doctor) and have your blood drawn. Glucose (sugar) levels are analyzed and reported to your doctor.

GOOD FOR: Detecting diabetes and most, but not all, prediabetes.

NOT GOOD FOR: People who already have diabetes. You'll get the information you need from daily self-checks and regular A1c tests (described below).

WHAT THE RESULTS MEAN:

FASTING BLOOD SUGAR	
HEALTHY	70 to 99 mg/dL
PREDIABETES	100 to 125 mg/dL
DIABETES	126 mg/dL and above

NOTE: Doctors usually test twice to confirm a diagnosis of diabetes.

WHEN TO RETEST: We recommend at least once a year if you're at risk for diabetes.

ORAL GLUCOSE TOLERANCE TEST This check, which tests your body's response to blood sugar immediately after a meal, takes longer than the fasting blood glucose test—more than 2 hours from start to finish. It can be a more sensitive way to detect some prediabetes, and to assess whether prediabetes is progressing toward diabetes. For these reasons, the American Diabetes Association says it can be used in place of a fasting blood sugar check. Some doctors use it in addition to a fasting check to look for high blood sugar levels after a meal that might be missed by a fasting test.

HOW IT WORKS: After an overnight fast (8 to 12 hours or so), you report to the doctor's office or lab. A blood sample is taken (to check fasting blood sugar), then you drink a very sweet beverage (sort of like a flat cola or orange soda, but thicker) containing 75 milligrams of glucose. Your blood is drawn after 1 hour and again after 2 hours. (Bring something to read—you'll be sitting in a waiting room between blood draws!) Blood glucose (blood sugar) levels of both blood samples will be checked.

Note: This test may sound familiar if you've ever had a diabetes test during pregnancy. Pregnant women are usually given a similar oral glucose challenge test for gestational diabetes. For that test, you may be checked just once an hour after sipping a smaller glucose drink or up to three times in 3 hours after drinking a larger drink. Testing positive for gestational diabetes doesn't mean you have lifelong diabetes, though it does raise your risk for later type 2 diabetes.

GOOD FOR: Catching some cases of prediabetes that would be missed by a fasting blood sugar test.

NOT GOOD FOR: People with diabetes. Read on for the checks that are right for you.

WHAT THE RESULTS MEAN:

ORAL GLUCOSE TOLERANCE TEST	
NORMAL	Less than 140 mg/dL
PREDIABETES	From 140 to 200 mg/dL
DIABETES	Over 200 mg/dL

NOTE: Doctors usually test twice to confirm a diagnosis of diabetes.

WHEN TO RETEST: We recommend rechecking once a year if you're at risk for diabetes.

Do I Have Metabolic Syndrome?

BE SURE YOU REVIEW all of your health numbers with your doctor—we also recommend knowing your current blood pressure, cholesterol, and triglyceride levels. You have metabolic syndrome if you have any three of the following:

- A waist measurement of 40 inches or more for men and 35 inches or more for women
- Triglyceride levels of 150 milligrams per deciliter (mg/dL) or above, or taking medication for elevated triglyceride levels
- HDL, or "good," cholesterol level below 40 mg/dL for men and below 50 mg/dL for women, or taking medication for low HDL levels
- Blood pressure levels of 130/85 or above, or taking medication for elevated blood pressure levels
- Fasting blood sugar levels of 100 mg/dL or above, or taking medication for elevated blood glucose levels[3]

WHY IT MATTERS: Metabolic syndrome may look like a bunch of little, unrelated health problems, but it's a sign that you have insulin resistance—the driving force behind type 2 diabetes. Don't ignore it. Even if your blood sugar is still in the normal range, it boosts your risk for eventually developing diabetes five times higher and your risk for cardiovascular disease 1.6 to 2 times higher than it is for people who do not have metabolic syndrome.[4] The more of this health condition's signature traits you have, the higher your risk. Compared to three traits, having five raised diabetes risk twice as high—to 10 times higher than normal—in one British study.[5, 6]

WHAT YOU AND YOUR DOCTOR CAN DO: Many experts say lifestyle changes like the ones we describe in the Flat Belly Diet Diabetes are usually the first choice for taming metabolic syndrome,[7] but be sure to get your doctor involved. She can advise you about the best ways to raise your HDLs, control blood pressure, and lower your triglycerides. Ask how often you should have these risk factors rechecked to see if they're returning to

"Hidden" High Blood Sugar: Not So Sweet

About 100 million Americans are stuck in a dangerous blood-sugar information gap. This includes 5.7 million with undiagnosed type 2 diabetes,[8] 57 million with prediabetes,[9] and 47 million with metabolic syndrome[10] (there's some overlap between the last two groups,[11] so the true total is impossible to pinpoint).

You may be among them if you're at risk for diabetes and haven't had a fasting blood sugar test in the past year—or if you have diabetes and haven't, for whatever reason, been monitoring your own blood sugar regularly or getting A1c checks—a test of long-term blood sugar control—every 3 to 6 months. Why the gap? We've found five reasons:

The diabetes epidemic is moving fast. Rates of diabetes climbed 50 percent between 1990 and 2000,[12] and then doubled between 2005 and 2009. In the past, keeping up with your health status meant asking about your blood pressure and your cholesterol levels. Now it's time to add, "How's my blood sugar?" to the list.

There's confusion about who needs to be screened for diabetes. Don't wait until you're age 45 or older! Get screened now if you're overweight and have even one of the diabetes risks mentioned earlier in this chapter. The American College of Endocrinology recommends starting in your thirties.[13] If type 2 diabetes runs strongly in your family, then it is never too early because teenage kids and younger are developing type 2 diabetes.

Your doctor might have overlooked your risk. In November of 2008, the Centers for Disease Control and Prevention (CDC) released a survey showing that just 4 percent of people with prediabetes have been told by their doctors that they have it.[14] Experts note that doctors sometimes downplay the importance of prediabetes—shrugging it off as a "borderline" or "mild" problem. Same goes for metabolic syndrome.

If you have diabetes, you may need a "refresher course" in the art of daily blood sugar monitoring. Today, 40 percent of people with diabetes don't check their blood sugar on a daily basis, according to a report from the CDC.[15] If you have diabetes, we recommend daily checks while you're on the Flat Belly Diet Diabetes so that you know how your new eating and exercise habits influence your blood sugar.

If you have diabetes, you may need more frequent A1c checks. In one survey of 157,000 diabetic women and men conducted by the American Academy of Clinical Endocrinologists, 85 percent *thought* they were keeping the lid on high blood sugar. But two out of three were actually experiencing dangerous blood sugar "highs" that can lead to serious complications. What went wrong? Study participants said they knew that *daily* sugar checks were vital. But half didn't know the results of their latest A1c test, and others weren't getting these checks as often as diabetes groups now recommend.[16]

healthier levels and whether you might be a candidate for medication.

WHAT ELSE YOU SHOULD KNOW: Women from some racial and ethnic backgrounds are at higher risk for metabolic syndrome than men from the same backgrounds. In one study that looked at metabolic syndrome rates among 8,814 people, African American women had a 57 percent higher risk than African American men and Hispanic American women had a 26 percent higher risk than Hispanic American men.[17] For everyone, risk rises with age, nearly doubling from your twenties to your thirties and tripling in your forties.[18] And while any combination of the five traits is risky, one study of postmenopausal women found that those who had the largest waistlines plus high triglycerides were five times more likely to have a fatal heart attack or stroke compared to women without metabolic syndrome.[19]

Do I Have Prediabetes?

YOU HAVE PREDIABETES—ALSO CALLED impaired fasting glucose or impaired glucose tolerance—if you have one of the following:

- A fasting blood sugar level of 100 to 125 mg/dL
- Oral glucose tolerance test results of 140 to 200 mg/dL

WHY IT MATTERS: One in four people with prediabetes develop full-blown, type 2 diabetes within 3 to 5 years and 8 out of 10 develop it over the course of their lifetimes—*if they don't take steps to prevent it*, says the CDC.[20] Your risk may be even higher if you're of African American, Latino, Asian, Pacific Islander, or Native American descent. Finding out you have prediabetes isn't a reason to panic. Think of it as major motivation: You have an important window of opportunity for making healthy changes to prevent diabetes.

WHAT YOU AND YOUR DOCTOR CAN DO: If you've had a fasting blood sugar test, ask your doctor about also doing an oral glucose tolerance test to get a better picture of what's going on with your prediabetes. If the results of both are elevated, your odds for developing diabetes are even higher. A healthy lifestyle is your number one priority. In one study, losing weight, flattening your belly, and becoming active cut risk for progressing from prediabetes to diabetes by 58 percent.[21] If you don't yet have prediabetes, the same steps can help prevent it.

Ask your doctor whether you should get a blood sugar meter for home blood sugar testing to uncover times of day when blood sugar is climbing toward the diabetic range. And make an appointment to have your blood sugar rechecked by your doctor in 6 months to a year. In addition to the healthy changes you'll make on the Flat Belly Diet Diabetes, your doctor may suggest a diabetes medication such as metformin, which helps improve the way your body absorbs blood sugar and cuts your risk for diabetes by 31 percent. While the FDA has not yet approved any medications for prediabetes, state-of-the-art treatment often includes this step for people younger than age 65 with impaired glucose tolerance, because some studies suggest it may help this group of people.

WHAT ELSE YOU SHOULD KNOW: Don't limit the conversation to blood sugar. Be sure your blood pressure, cholesterol levels, and triglycerides are also within healthy ranges to protect your cardiovascular system.

If You Have Diabetes

IF YOU'VE ALREADY BEEN diagnosed with type 2 diabetes, your "prepare for success" plan focuses on daily self-checks with a blood sugar meter plus regular tests of your long-term blood sugar control with an A1c test. (In contrast, the fasting blood sugar test and oral glucose challenge described above are good at *diagnosing* diabetes and prediabetes, but aren't useful for *monitoring* blood sugar once you have diabetes.)

It's also important to know how to check your blood sugar once you've started the Flat Belly Diet Diabetes—to see where you're succeeding, to pinpoint foods that raise your blood sugar more than others, and to monitor for low blood sugar situations if you use insulin or other blood sugar–lowering medications. We also have advice on getting your doctor's okay to start exercising and on avoiding blood sugar lows during and after your workout.

How's My Daily Blood Sugar?

GLUCOSE MONITORING To use your glucose monitor—also called a blood sugar meter or glucometer—just prick your finger for a blood sample and you get nearly instant feedback about your blood sugar level. These checks are a cornerstone of stellar blood sugar control because they give you immediate, real-time information about how the sandwich you just ate for lunch, the medication you took 2 hours ago, the walk you just enjoyed, or even the relaxation exercise you'll soon learn in Phase 1 of the Flat Belly Diet Diabetes affects your blood sugar. This information empowers you to make smart decisions that help keep your blood sugar within a healthy range.

GOOD FOR: Revealing your blood sugar level at one moment in time. Daily tests are like snapshots and are extremely useful for finding out how high your blood sugar is at key times of the day: first thing in the morning before you eat, before a meal, and before and after exercise. They also let you see how well your body handles the natural rise in blood sugar after you eat. These checks give you up-to-the-minute info on how your meal choices and portions, physical activity, stress levels, and medications affect your blood sugar. Regular checks are vital if you take insulin or other diabetes medications, have low blood sugar episodes without warning signs, or have a difficult time controlling your diabetes.

NOT GOOD FOR: Knowing with certainty whether your blood sugar was in control all day and all night—simply because you can't test 24/7, and therefore, you can't catch every rise and fall.

WHAT THE RESULTS MEAN:

GLUCOSE MONITORING	
IDEAL ON A FASTING TEST OR BEFORE A MEAL	90 to 130 mg/dL
IDEAL 2 HOURS AFTER THE BEGINNING OF A MEAL	Less than 180 mg/dL

WHEN TO RETEST: As recommended by your doctor. Some people test many times each day; others with well-controlled blood sugar test just a few times a week.

How's My Long-Term Blood Sugar Control?

A1C LEVELS An A1c check, usually done in your doctor's office, tells you what your blood sugar "batting average" is. It's a sign of your overall blood sugar level for the past 2 to 3 months and clues you in about how well your blood sugar was controlled around the clock, every day. High levels over many years increase your odds for diabetes complications; in-control levels reduce them. The A1c tells you how much blood sugar has attached itself to hemoglobin molecules in your red blood cells. The more sugar coated hemoglobin you have, the higher your A1c percentage is. Home tests are available and can be convenient, but always share the results with your doctor and your diabetes care team, so that changes can be made in your diabetes management plan if needed.

GOOD FOR: Seeing whether your diabetes management plan is really working.

NOT GOOD FOR: Judging how your blood sugar responds to specific meals, foods, exercise sessions, or to a single dose of medication.

WHAT THE RESULTS MEAN:

A1C LEVELS	
IDEAL	Below 6.5% if recommended by your doctor
HEALTHY	Below 7 percent
HIGH	Above 7 percent for most people with diabetes

NOTE: Each person's goal may be different, so be sure to discuss it with your doctor.

WHEN TO TEST: Two to four times a year or as recommended by your doctor.

How Should I Monitor My Blood Sugar While I'm on the Flat Belly Diet Diabetes?

EVEN IF YOUR BLOOD sugar is so well controlled that you only have to double-check with your blood sugar monitor a few times a week, we recommend talking with your doctor about increasing your self-checks as you begin the Flat

Belly Diet Diabetes. Why? For several reasons: First, there's no doubt that altering your diet and physical activity patterns will have an impact on your blood sugar. You may find that your blood sugar becomes easier to control or that levels are dipping lower more often—a situation that, if you take medication, will require a phone call to or visit with your doctor to discuss your diabetes drugs and doses. Getting into the habit of regular blood sugar monitoring will help you pinpoint personal trigger foods that raise your blood sugar and that you'll want to eat sparingly or avoid.

If you don't have a blood sugar meter, we recommend shopping the smart way. Meters can be inexpensive or even free, and insurance sometimes covers the full cost. A bigger expense: test strips and lancets for getting a blood sample. Before you buy, check to see which supplies your insurance company covers so that testing is as economically painless as possible. (More on reducing the pain of getting a blood sample in a minute!)

You need one more important tool: a blood sugar logbook. Some monitors

The Perfect Diabetes Checkup

If you have diabetes, you should plan to see your doctor about every 3 to 6 months—every 3 to 4 months if you're using insulin. You may need to be seen more often if your blood sugar is not under tight control, a little less often if your blood sugar is staying within your target ranges.

Staying healthy with diabetes means working with a "diabetes care team"—a group of practitioners who understand that you have diabetes and have special needs. That team will include your family doctor, eye doctor, and dentist. It may also include an endocrinologist (a diabetes specialist) to help you achieve the best blood sugar control possible, a registered dietitian to help with healthy eating, a certified diabetes educator (who could be a registered dietitian or a nurse) to help you fit healthy changes into your life, a podiatrist if you're having nerve or circulation problems due to diabetes, and even an exercise physiologist to help you develop a custom-tailored exercise program and a therapist or social worker to help you cope with emotional and relationship issues raised by living with diabetes.

store data and allow you to download it into a blood sugar–monitoring computer program. If you don't have a logbook, ask your doctor for one—or use the journal pages in this book, which include space for daily checks. Be sure to bring your logbook to all appointments with your doctor and other members of your diabetes care team. If your meter stores readings and allows you to download them into your computer, that works, too. Just be sure to make printouts.

Your doctor can help you set up a monitoring strategy that's right for you. Here are some considerations:

KNOW YOUR TARGET LEVELS. For people with diabetes, recommended blood sugar levels at different times of day are:

- **BEFORE MEALS:** 90 to 130 mg/dL
- **TWO HOURS AFTER MEALS:** Below 180 mg/dL
- **BEDTIME:** 110 to 150 mg/dL

However, your personal targets may be slightly different. Talk with your doctor about your personal blood sugar goals for pre-meal and post-meal readings.

Several times a year, your doctor and/or diabetes care team should:

- Review successes and challenges of your diabetes care plan
- Review your blood sugar monitoring logbook
- Ask about episodes of high and low blood sugar since your last visit
- Ask how your diabetes care plan is working in everyday life
- Discuss any symptoms you have that might indicate a diabetes complication
- Review all of the medications you take (not just diabetes medications)
- Check your height, weight, and blood pressure
- Examine your feet
- Take blood for an A1c test (at most visits)

You should have the following checks:

- Eye exam—once a year
- Dental exam—twice a year
- Blood tests for cholesterol and triglycerides—once a year
- Urine test for a protein called albumin that can indicate kidney problems—once a year

REVIEW YOUR TESTING PROCEDURE. Ask your doctor, nurse, or certified diabetes educator to watch you take a sample reading. Clean up and boost circulation (it makes getting a good sample droplet easier!) by washing your hands in warm water, then shake your hand below your waist to increase blood circulation. Learn how to check your glucose. Use a fresh lancet in your meter to do the finger stick, and put the drop directly onto the test strip.

SCHEDULE YOUR SUGAR CHECKS. Discuss the best times of day with your doctor or team. Testing before and then 2 hours after a meal is important, because it gives you a picture of how well your body is processing blood sugar. You'll also want to test before, after, and even during exercise and at any time when you think your levels may be high or low.

LOOK FOR PATTERNS. Look through your log every week or so to see if you're reaching your goals—or if you're experiencing highs or lows. This information will help you and your doctor further customize your diabetes management plan and make adjustments as you move through the 35 days of the Flat Belly Diet Diabetes—and beyond.

STAY IN TOUCH WITH YOUR DOCTOR AND/OR TEAM. Ask your doctor when you should check in to discuss your blood sugar patterns. If you take medication, for example, your doctor may have to adjust the dose or even the drugs you take if your blood sugar levels begin to drop.

How Can I Avoid Low Blood Sugar on the Flat Belly Diet Diabetes?

IF YOU HAVE DIABETES and use insulin or one of a handful of other medications (listed below) to help control your blood sugar, it is important to talk with your doctor about how to avoid episodes of *low* blood sugar, or hypoglycemia. Signs of low blood sugar include sweating, lightheadedness, shakiness, weakness, anxiety, hunger, headache, problems concentrating, and confusion. More severe cases can cause fainting or seizures. Use of diabetes medication is the most common cause of hypoglycemia. (People who don't use these medications—and who don't have diabetes—may also develop hypoglycemia due to missed meals, release of too much insulin after a meal, or, even more rarely, due to disorders of the pancreas or adrenal or pituitary glands. These types of hypoglycemia need medical attention, but probably wouldn't be affected by the Flat Belly Diet Diabetes eating plan or exercise program.)

If you take medications that act to increase the insulin in your bloodstream, your blood sugar could drop too low if you eat significantly less food than usual, if you cut back on carbohydrates such as grains, sweets, and fruits, or if you increase your physical activity. Since you'll be doing all of these things on the Flat Belly Diet Diabetes, knowing how to prevent hypoglycemia, how to recognize it, and how to fix it are essential. Your strategy may involve altering your medication schedule or doses, extra blood sugar checks, or even adjusting your eating plan or exercise routine—steps you can only take with the guidance of your doctor and/or other members of your diabetes care team.

Here's how to work with your team to minimize hypoglycemia risk:

REVIEW YOUR MEDICATIONS AND DOSES. Insulin users have a higher risk for hypoglycemia, but the other diabetes drugs that increase your body's insulin production can also lead to "lows." These include chlorpropamide (Diabinese), glyburide drugs (including DiaBeta, Glynase, Micronase), glipizide drugs (such as Glucotrol, Glucotrol XL), glimepiride (Amaryl), nateglinide (Starlix), repaglinide (Prandin), tolbutamide (Orinase), and tolazamide (Tolinase).

The injected drug exenatide (Byetta) can also cause hypoglycemia if used in combination with chlorpropamide, glimepiride, glipizide, glyburide, tolazamide, and tolbutamide. Some combination drugs can also contribute to "lows," including glipizide + metformin (Metaglip); glyburide + metformin (Glucovance); pioglitazone + glimepiride (Duetact); and rosiglitazone + glimepiride (Avandaryl).

DISCUSS THE BEST STRATEGIES FOR YOU FOR AVOIDING "LOWS." Since medications, doses, and schedules are so individual, it's important to custom-tailor this approach with your doctor, certified diabetes educator, or another member of your diabetes care team. It's not something to do on your own. Some ways to avoid lows include:

■ Whether you can adjust your medication dosages to reduce your odds for lows during exercise. For example, if you use insulin, your doctor may suggest slightly lowering the dose of fast-acting insulin at the meal before your workout.

■ Picking the best injection site for insulin. Should you avoid injecting in your leg before you walk or in your arm before you use resistance bands? Maybe. Exercising a muscle that's near an injection site could lead to faster absorption and lower blood sugar.

■ Checking your blood sugar before you exercise. If you use insulin or some types of oral diabetes medications, consider having part of your snack before you work out if your blood sugar level is below 100 mg/dL.

■ Rechecking during exercise during your first week or two on the Flat Belly Diet Diabetes, to see how your body responds to physical activity.

■ Recheck after you're done . . . and a few more times during the day. (Ask your doctor how often and when.) Exercise can keep your blood sugar levels lower for up to 24 hours afterward, as your muscles continue to absorb extra blood sugar.

KNOW THE SYMPTOMS OF HYPOGLYCEMIA—AND WHAT TO DO. Review the warning signs with your doctor, as well as the strategies outlined below for treating it.

SYMPTOMS: These can be a little different for each person, and include nervousness, shakiness, hunger, lightheadedness, sweating, irritability, impatience, chills, fast heartbeat, anxiety, anger, sadness, clumsiness, blurred vision, sleepiness, stubbornness, nausea, tingly or numb tongue or lips, nightmares, headaches, unusual behavior, and confusion. When blood glucose falls low enough, unconsciousness and seizures may occur.

WHAT TO DO: If you use insulin or any other diabetes medication that can cause hypoglycemia, these steps are essential:

Be prepared. Have a blood sugar meter handy so that you can check your sugar level before, during, and after exercise—and right away if you have any signs of low blood sugar. Generally, a reading below 70 mg/dL is considered hypoglycemia. Don't have your meter? If you suspect your blood sugar is dropping, treat the situation as hypoglycemia and act accordingly. It's the safe thing to do.

Keep a supply of "fast acting" carbohydrates with you, such as hard candy, a can of sweetened soda (not diet or sugar-free) or orange juice, or glucose tablets or gel. (Chocolate and candies with nuts aren't a good idea—the fat slows absorption of blood sugar, which isn't what you need during hypoglycemia.) If your blood sugar drops, eating or drinking something that raises it quickly is essential.

Use the 15–15 rule. To take care of mild to moderate hypoglycemia, eat or drink something containing 15 grams of carbohydrate, wait 15 minutes, and test your blood sugar to see if it has risen above about 80 mg/dL. (Ask your doctor what your target should be.) If your blood sugar is still too low, have another 15 grams of carbohydrates. Wait another 15 minutes and test again. Recommended carbs, in 15-gram portions, are:

- Four to five glucose tablets (dosage varies by product)
- Two teaspoons of sugar, honey, or corn syrup
- One 0.68-ounce tube of decorating gel, such as Cake Mate
- One serving of glucose gel (e.g., Glutose)
- Six to 8 ounces of fat-free or 1% milk
- Four ounces of orange juice
- Five to seven Life Savers
- One-half can of sweetened soft drink (not diet or sugar free)

Important note: If you also take the medications acarbose (Precose) or miglitol (Glyset), be sure to carry glucose tablets or glucose gel. Only pure glucose (also called dextrose) will raise your blood sugar sufficiently. Foods and drinks won't work quickly enough because these medications slow the digestion of carbohydrates.

ASK IF YOU'RE AT RISK FOR SEVERE HYPOGLYCEMIA. If you are, be sure your family and exercise partners know how to recognize the signs of a blood sugar "low." They can help you eat or drink something, or can call 9-1-1 if necessary. Ask your doctor whether you need a glucagon emergency kit, which can be used in extreme hypoglycemia.

KNOW WHEN TO CALL YOUR DOCTOR ABOUT LOW BLOOD SUGAR. If you are taking insulin, the general rule is to contact your doctor if you have hypoglycemia more than three times in a week or if you have severe low blood sugar (less than 40 mg/dL or if you needed help). If you take other medications, contact your doctor, certified diabetes educator, or nurse if your blood sugar is often below 80 mg/dL or if you've had an episode of severe low blood sugar. It may be time to change your medication doses, switch drugs, set up a new medication schedule, tweak the timing of your exercise, or review the effects of your meal plan on your blood sugar.

What Do I Need to Know about Exercising Safely?

THE FLAT BELLY DIET Diabetes exercise plan includes walking, gentle resistance training, and belly-flattening exercises. No sprinting, no gearing up for a marathon, and no Olympic-style weight lifting is involved! But be sure to discuss it with your health-care practitioner and get her okay—particularly if you're over age 35; have had type 2 diabetes for more than 10 years; have heart disease or a strong family history of heart disease, high cholesterol, or high blood pressure; or have diabetes-related eye problems, nerve damage, foot injuries, or circulation problems. Your health-care practitioner may want you to take an exercise stress test to evaluate how healthy your heart is first before you embark on an exercise program.

Discuss these exercise-related issues:

FOOT CARE: One in four people with diabetes develops foot complications, thanks to reduced blood circulation and nerve damage that allow "little" problems like blisters to become major infections. Be sure to inspect your feet every day, looking for even tiny skin problems such as redness, chafing, blisters, sores, or cuts. Ask your doctor what to look for, how to treat little problems, and when a foot problem deserves a trip to the doctor's office. You should also wash and dry your feet carefully every day, then apply a moisturizer made for people with diabetes. Ask your doctor for a recommendation. And ask how often you should have your feet examined by your doctor; once a year is the general rule, but you may need more frequent checks as you become physically active.

STAYING HYDRATED WHILE EXERCISING: Hot-weather exercising could raise your risk for dehydration, especially if your blood sugar isn't well controlled. The reason: High blood sugar levels lead to more urination and to a reduced sense of thirst, so you end up with more fluid leaving your body and less coming in. But the opposite is also true: Dehydration can cause your blood sugar level to rise. It's smart to sip 12 to 16 ounces of water before you begin exercising and another 4 ounces (that's a half-cup) every 15 to 20 minutes while you're exercising. Ask your doctor how you can recognize signs of dehydration.

WEARING A MEDICAL ID BRACELET: If you're exercising alone, a medical ID could save your life in the event of an emergency. Ask your doctor what it should say.

READ A FLAT BELLY
SUCCESS
STORY

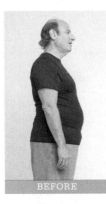

BEFORE

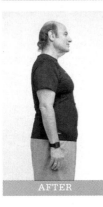

AFTER

Steve Lipman

AGE: 63

POUNDS LOST:

10.4

IN 35 DAYS

ALL-OVER INCHES LOST:

2

✳ **BLOOD SUGAR: A1C FELL FROM 6.2 TO**

6.1

PERCENT

* The A1c is a check of long-term blood sugar control; for most people with diabetes, a reading below 7 percent is considered ideal.

"I LOST MORE THAN 10 POUNDS! I DON'T HAVE THE KIND OF metabolism that lets me cheat," Steve says. "If I eat the wrong foods or slack off on exercise, I get a real reversal of fortune. Lucky for me, I love nuts, I love avocado, and whenever I got a chance to have 10 olives as part of a Flat Belly Diet Diabetes meal, I would pop them in my mouth like M&Ms! When I heard I could eat an ounce of chocolate, I was excited. And I lost more than 10 pounds!"

Diagnosed with type 2 diabetes 12 years ago, Steve says he ignored early warning signals that had emerged years earlier. "Four years before my diagnosis, my doctor told me I was gaining weight and that my blood pressure and cholesterol were creeping up, but I didn't really pay attention," he says. "I didn't realize what was coming my way. When I found out I had diabetes, it hit me like a ton of bricks. I didn't know anyone with diabetes; I didn't know what the long-term repercussions were—but I just didn't like the sound of the word."

The news changed his life forever. "I began losing weight and exercising," he says. "I quickly discovered battling weight and adding diabetes to the equation is practically the hardest thing I've ever had to do. It's a job that never ends. What I've learned is that losing weight isn't rocket science. It just takes commitment and hard work."

Steve's Flat Belly Diet Diabetes experience has added some new meals and strategies to his weight-control arsenal. "The whole wheat tortilla roll-up with hummus and pine nuts, with deli turkey on the side, is a snack I adored. It's like pizza—very filling, tasty, and the pine nuts add a nice crunch."

Blood sugar control is something Steve had already mastered—thanks to a long-standing exercise routine (he works out at a local gym), healthy eating, and daily medication (metformin). "My A1c was already at a very healthy 6.2—a good level for someone with type 2 diabetes that can help lower my risk for diabetes complications," he says. "It was great seeing that I could add some delicious foods and see it fall a little bit further in just 5 weeks."

The icing on the cake? Steve took his Flat Belly Diet Diabetes habits along during a 5-day stay at an island resort in Barbados and didn't gain an ounce. "I took meal replacement bars and little bags of almonds and sunflower seeds with me and ate carefully," says Steve, a student affairs administrator for a music college. "Amazingly, I didn't gain any weight at all. This diet can go anywhere."

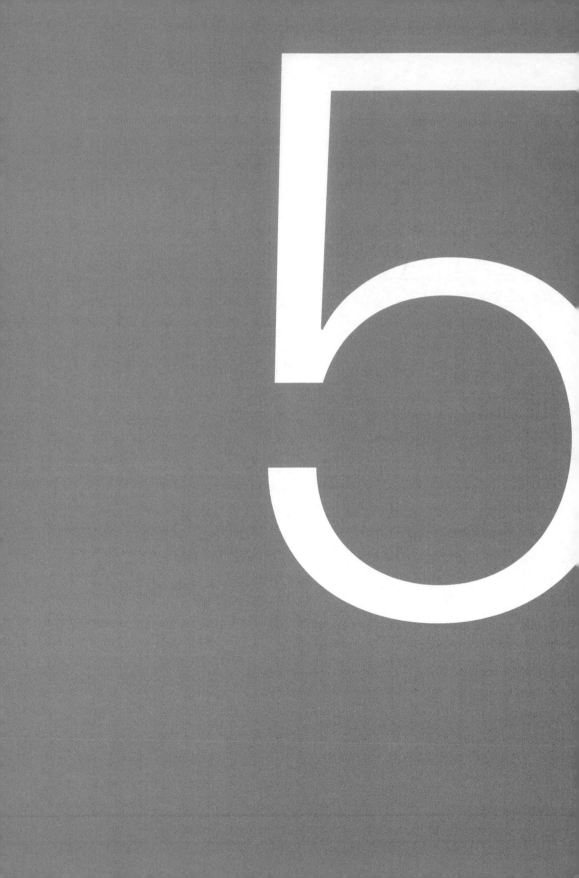

TOOLS FOR
FLAT BELLY DIET
DIABETES
LIVING

A FLAT BELLY and normal blood sugar levels aren't just about food—they're about attitude and lifestyle, too. Your emotions, your stress level, and your self-confidence all play roles in how and when you eat, whether you make time for exercise—and as a result, in how and where you put on weight. That's right. Your emotional state can actually cause you to store belly fat!

Stress and emotions are definitely factors in blood sugar control, too. "I have absolutely seen my patients achieve better blood glucose control when they work on stress reduction," Gillian told me in describing her work as a registered dietitian and certified diabetes educator at the Joslin Diabetes Center in Boston. She makes sure that in addition to talking about food and blood sugar testing, her sessions also focus on this mind-body connection. What works? "Many patients have told me that exercise and meditation help," she says. "And we work a lot on emotional eating—not just strategies for avoiding it, but also finding out what people are really hungry for in their lives."

At the Veterans Affairs San Diego Healthcare Center in California, Dr. Edelman's patients with diabetes are having similar experiences. "The way you take care of your health and your body when you're under stress can help you—or mess you up," he notes. "If your life gets hectic and you fall off your food plan, stop exercising, stop taking medications, or get off-schedule with them, it shows in your blood sugar, your weight, and your outlook. It happens to everybody; it just has bigger effects if you have diabetes."

The Stress-Less Rx

IN CHAPTER 2, YOU learned about the latest thinking about links between the human stress response and weight gain, belly fat buildup, and diabetes risk. When stress strikes, "fight-or-flight" hormones boost blood sugar and increase alertness. One, called cortisol, even triggers cravings for high-calorie foods and directs your body to store the excess calories as an "emergency fuel supply" in . . . you guessed it . . . belly fat.

In prehistoric days, this system helped cavemen outrun marauding predators and successfully bring home dinner after hunting. But it's no asset in the 21st century, when everything from a flat tire to a family emergency to a demanding boss leads to *chronic* stress and all of its negative health consequences. Lucky for us, scientists have also discovered an equal-and-opposite force that counteracts stress. In amazing real-world medical studies with real people (we're not talking test tubes or mice!), this "relaxation response" has reversed some of the worst effects of stress.

You've experienced this profoundly serene *Ahhh* if you've ever had a terrific massage, spent a week of perfect vacation time at the beach, or awakened after a night of long, peaceful slumber. Deep relaxation may steal upon you while cuddling in front of a fire with your kids, while petting a beloved dog or cat, holding hands with a loved one, or praying—doing anything that brings bliss and contentment. The good news? You don't have to wait for it. You can invoke this level of deep, restoring calm whenever you need it.

Here's how vaporizing stress benefits your belly, your weight, your health:

HEALTHIER BLOOD SUGAR. In a breakthrough study conducted at Duke University, 108 women and men with type 2 diabetes took diabetes-education classes with or without stress-management training. After a year, whereas A1c levels rose slightly in the control group, more than half of the stress-relief group improved their blood sugar levels by at least 0.5 percent on an A1c test—a check of long-term blood sugar control. One-third reduced their A1c test result by 1 percentage point or more. That's huge: Lowering your A1c levels that much cuts risk for diabetes-related complications such as heart disease, kidney failure, nerve damage, and vision problems by 17 to 35 percent. Study participants soothed their stress with muscle relaxation, deep breathing, and positive mental imagery.[1]

LESS INSULIN RESISTANCE. When researchers at the University of Virginia Health System in Charlottesville reviewed 70 studies on the health benefits of yoga—one of the ultimate relaxation exercises!—they discovered that this stress-reducer can reverse insulin resistance. How much? Lead researcher Kim Innes, PhD, an assistant professor of research in the university's school of nursing, found that yoga improved insulin sensitivity by about 19 percent. And it worked for a wide variety of people with and without diabetes, women and men, young and older.[2]

HELP FOR STRESS EATING. A recent British study confirms something most of us already know up close and personal. It's easy... almost automatic... to reach for a snack when daily life becomes overwhelming or just plain annoying.[3] Researchers at University College London found that stress-snackers don't reach for baby carrots. They head for high-sugar, high-fat, high-calorie foods (that explains why it's so easy to head for the vending machine—and totally forget the apple in your purse—when anxiety levels rise at work!).[4] Practicing stress reduction lets you defuse rising tensions in the moment, leaving you feeling more relaxed and in control, and less likely to reach for the M&Ms to feel better.

▨ EASIER WEIGHT LOSS. In a study of 225 overweight New Zealand women who followed one of three healthy lifestyle programs, only those who learned stress-management strategies lost weight—5½ pounds.[5] The women used a tension-melting progressive muscle relaxation technique like the one in this book—deep and slow abdominal breathing and soothing visualizations.

▨ HOPE FOR LESS BELLY FAT. We're eagerly awaiting the results of an ongoing University of California, San Francisco, study looking at the effects of stress reduction on weight loss and belly fat. Called CALMM—Craving and Lifestyle Management through Mindfulness—it's the first of its kind and is conducted by researchers who've already done pioneering work on the links between stress, abdominal fat, and food cravings.

Lifestyle Tools for Lasting Weight Loss

MASTERING THE STRATEGIES IN this chapter will equip you with a variety of tools guaranteed to help you stick with the Flat Belly Diet Diabetes for the long haul. I know that no diet-and-exercise plan truly works if it can't help you overcome personal obstacles to healthy, active living. (Otherwise, we'd all be slender and automatically order the salad every time we go out to eat!)

I don't want you to have to fight off your personal demons, but to learn how to cope with them, even honor them, as you find your way to a healthier lifestyle. Your own challenge may be a high-stress life, a penchant for emotional eating (who hasn't reached for a doughnut when feeling down?), a distaste for exercise (not everyone pops out of bed at 5:00 a.m. to walk 5 miles, I know!), or sleep problems that leave you tired, irritable, and fighting larger-than-life food cravings.

If you're a member of today's Sandwich Generation, you may be coping with all of these at once. You're a member of this club if one minute you're taxiing kids to soccer practice and ballet lessons and the next you're fielding phone calls about the health and well-being of an aging parent or in-law. In between, you're squeezing in a job, a relationship with a significant other, and maybe, just maybe, a little time for yourself. *Maybe!*

Regardless of your personal situation, the Flat Belly Diet Diabetes tool kit can help you find success. Let's get started!

LIFESTYLE TOOL #1: **10 Minutes of "Me" Time**

WE KNOW THAT THE stresses in your life—and the ways you respond to them—are as unique as you are. And your stress-less strategy has to reflect that. It's true for me: I manage the day-to-day pressures of running a magazine, raising two wonderful daughters, and taking on hundreds of other projects (like writing this sequel to the *Flat Belly Diet!*) by going on hikes with my family, calling my parents as often as I can, and laughing a lot.

Your path needs to be equally personal and unique—and by using a little trial and error, you'll discover what truly works best for you. There are no rules. You may be surprised by what you find. Gillian discovered a few years ago, much to her surprise, that yoga felt good but didn't really ease her stress. What does work for her: regular exercise and getting enough sleep.

Dr. Edelman turns to exercise, too—and knows from experience that hiding from stress doesn't work for him; facing it head-on does. "Avoiding the situation, by trying to do nothing—watching TV or a movie—does not help at all!" he says. "To be honest, if I am stressed out because I'm behind on my work, my e-mail, etc., the best thing for me is working late to get it done and having a clean slate." Of course, he adds, it's also important to give yourself downtime for rest and relaxation!

In Phase 1 of the Flat Belly Diet Diabetes, we want you to spend 10 minutes a day practicing progressive muscle relaxation as your introduction to the relaxation response. In Phase 2, use the time to pursue the stress-soothing path of your own choice. What follows are five specific, stress-busting strategies you might want to explore. Consider it a tool kit—the more strategies you have, the more effectively you'll stop stress in its tracks.

GET CALM! FIVE WAYS TO STRESS LESS

1. PROGRESSIVE MUSCLE RELAXATION. So simple and easy to learn that all the instructions are right there in the name: Progressive muscle relaxation involves systematically tensing and relaxing the muscle groups in your body. Studies show it's as effective as biofeedback and meditation for lowering blood sugar and has the advantage of needing no special equipment or training with a therapist, psychologist, or other expert. And you can do a mini-version any time, any place.

You'll find directions for a 10-minute progressive muscle relaxation exercise in Chapter 7. While you perform this exercise, remember to, well, relax! Just let it happen, even if it doesn't seem to be working perfectly at first. (Trying harder will only make you tense!) Choose a quiet place for practice—not in front of the TV or in a room full of people. If you find that your mind keeps spinning with to-do lists and worries, try doing this exercise just after your daily walk—when you'll already be feeling relaxed.

2. A "MEDITATIVE" HOBBY. Knitting, woodworking, gardening, playing that clarinet you haven't tooted since high school—any hobby that's creative and absorbing—can be a powerful stress stopper. And there's research to back it up. In a study commissioned by the Home Sewing Association, a New York University psychiatrist measured signs of stress in 30 women before and after they performed three different activities: sewing, reading the newspaper or playing cards, or playing a video game. Sewing was the clear winner: It lowered heart rates by 7 to 11 beats per minute, while the other pastimes raised heartbeats by about 4 to 8 beats per minute, reports study author Robert H. Reiner, PhD. "The importance of a hobby or creative pursuit cannot be overemphasized," he notes. "If we don't allow our bodies to rest from the pressures of everyday life, we are placing ourselves at risk for heart disease or other illnesses. Creative activities and hobbies—like sewing—can help a person focus on something productive and get away from their worries for a while."

Why is an absorbing hobby such a great stress reducer? Simply because it takes you away from everyday thoughts and cares and delivers you into a quieter state. Hobbies that include repetitive, rhythmic actions—whether it's the knit-one, purl-one of creating a sweater, digging holes for daffodils, or rubbing stain into the surface of a refinished table—literally move your body and mind into a quieter state.

3. CONNECTIONS. *You've gotta have friends* is more than a catchy song lyric. We're social creatures and have been for millennia. Being alone too much (how much is too much? That's individual!) actually raises cortisol levels.[6] In one UCLA study, brain scans showed that our brains register social isolation in the same way we register physical pain.[7]

But in case you hadn't noticed, having a social life is going the way of public telephones and thank-you notes: When Duke University researchers studied the social lives of 1,467 women and men in 1985 and again in 2004, they found that the number of people who had no close companions at all doubled—to 25 percent. And the number of friends in whom study volunteers said they could really confide in fell by one-third.

If you can't remember the last time you shared a laugh or a confidence with a friend, it's time. One caveat: Spend time with people who leave you feeling energized, not emotionally tapped-out. Real friends are people you have a genuine connection with. If your social life is so full that it's stressing you out, consider saying "no thanks" a little more often—simply networking or brushing up against acquaintances at yet another party or committee meeting won't bring you the heart-to-heart benefits I'm talking about!

4. BREATHING. Bring yourself into the present moment—not worried about the future or mulling over an event from hours, days, or weeks ago—with a few minutes of quiet, calm breathing. Breathing exercises like this can restore healthier levels of stress hormones, Canadian researchers report.[8] Here's how to get there: In a quiet room, sit in a comfortable chair with both feet planted on the floor (in other words, don't cross your legs), your arms relaxed, and your hands in your lap. Now just follow your inhalations and exhalations as you breathe normally—in and out, in and out. If your thoughts wander (and they will—it's only natural!), simply invite your attention to refocus on your breath. As you relax, try deeper breaths—inhale as you count to four. Let your breath fill your abdomen. Pause for a second, then exhale for a count of four. Pause for a second, then repeat.

This type of breathing exercise was associated with healthier stress hormone levels in one Canadian study. And when 38 doctors, nurses, and other busy health-care professionals tried it in a study published in the *International Journal of Stress Management*, 88 percent felt less stressed and burned-out.[9]

■ **5. VISUALIZATION.** Visualizing is a good way to remove yourself mentally from a stressful situation. It can also help you imagine future successes—for weight loss, a slimmer torso, or healthier blood sugar levels—and boost your motivation to reach your goals. Sit or lie somewhere comfortable. Close your eyes. Practice the progressive muscle relaxation exercise mentioned earlier in this chapter and described in Chapter 7. Allow thoughts to pass through your mind without actually "thinking" about them. Imagine

Have You Laughed Today?

Rent a funny video, read the comics, or ask everyone in your family to tell their funniest joke. Laughter is good medicine for better blood sugar. Japanese researchers report that people with diabetes had a smaller, healthier rise in blood sugar after a meal if they watched a live comedy show and a larger blood sugar rise when they attended a boring lecture. It worked for people without diabetes, too.

DID YOU KNOW ?

you are somewhere that makes you feel good, such as the beach, the woods, a spot where you have spent a restful vacation, or a beautiful place you can picture even if you have never visited. Breathe slowly and deeply until you feel relaxed. Focus on all five senses. Imagine what you see, feel, hear, taste, and smell. Continue to visualize yourself in this place for 5 to 10 minutes. Then gradually return your focus to the room you are in and end the visualization exercise.

LIFESTYLE TOOL #2: Mindful Attention to Stop Emotional Eating

PHYSICAL HUNGER IS A matter of physiological cause and effect. Your brain constantly monitors your blood sugar level, the relative fullness or emptiness of your stomach and intestines, and levels of appetite stimulating and muting hormones in your bloodstream. When levels dip, your brain tells your tummy to ring the dinner bell. The next thing you know, it's growling loudly and contracting with impossible-to-ignore hunger pangs. So you eat—until your stomach and brain decide you're full and send signals to stop. But that's not all there is to hunger. We eat not only to fill physical need, but in response to *emotional* hunger. And to do so, we've taught ourselves how to override the body's natural "I'm full" and "I'm not hungry yet" signals.

Coming to grips with emotional eating means understanding why you do it. For most of us, it's rooted in childhood, when everything from a cake on your birthday to a piece of candy when you skinned your knee equated food with love, comfort, and celebration. As adults, most of us have turned this into a grown-up equation: We snack and overeat in response to stress, boredom, happiness, sadness, anxiety, anger, fear, and loneliness. It can be a difficult connection to break, because our minds quickly fill in compelling reasons why we need spoonfuls of peanut butter while on deadline finishing a book; a handful of chocolate chips after a long and difficult day at work; a gooey, cheesy plate of nachos just because it's Monday . . . or Wednesday . . . or Friday. Years of eating in response to everything except physical hunger mean we need to relearn what true hunger feels like—and to find the emotions fueling psychological hunger.

The line between true hunger and emotional hunger is actually very distinct. According to the University of Texas at Austin Counseling and Mental Health Center, there are five key ways to tell the difference between emotional eating and real hunger for food:

1. EMOTIONAL HUNGER COMES ON SUDDENLY. Physical hunger is gradual.

2. PHYSICAL HUNGER IS FELT BELOW THE NECK (THAT GROWLING TUMMY!). Emotional hunger is felt above the neck (that craving for carrot cake or mint chocolate chip ice cream).

3. PHYSICAL HUNGER IS SATISFIED WITH FUEL—many types of food will do the trick. Emotional hunger can be satisfied by just one food—at the moment it might be pizza or a glazed doughnut or a banana split.

4. EMOTIONAL HUNGER DEMANDS IMMEDIATE SATISFACTION. Physical hunger can usually wait.

5. PHYSICAL HUNGER LEAVES NO GUILT BEHIND. Emotional hunger leaves plenty of guilt in its wake.

The ability to distinguish between these two types of hunger is your first strategy for overcoming emotional eating. How to use it wisely? The next time a craving strikes, try this: Tune out any signals coming from the neck up. Now ask yourself: Am I physically hungry? If not, what's going on?

This second step involves *feeling* the emotions hidden behind the craving. We'll be honest—that isn't always easy. There are good reasons why we wash down feelings with chocolate-chip cookies and Kit Kat bars. We may feel unworthy of what we desire. Or think there's no time or place for our needs. For many women, emotional eating puts down strong roots when our days are filled with taking care of the needs of others—at home, at work, and in our communities. It's easier to stop off for fries on the way home from the kids' swim practice than to investigate the pang that's really a little voice inside saying, "Hey, I need time to exercise, too!"

How does all of this tie in to belly fat and blood sugar? In one cutting-edge area of research, scientists are beginning to suspect that people with heightened responses to stress are more likely to engage in emotional eating. In one University of California, San Francisco, study of college students, psychologists found that stress eaters gained weight and showed signs of growing insulin resistance during the most high-anxiety time of year: final exams. The scientists speculate that stress eaters may be at greater risk for metabolic syndrome, prediabetes, and diabetes.[10]

BREAKING FREE

These steps can help you recognize and overcome emotional eating:

PAUSE AND REFLECT. If you've determined that you're dealing with emotional hunger, wait 5 minutes before eating. During that time, take a break from whatever you've been doing. Sit quietly and relax. Then ask yourself what you're really feeling. Think back over the past few hours to find clues. Ask yourself what you need, on an emotional level. Are your muscles tight from sitting at your desk—something a brief walk would fix? Are you feeling worried about a project or a situation—something that calling a friend or consulting with a co-worker might help? Do you simply need a mental break—like a brief relaxation exercise? Ask yourself what the best thing is that you could do for yourself right now.

RATE YOUR HUNGER BEFORE, DURING, AND AFTER A MEAL OR SNACK. Getting in touch with physical hunger and physical satisfaction can help you avoid the kind of overeating at meals and snacks that's actually fueled by emotional hunger. Use a "hunger scale"—with 1 being "so hungry I could eat a horse" and 10 being "the stuffed feeling I get after Thanksgiving dinner." Aim to eat when you're at about zero—mildly to moderately hungry (when you have some physical symptoms of hunger like a growling tummy and that "I need to eat soon" feeling, but you aren't starving or experiencing any unpleasant symptoms such as a headache or shaking). Stop when you're at a 5 or 6—comfortably full. This exercise in hunger awareness can help you enjoy food to the fullest—by focusing on the best foods for satisfying real, physical hunger. It can also help you learn to recognize the feeling of physical satisfaction—the warm, cozy, "I've had just enough" feeling that truly tells you that you're filling your body's real needs with healthy food.

To help you achieve this crucial hunger and satisfaction awareness, you'll use the hunger scale while filling out your daily Flat Belly Diet Diabetes journal.

THINK ABOUT WHAT YOUR EMOTIONAL HUNGER MEANS. Do you have no time to stop and relax or feel there's not enough pleasure or fun or *zing* in your life? Or do you need comfort and support that may be missing? How can you begin to meet these needs? The real point of overcoming emotional eating is to find ways to nourish these deep needs—not deny them. Sometimes, identifying these needs is as simple as asking yourself how a gorgeous, perfect chocolate brownie or a bowl of crunchy, salty tortilla chips makes you feel. Those feelings may be what you're really missing in your life—and entirely deserve to have for real. Just knowing what you desire is important—it means you're listening to yourself.

LIFESTYLE TOOL #3: Physical Activity

IF I TOLD YOU that in about 30 minutes a day, you could do something that would make your skin glow, tone your torso, rev your energy—and make you feel absolutely happy—wouldn't you do it? Of course, that something is exercise. We've made it another integral part of the Flat Belly Diet Diabetes because we've seen, firsthand, how effective it is for targeting the three areas this program aims to improve: your weight, your belly fat, and your blood sugar.

What we really, really love about exercise, though, is how great it makes us feel. Remember hearing about the "runner's high" that long-distance runners say they feel? I'm here to tell you that your brain starts releasing "happy chemicals"—endorphins and feel-good brain chemicals such as serotonin—less than 20 minutes after exercise begins. That means that the feel-good benefits of exercise aren't reserved for elite athletes. They're for everyone. And there's more. Here's a rundown of the top six reasons why we want you to move your body, 6 out of 7 days a week:

■ EXERCISE BOOSTS WEIGHT LOSS TWO WAYS. Every time you move—whether you're strolling, swimming, gardening, or washing the car—you're burning calories. For example, walking for just 15 to 20 minutes can burn off 85 to 100 calories. As you control the calories you're taking in and burning more off, you'll begin losing body fat. Add gentle strength-training moves to the equation and you also bolster muscle mass—giving your metabolism an important boost. When women at the South Shore YMCA in Quincy, Massachusetts, strength-trained for 30 minutes, twice a week, for 6 weeks, they added 3 pounds of calorie-hungry muscle mass and lost 2.7 pounds of fat. That little bit of extra muscle boosts metabolic rate—the calories your body burns 'round the clock—by about 7 percent.

■ EXERCISE TARGETS VISCERAL FAT BETTER THAN DIET ALONE. When Japanese researchers put 209 overweight women and men on low-calorie diets, those who also exercised lost 30 percent more visceral fat than those who didn't.[11]

Armed and Ready:
Affirmations for Inspiration

Before you embark on Phase 1 of the Flat Belly Diet Diabetes, we want you to take a few moments to reflect on these vital, change-inspiring "mantras." Repeat as necessary along your journey over the next 35 days:

◼ **The past is past. Today I will love, honor, and care for my body, my health, my well-being.** If you're carrying an emotional burden related to your weight, worries about your future health, or the day-to-day stress of managing diabetes, we're here to assure you that you are not alone. You may feel guilty or ashamed, blame yourself, deny your own needs by putting everybody else in your life first, or be frustrated if previous diets and exercise programs haven't gone quite the way you planned. In surveys of more than 600 people with diabetes, Dr. Edelman and his colleagues have found that most live with difficult feelings related to their health—82 percent felt worried, 69 percent felt hopeless about future complications, 66 percent felt caring for their health took too much time, and 58 percent felt angry, afraid, or depressed. And even if you don't have diabetes, you may be coping with some similar feelings about your weight or health.

It's time for a fresh start—one that puts *you* at the center of your life and gives you the conviction that you're worth it. This deep level of self-caring can help you stay motivated. And it goes deeper: Knowing in your heart and deep down in your bones that you're worth taking care of is the core of true self-confidence. This isn't the "shiny on the surface, shaky on the inside" kind. It's rock-solid self-confidence that builds even further as you see the results of your efforts, that takes setbacks in stride, and that learns from everything you experience. To build confidence in yourself and your ability to take the small, daily steps that will add up to big benefits, consider these affirmations:

◼ **I make time for myself and my needs.** You may be more comfortable doing things for others, but how often do you nurture yourself? Go ahead and put your exercise time and stress-reducing "me time" on your calendar, fill the kitchen cabinets with good-for-you Flat Belly Diet Diabetes foods, and treat yourself to new sneakers or walking shoes if you need them. (Splurge on comfy socks, too.) Remember, you deserve it!

I surround myself with love and support. Don't go it alone. Before you begin, consider having a serious heart-to-heart with everyone in your immediate circle. Tell them why you're doing this, why it's so important to you, what you need from them, and how you think it might affect your relationship. You might need to swap your family's Sunday IHOP stop with a healthier breakfast at home or happy hour with the girls for a cup of tea at a local café. When they realize how important this is to you, they'll listen, and I'll bet some of them will even want to join in!

If people in your life have fallen into the habit of nagging you about your health or your weight, realize they mean well—but find time for a calm, quiet chat. You could say that you understand that they love you, but you're in charge of your health. Of course, they'll still want to be helpful. So give them an assignment: You might sign one or more up as exercise buddies or take turns preparing the meals in this book, for example.

I give myself permission to make mistakes. We've all fallen off the weight-loss wagon. It's what you do *next* that spells the difference between success and, well, staying off the wagon. Decide here and now to adopt a "no-fault" stance with regard to slipups such as indulging in an extra piece of pizza, skipping an exercise routine, or not finding time for relaxation. No harm, no foul. When you eliminate guilt and self-criticism, it's easier to get right back on the program rather than giving up or slipping back into old emotional-eating habits. In fact, when you really believe that your health, your body, your total well-being are worth pampering, you can see setbacks for what they really are: vital tidbits of information that can help you tweak your plan so that it really works for you. You couldn't resist the office birthday cake for a co-worker? You're only human—and maybe you could bring part of your Flat Belly Diet Diabetes snack to the next celebration, so you can have a treat along with everybody else!

■ **EXERCISE IMPROVES INSULIN SENSITIVITY.** When researchers at the University of South Carolina asked 1,467 people about their activity levels and then did blood tests to check their sensitivity to insulin—the key blood sugar control hormone—they found an important link. Those who were the most active—moving 5 days a week as they exercised, did housework or yard work, or performed an active job—were 70 percent more insulin-sensitive than those who were almost never active.[12] That's good news for everyone, because improving insulin sensitivity is crucial for lowering diabetes risk and for improving blood sugar control if you have diabetes. No wonder a Harvard School of Public Health study of 40,000 women found that 30 minutes a day of brisk walking cut diabetes risk by 43 percent. In contrast, inactivity is big trouble: Each 2 hours a day you spend in front of the TV could raise your risk for insulin resistance by 23 percent.[13]

■ **EXERCISE LOWERS HIGH BLOOD SUGAR.** When 31 people with type 2 diabetes performed an easy, 45-minute strength-training routine three times a week for 16 weeks, 72 percent were able to reduce their doses of diabetes medications because their blood sugar levels fell to healthier levels, according to researchers at Tufts University. The scientists found that physical activity prompted the participants' muscle cells to absorb 33 percent more blood sugar. And their scores on an A1c test—a measure of long-term blood sugar control—fell from 8.7 to a healthier 7.6. Sounds small, but this change significantly reduced their odds for diabetes-related complications in the future.[14]

Combining cardiovascular exercise (like walking, riding a bike, or swimming) with strength training—as you will on the Flat Belly Diet Diabetes—yields a bigger blood sugar bonus than doing just one or the other. In a study from Canada's University of Calgary, 251 people with type 2 diabetes followed one of four programs: an all-cardiovascular workout on a treadmill or exercise bike, an all–strength-training workout in a gym, a routine that combined cardiovascular exercise with strength training, or doing nothing at all. After 6 months, blood sugar improved the most on the combined program.

A1c scores for this group declined from an average of 7.4 to 6.5—twice the improvement seen in people who did just a cardiovascular routine or just strength training. The winning combo included 20 to 45 minutes of walking or riding an exercise bike, three times a week, plus two to three strength-training sessions a week.[15]

Physical activity improves blood sugar levels in two ways: First, as we've shown you, it makes your body more sensitive to insulin, the hormone that tells cells to absorb blood sugar. It does this by increasing the number of insulin receptors on the surface of your cells. Second, physical activity prompts muscle cells to absorb blood sugar without the help of insulin and to go on absorbing it for hours after you're done walking, swimming, or playing with the kids. In fact, this effect is so dramatic that people with diabetes who use insulin or some other diabetes medications should take steps to avoid low blood sugar levels during and after exercise. (Turn to Chapter 4 for more information.)

■ EXERCISE COOLS CHRONIC INFLAMMATION. Researchers now suspect that physical activity helps lower the risk for inflammation-related health conditions—such as diabetes—in ways that go beyond controlling body weight, body fat, and blood sugar. The new thinking: Exercise seems to tackle inflammation head-on—perhaps by releasing compounds called heat shock proteins that repair damage inside cells or by preventing white blood cells called macrophages from invading fat cells (a situation that revs up inflammation). What does it all mean? Simply that exercise is an even more powerful health tool than experts ever realized.[16]

■ EXERCISE BOOSTS YOUR MOOD. We would love exercise even if it weren't such a powerful supporter of good health and a flat belly—simply because it's a surefire way to boost your mood and brighten your attitude. The benefits reach deep into your brain, increasing levels of the feel-good brain chemicals serotonin, dopamine, and norepinephrine, as well as endorphins, with as little as 10 minutes of activity![17]

In one study from Finland, people who exercised just two or three times a week felt significantly less angry, stressed, cynical, and distrustful.[18] Plenty of other research has found links between exercise and a rise in self-confidence. How can you *not* love an activity that gives your skin a healthy glow, keeps your body trim and strong, pampers your health—and leaves you feeling happy, relaxed, open to all of life's wonderful possibilities, and deeply appreciative of your own self-worth and abilities? And when you're feeling good, following a healthy diet is so much easier!

THE FLAT BELLY DIET DIABETES EXERCISE PLAN

Now THAT YOU UNDERSTAND exactly why exercise is an essential element of the Flat Belly Diet Diabetes, we're happy to tell you that incorporating it into your life won't require you to live at the gym, get up before dawn for triathlon-style intensive training, or pack your house with oversize and expensive home exercise equipment!

We knew that for this plan to work, it had to fit into real life—and to be what we like to call "life proof." That means that even on the busiest day, you can fit something in. And when you do have time to exercise, getting it done won't require driving to a health club or fussing with gadgets or even putting on special clothing (absolutely no Spandex is required, we promise!). All you need: supportive sneakers, good socks, clothes in which you can walk and do a few exercise moves, a water bottle, and a few lightweight dumbbells.

You'll find a detailed description of our Fat Blast Walk and Calorie Torch Walk, easy Metabolism Boost strength-training exercises, and Belly Routine tummy-toning plan in Chapter 11. And you'll find a day-by-day breakdown of what to do, when, how often, and for how long in Chapter 7: Phase 1 and Chapter 8: Phase 2.

This exercise plan is based on the successful Flat Belly Diet Workout from our original book. We asked Gillian, Dr. Edelman, and *Prevention*'s fitness director, Michele Stanten, to review it, and sure enough, everyone agreed that it's the perfect plan for people with or at risk for diabetes. Michele based this workout on the most current research—not only of the benefits of exercise, but of what types delivered those benefits in a doable way that fits into your real life—into the time you can squeeze from your busy and demanding schedule. And I had one more request: *No crunches!*

Having taken many exercise classes and having talked to hundreds of women, I can say with certainty that nobody loves crunches. Not only do they strain your neck and lower back and require a lot of huffing and puffing, they often just don't seem to work! The consensus coming out of exercise labs is that the crunch is never the top-recommended move for targeting abdominal muscles. And fitness trainers—the ones with the most gorgeously toned midsections I've ever seen—say they've gone beyond this one-time aerobics studio darling to a more holistic, results-oriented approach that targets your entire core—front, back, and sides.

The basics of the Flat Belly Diet Diabetes workout plan:

- Cardio exercise—walking—to burn calories, shed fat, and improve blood sugar
- Strength training with weights to build muscle, boost metabolism, and, again, improve blood sugar
- Core-focused moves to tone and tighten your torso

Your time commitment? Just 15 minutes of walking a day if you haven't been exercising until now, 30 minutes a day if you have. As the plan progresses, you'll add in the strength-training Metabolism Boost and Belly Routine torso-tighteners on alternate days. These routines contain just four and five moves, respectively, and take less than 10 minutes each. That means they'll fit easily into little pockets of "downtime" you may have. You'll learn all the details in Chapter 11.

LIFESTYLE TOOL #4: Deep, Restorative Sleep

THE CONNECTION BETWEEN SLEEP and blood sugar is solid. A growing stack of medical studies shows that a good night's sleep not only makes you feel deliciously refreshed and energetic, it can also help keep blood sugar under better control—and reduce food cravings, help whittle extra pounds, and fight high blood pressure and heart disease.

When sleep researcher James Gangwisch, PhD, an assistant professor of psychiatry at Columbia University in New York City, analyzed the health and lifestyle habits of 8,992 women and men recently, he found that those who averaged 5 or fewer hours of sleep a night were twice as likely to develop type 2 diabetes as those who got 7 to 8 hours. (Getting 9 or more hours of shut-eye also raised risk; researchers suspect it's due to poor-quality sleep.)[19]

And in a recent study presented at the American Heart Association's Annual Conference on Cardiovascular Disease Epidemiology and Prevention, researchers from the University at Buffalo reported that people who sleep less than 6 hours per night may be 4.5 times more likely to develop prediabetes as those who get 6 to 8 hours per night. The study followed 1,500 people for 6 years.

For people who already have diabetes, a sleep deficit can make long-term blood sugar control more difficult. In a University of Chicago study of 161 people with type 2 diabetes, researchers recently found that those who slept poorly or rarely got enough sleep had significantly higher A1c levels (an important measure of long-term blood sugar control) than those who slumbered well.[20]

Ever notice that doughnuts, muffins, and pastries are so much harder to resist when you're running on not quite enough sleep? You're not alone. In studies from the University of Chicago, it was found that sleep deprivation increases insulin resistance quickly and boosts serious cravings for high-fat, high-carb sweets like pies, cakes, and cookies![21, 22]

Why does a sleep deficit lead to a sugar glut? Experts believe shorting yourself on shut-eye reduces insulin sensitivity (so cells don't respond to insulin's signals to absorb blood sugar), raises levels of the stress hormone cortisol, and cranks up levels of the hunger hormone ghrelin, while depressing levels of the satisfaction hormone leptin. Translation: The cravings you're battling today may be the direct consequence of the sleep you missed last night.

Most of us truly need $7\frac{1}{2}$ to 8 hours of sleep per night—it's the rare and lucky few whose bodies and minds are nourished by 5 to 6 hours of shut-eye. But as the national nightly sleep average drops to 6 hours, 40 minutes, it's clear that more and more of us are trying to live as if we were "short sleepers." If you struggle to get a good night's sleep, these steps can help you enjoy more hours in dreamland:

FIND YOUR "SNOOZE NUMBER." How much sleep do you really need? Keep a sleep diary for a week and find out. (You'll find one at the National Sleep Foundation Web site, www.sleepfoundation.org.)

Note how long you spent under the covers and how awake and alert you felt when you woke up. If you're getting less than $7\frac{1}{2}$ to 8 hours a night and are dragging during the day, hit the hay a half-hour earlier and see how you feel. Still tired? Add another half-hour. Keep adding to your sleep time every night until you're able to wake up refreshed.

Another way to find out how much sleep you need is to simply spend 8 hours in bed every night for a week. Turn in at the same time and get up at the same time each day. It may take your body and mind a few days to grow accustomed to this new schedule and a few more to "pay back" the sleep debt you've run up. After that, notice if you're sleeping the full 8 hours. If you are, you need 8 hours. If you're taking longer to fall asleep or find yourself popping out of bed earlier, your body naturally needs a little less. If you're still tired, you may need a bit more. Your body will tell you.

If you're tired despite getting 8 to 9 hours of shut-eye per night, you may have obstructive sleep apnea (especially if you're snoring or your bed partner says you momentarily stop breathing, then start again, possibly with a loud snort or gasp, multiple times through the night). See your doctor for an evaluation.

CREATE A BEDTIME RITUAL. It works for our kids—and it works for adults, too! Take a bath or shower, slip into your favorite PJs, and slip between the sheets for a few minutes of light reading or relaxing music. Done regularly, this ritual tells your brain that the next stop is dreamland.

GIVE YOUR BEDROOM A SLEEP-FRIENDLY MAKEOVER. This inner sanctum should be cool, dark, and cozy at bedtime. Moonlight, streetlights, early dawns, and late sunsets can all interfere with your body's natural circadian rhythms, throwing off your attempts to sleep. Invest in light-blocking window coverings.

Turn down the thermostat or open a window slightly to let in cool, fresh air. And treat yourself to comfortable pillows, blankets, and sheets.

Use your bedroom and your bed as an oasis. Reserve your bed and your bedroom exclusively for sleep and sex—banish stimulating and stressful activities such as late-night TV or Internet surfing, bill paying, and catching up on work.

Diabetes and Sleep Apnea

As many as one in three people with diabetes may also have sleep apnea[23]—when tissue in the throat blocks airways and halts normal breathing dozens or even hundreds of times each night. Linked with higher blood sugar as well as high blood pressure, heart disease, and overweight, apnea can be diagnosed at a sleep clinic and fixed in one of several ways. These include surgery, wearing an "oral appliance" that helps keep airways open, or sleeping with a continuous positive air pressure (CPAP) machine that uses gentle air pressure to keep airways open.

You may have apnea if your bed partner notices that you snore loudly and/or seem to stop breathing at night or if you wake up feeling dead-tired. Reversing apnea has been shown to help lower blood sugar and blood pressure and improve heart function. And you'll feel well rested and energetic in the morning!

DID YOU KNOW?

A practical, solutions-oriented type of therapy called cognitive behavioral therapy for insomnia (CBT-I) works as well as or better than sleeping pills for overcoming insomnia. To find a trained CBT-I practitioner, start by contacting a sleep center near you. You'll find a list of sleep centers in the United States on the Web site of the American Academy of Sleep Medicine—at www.sleepcenters.org.

DON'T WATCH THE CLOCK. If your bedside clock has a light-up display, switch it off, cover it up, or turn it to face the wall.

SHUSH THE SNORER BESIDE YOU. Sleeping with a chronic snorer is bad news for your sleep quality. In the Married Couples Sleep Study conducted by researchers at Chicago's Rush University Medical Center, the spouse of one snorer was awakened eight times an hour by her husband's rasping snores! Move to another room, wear earplugs, or ask your mate to seek medical help. When the snorer in the Rush study got help, his mate's daytime sleepiness was cut in half—and her marital satisfaction soared![24] Adhesive strips that hold the nose open wider help some people, as do pillows that reposition the snorer's head.

EXERCISE FOR BETTER SLEEP. People who exercise regularly fall asleep faster, sleep more deeply, awaken less often, and sleep longer, according to the Centers for Disease Control and Prevention. If exercise close to bedtime keeps you awake, work out before dinner.

SAY "NO THANKS" TO CAFFEINE AFTER NOON. Caffeine blocks the action of a sleep-inducing brain chemical called adenosine.[25] It takes 3 to 7 hours for your body to metabolize half the caffeine in a cup of tea or coffee,[26] so it's smart to make noon your "last call" for caffeinated drinks. In an Australian study of 4,558 people, those who got 240 milligrams of caffeine a day—about the amount in two 8-ounce cups of coffee or 2½ "shots" of espresso—had a 40 percent higher risk for insomnia than those who avoided caffeine.[27]

READ A FLAT BELLY
SUCCESS STORY

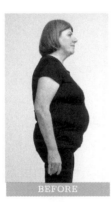

BEFORE

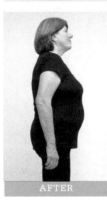

AFTER

Susan Hoar

AGE: 60

POUNDS LOST:

2.4
IN 35 DAYS

ALL-OVER INCHES LOST:

2.75

> **✱ BLOOD SUGAR: A1C FELL FROM 7 TO**
> # 6.6
> **PERCENT**

* The A1c is a test of long-term blood-sugar control; levels below 7 percent are considered ideal for most people with diabetes.

"PEOPLE KEEP TELLING ME HOW GREAT I LOOK! MY WAIST IS smaller, my hips are smaller, and my body fat percentage dropped by 2.5 percent, too," Susan says. "My whole body seemed to change shape! People even tell me my skin looks wonderful! I didn't get this kind of reaction when I lost 30 pounds a while back! I feel better, I look better, and everyone keeps saying these wonderful things to me about it."

But the really big news? "I would say the very best thing was that my blood glucose numbers dropped significantly. In just 5 weeks, my A1c levels went from 7 to 6.6, which is a remarkable change and a remarkably healthy number for someone with diabetes. This pleases me more than anything else, because a healthy A1c means I'm at lower risk for the complications of diabetes—nerve problems, eye problems, kidney problems—in the years ahead. That's a good feeling."

And the food! "It's fabulous," Susan says. "The red snapper fish dinner was truly delicious and became a favorite in my house. In fact, it's so good I'm planning to serve it to company. The chicken piccata was delicious and so easy that if I came in late from work, I could make it, and we'd be sitting down to eat in just 15 minutes. The salad is amazing—goat cheese, pears, raisins, and spinach, with a dressing of olive oil, honey, and lemon juice. Wow!

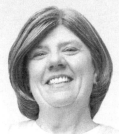

"I'm a high-energy person. I really appreciated the fact that I never got that underlying tired feeling I've felt on other diets. The meals were so satisfying and stayed with you. Maybe it was those MUFAs at every meal. They were such a treat. I hadn't had a cream cheese and olive sandwich since college! I love all this food—the avocados, the nuts, the olives. And chocolate. It's a little bit of heaven to know you can eat some and your blood sugar numbers won't go crazy as a result. In the past, I kind of felt I couldn't really have it. I haven't enjoyed guilt-free chocolate in years!

"I'm wearing belts now. I need to wear belts with my pants now, and I didn't before. My other clothes are fitting better, too. I'm a pants and sweater girl, and my sweaters look better. We recently went on vacation to Boston and did a lot of walking. It felt good to be able to do it—the exercise portion of the program helped me feel stronger—and I just felt good that my clothes were fitting me better!"

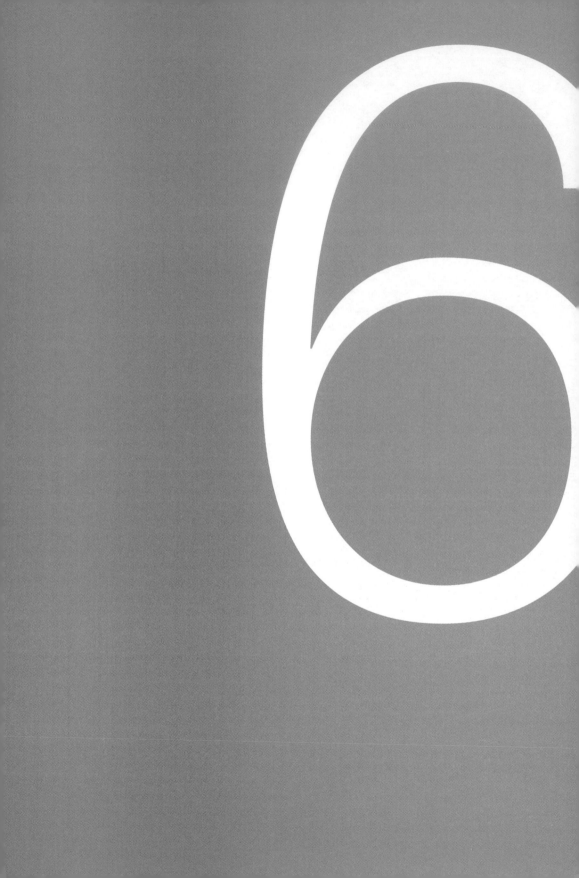

THE FLAT BELLY DIET
DIABETES
RULES

FOR NEARLY EVERYONE who's ever tried to lose weight, the word *diet* means long lists of forbidden foods, nonstop hunger, cravings, gargantuan willpower struggles—and eventually, a return to your pre-diet "normal" eating habits once you've reached your goal. But for Gillian, Dr. Edelman, and me, the word *diet* has a different meaning. The Flat Belly Diet Diabetes is a way of eating—one that allows you to reach and maintain a healthy weight while optimizing your health, making blood sugar control easier, and lowering your odds for diabetes and nearly every other chronic disease.

Our plan makes specific promises: less belly fat and better blood sugar control. But even after we'd found exciting new research supporting the notion that MUFAs—those glorious monounsaturated fats—could accomplish that, our work wasn't done. I knew that to stand out amid the shelves and shelves of popular weight-loss plans out there, our plan had to offer something—or several things—that other diets didn't deliver. In addition, it absolutely had to meet the specific needs of people with diabetes or at risk for this serious blood sugar problem.

And, oh yes, it had to be delicious. Flexible. And realistic.

That's a tall order. So I turned to a true expert: Gillian. As a registered dietitian and certified diabetes educator, she knows what people with blood sugar issues need in terms of nutrition. And she has penetrating and compassionate insight into the ways that translates—and fails to translate—into what we actually put on our plates and into our bodies.

Gillian worked out the calorie counts and nutrient balance of every meal and snack. She calculated carbohydrate content and included a healthy mix of produce, whole grains, lean protein, dairy products, and good fats so that this plan is easy on your blood sugar. But she didn't stop there. She fit in our beloved MUFAs without sacrificing the satisfaction and fill-you-up power of breakfast, lunch, and dinner. She scoured supermarket shelves and nutrition databases for the healthiest convenience foods so that you can follow the Flat Belly Diet Diabetes even on your busiest days. She analyzed restaurant menus, identifying healthy choices so that you can eat out without regrets. And she pulled off a feat that made us cheer by fitting nuts, olives, and—hooray!—*chocolate* into a 100 percent healthy eating plan, so that you can enjoy these decadent delights without worry, fear, or guilt.

Then we added one more thing. When Gillian, Dr. Edelman, and I reviewed all the evidence about the big health benefits and fat-blasting potential of exercise, we knew immediately that physical activity had to be an integral part of this plan. We also knew that for exercise to work, it had to fit seamlessly into your day. The best exercise routine on the planet won't help you burn calories, control blood sugar, or reduce stress if it requires you to get up at 4:30 in the morning, spend 2 hours at the gym every night, or give up your lunch hour!

Prevention magazine's fitness director, Michele Stanten, reviewed and "tweaked" the easy and effective workout we introduced in the original Flat Belly Diet. With input from Gillian and Dr. Edelman, we updated this routine so that it will work for you, whether you have diabetes or are at risk. That means we've included comprehensive advice for avoiding blood sugar lows that can happen if you use insulin or some other blood sugar–lowering diabetes medications. We've added options for you if nerve damage or other foot problems make walking difficult. But the big news is that this workout packs a lot of benefits into a small time commitment, which for me is an absolute "must" for any exercise program. You'll need a mere 15 to 30 minutes for walking or another aerobic exercise and less than 10 minutes more for two important toning routines, and the results are nothing short of amazing.

Four Rules to Live By

OVER THE NEXT 35 days—and beyond—you're going to live well. How do Strawberry-Almond Topped French Toast for breakfast, Spinach Salad with Avocado, Fresh Mozzarella, and Strawberry Dressing for lunch, and Filet Mignon with Mustard-Horseradish Sauce and Roasted Potatoes for dinner sound? You also get snacks—like Chocolate-Zucchini Snack Cake and Spicy Snack Mix. These are just a few of the blood sugar–friendly, belly-flattening "anti-diet" dishes you'll be eating. And it won't be a lot of work. Our quick and easy meals, which you'll find in Chapter 9, come together in a snap. Perfect if you don't like to cook or simply don't have time. We've made it easy. All of the information and ingredients are laid out for you. And you don't have to worry about portion sizes, because everything is preportioned. Chapter 10 is loaded with MUFA-packed recipes and meal additions that will allow you to follow the Flat Belly Diet Diabetes at times when you want or need to cook—such as for family meals and when entertaining. Both meal types adhere to three very important Flat Belly Diet Diabetes rules. The fourth rule? Fitting in time for physical activity, which is as simple as taking an enjoyable stroll after dinner, after work, or for part of your lunch break. You must follow these rules to reap the health and weight-loss rewards of this plan. The rules are:

▪ **RULE #1: STICK TO 400 CALORIES PER MEAL.**
▪ **RULE #2: NEVER GO MORE THAN 4 HOURS WITHOUT EATING.**
▪ **RULE #3: EAT A MUFA AT EVERY MEAL.**
▪ **RULE #4: EXERCISE MOST DAYS OF THE WEEK.**

RULE #1: STICK TO 400 CALORIES PER MEAL

You've probably noticed by now that infusing your diet with MUFAs is a balancing act—one that pits the belly-flattening, blood-sugar-pampering benefits of this amazing nutrient against the unavoidable fact that MUFA-rich foods aren't exactly low-calorie choices. That's why most diets tell you to avoid nuts, oils, and chocolate. But because these MUFAs are so essential for belly fat and blood sugar control—and because they also provide a unique satisfaction factor—we put them front and center. And that means calorie control in what surrounds them takes on extra importance.

All of the meals in the Flat Belly Diet Diabetes provide a total of about 400 calories (there's an optional 200-calorie extra snack for those who need a few more calories!). This means you can substitute one whole meal for another. You can eat breakfast for dinner or lunch for breakfast. If you like, you can even eat four breakfast meals in one day. That's part of the ease of this plan. We don't expect that you'll love every single meal. But on the other hand, if you find a few you absolutely adore, it's perfectly okay to enjoy them to your heart's content—with one important exception: Choose meals containing chocolate or olives just once a day, so the rest of your meals can balance the slightly higher sugar content in chocolate and the higher sodium levels found in most olives.

This diet is 1,600 calories per day because that's how much it takes for a woman (as well as most men) of average height, frame size, and activity level to get to and stay at an ideal body weight. Men who are more active or who have a larger frame, as well as women who exercise vigorously most days of the week, will find advice for fitting in an extra 200-calorie snack.

So 1,600 to 1,800 calories is not a starvation plan—it's enough to keep up your energy level, support your immune system, and maintain your precious calorie-burning muscle. That means you won't feel run-down, cranky, irritable, moody, or hungry. But you also won't be eating enough calories to hang on to your belly.

RULE #2: NEVER GO MORE THAN 4 HOURS WITHOUT EATING

We don't have to tell you that a diet that makes you feel hungry, cranky, or tired simply won't work. That's why on the Flat Belly Diet Diabetes, you're *required* to eat every 4 hours. Waiting too long can leave you so hungry it's hard to think straight—and harder to stick with healthy foods and portions when you finally sit down to eat something! You won't have the energy or patience to think through the healthiest meal choice, let alone prepare one. And you'll probably have a hard time slowing down while you eat and not reaching for seconds.

If you have diabetes, spacing your meals at regular intervals also helps with blood sugar control. Topping off your tank with a healthy portion of carbohydrates on a consistent schedule helps you avoid blood sugar highs and lows that can happen if you skip a meal or wait a long time between meals, then devour a lot of food. If you use insulin to control your blood sugar, eating set amounts on a regular basis is a "must," but the same strategy can help any medication work better because your blood sugar levels won't have roller-coaster highs and lows.

Snacks are especially important, but when you eat them is entirely up to you. You may prefer a nighttime snack or find that you really need something to fill the empty corners in your stomach at midafternoon. Your snack time is entirely personal and entirely essential. To help you include your snack every day, Gillian has included a variety of Snack Packs that you can prepare ahead of time and take with you each morning. They're portable and MUFA-loaded. Use the Snack Pack as a floating meal. Same goes for the additional 200-calorie snack—fit it into the times of day when you feel hungry or know you're going to need energy, such as a half-hour or so before exercising.

RULE #3: EAT A MUFA AT EVERY MEAL

"A MUFA at every meal" has almost become a mantra for us. As you know, "MUFA" (MOO-fah) stands for "monounsaturated fatty acid," a type of heart-healthy, disease-fighting, "good" fat found in foods like almonds, peanut butter, olive oil, avocados, and even chocolate. MUFAs are an unsaturated fat and have the exact opposite effect of the unhealthy saturated and trans fats you've heard about in the news.

But there's more! MUFAs are delicious in and of themselves. Who doesn't love drizzling olive oil over a salad or crunching on almonds or walnuts? You'll find these MUFA-rich foods incorporated into every meal and every 400-calorie Snack Pack on the plan. MUFAs even star in some of our optional 200-calorie snacks, too! You can substitute most MUFAs for one another within meals and within snacks as long as the calorie counts are nearly equivalent. (Just remember, to help control blood sugar and blood pressure, we recommend having chocolate and olives only once a day.) For precise MUFA serving sizes per meal, consult the chart on page 127. Better yet, copy this chart and post it on the inside door of your pantry.

RULE #4: EXERCISE MOST DAYS OF THE WEEK

We start you off slowly. In Phase 1, you'll do a daily Fat Blast Walk that combines a warm-up, brisk stroll, and cooldown. The plan then gradually introduces an easy strength-training routine we call the Metabolism Boost and torso-tightening moves we call the Belly Routine. You could easily fit one of these into the commercial breaks in your favorite TV show, and the results are amazing: a leaner, stronger body, a toned midsection, and a metabolism that burns more calories around the clock. As you move through the program, you'll also be introduced to intervals—short bursts of faster, more intense walking proven to burn more calories. That's why we call it the Calorie Torch Walk.

Even our exercise plan is flexible. If diabetes foot complications—such as poor circulation or nerve damage—make walking difficult, there's a second easy and affordable option: using a "pedal exerciser." Available online and in stores for as little as $20, this very small piece of exercise equipment is simply a set of bicycle pedals. You use it while seated in a chair or on a sofa—so it keeps pressure and weight off your feet while giving your leg muscles a workout.

You'll find complete workout details in Chapter 11 and a breakdown of what to do each day of Phase 1 and 2 on the journal pages in Chapters 7 and 12.

And Beyond . . .

WE WANT TO ARM you with every winning strategy so that your time on the Flat Belly Diet Diabetes is not only successful, but also empowering and eye-opening. To stay on track and to put you in a frame of mind that's open to deeply appreciating the deeply pleasurable and nurturing effects of good food and gentle exercise, we've come up with two more recommendations:

▪ RELAX AND RECHARGE. By now you're aware that reducing stress and giving yourself the gift of deep, restorative sleep have a synergistic effect—they work together to help you overcome emotional eating and stress eating, lose weight, and bring your blood sugar into a healthier range. Setting aside 10 minutes of daily "me time" for stress reduction can help you reach all of these goals.

You'll find a progressive muscle relaxation exercise in Phase 1; in Phase 2 you may choose to continue practicing it or to relax in any way you choose.

■ TRACK YOUR PROGRESS DAILY IN THE FLAT BELLY DIET DIABETES JOURNAL. In one recent study that followed 1,700 dieters for 6 months, researchers at the Kaiser Permanente Center for Health Research found that those who kept food journals lost twice as much weight as those who didn't.[1] Journaling keeps you honest and aware of what you're eating, what you're doing, and what you're feeling as you take this journey. By completing the "core confidence" exercises on each day's journal page, you'll also continue adding to your box of tools that support your efforts to flatten your belly and manage your blood sugar.

YOUR MUFA SERVING CHART

FOOD	SERVING	CALORIES
SOYBEANS (EDAMAME), SHELLED AND BOILED	1 cup	244
SEMISWEET CHOCOLATE CHIPS	¼ cup	207
ALMOND BUTTER	2 Tbsp	200
CASHEW BUTTER	2 Tbsp	190
SUNFLOWER SEED BUTTER	2 Tbsp	190
NATURAL PEANUT BUTTER, CRUNCHY	2 Tbsp	188
NATURAL PEANUT BUTTER, SMOOTH	2 Tbsp	188
TAHINI (SESAME SEED PASTE)	2 Tbsp	178
PUMPKIN SEEDS	2 Tbsp	148
CANOLA OIL	1 Tbsp	124
FLAXSEED OIL (COLD-PRESSED ORGANIC)	1 Tbsp	120
MACADAMIA NUTS	2 Tbsp	120
SAFFLOWER OIL (HIGH OLEIC)	1 Tbsp	120
SESAME OR SOYBEAN OIL	1 Tbsp	120
SUNFLOWER OIL (HIGH OLEIC)	1 Tbsp	120
WALNUT OIL	1 Tbsp	120
OLIVE OIL	1 Tbsp	119
PEANUT OIL	1 Tbsp	119
PINE NUTS	2 Tbsp	113
BRAZIL NUTS	2 Tbsp	110
HAZELNUTS	2 Tbsp	110
PEANUTS	2 Tbsp	110
ALMONDS	2 Tbsp	109
CASHEWS	2 Tbsp	100
AVOCADO, CALIFORNIA (HASS)	¼ cup	96
PECANS	2 Tbsp	90
SUNFLOWER SEEDS	2 Tbsp	90
BLACK OLIVE TAPENADE	2 Tbsp	88
PISTACHIOS	2 Tbsp	88
WALNUTS	2 Tbsp	82
PESTO SAUCE	1 Tbsp	80
AVOCADO, FLORIDA	¼ cup	69
GREEN OLIVE TAPENADE	2 Tbsp	54
GREEN OR BLACK OLIVES	10 large	50

PHASE 1: THE 7-DAY START-UP PLAN

THE FLAT BELLY Diet Diabetes has two phases—and you're about to embark on Phase 1, the 7-Day Start-Up Plan. We've made it simple . . . and, we promise, delicious! (How about a hot breakfast sandwich featuring egg, cheese, and avocado on an English muffin, roast pork with sweet potatoes and a side of broccoli for dinner, and filling snacks that are as big as a full meal?)

In Phase 1, you'll:

■ **1. EAT:** You'll follow a set meal and snack plan, during which you eat four times a day. Never go more than 4 hours between meals.

■ **2. MOVE:** You'll walk for 6 out of the 7 days. There is a beginner and an advanced level of exercise throughout the plan.

■ **3. RELAX:** You'll do a progressive relaxation exercise every day, which should take no more than 10 minutes.

4. TRACK: You'll log what you eat and do (it's easy with our check-off system!), as well as your hunger level, your blood sugar (if you monitor on a daily basis), and your thoughts and feelings. In addition, you'll practice a fun Mind Trick at one meal per day, aimed at honing your awareness of what you're eating and how it makes you feel—a technique proven to boost satisfaction and reduce overeating.

Let's get started!

Phase 1 Meals

THE PHASE 1 MEAL Plan gives you breakfast, lunch, snack, and dinner. Each provides 400 calories and contains a food rich in monounsaturated fats

Seasoning Suggestions

Use these suggestions to add flavor and seasonings to your Phase I and Phase II meals. Or experiment for yourself with these herbs and spices.

FISH: bay leaf, curry powder, dill, dry mustard, lemon juice, marjoram, onion powder, paprika

POULTRY: curry powder, garlic, ginger, lemon juice, paprika, parsley, poultry seasoning, rosemary, sage, thyme

RED MEAT: basil, chili powder, coriander, dry mustard, garlic, marjoram, pepper, red wine vinegar, thyme

DRIED BEANS: balsamic vinegar, basil, chili powder, cumin, pepper

TOFU: balsamic vinegar, celery seeds, garlic, ginger, mustard

ASPARAGUS: dry mustard, garlic, nutmeg, paprika, tarragon

BROCCOLI: basil, garlic, marjoram, onion powder, oregano, tarragon

CABBAGE: caraway seeds, dill, lemon juice, marjoram

CARROTS: cinnamon, dry mustard, ginger, nutmeg

CORN: chili powder, cumin, parsley, pepper

GREEN BEANS: dill, lemon juice, marjoram, nutmeg, tarragon

PEAS: basil, garlic, mint, oregano, parsley, tarragon

TOMATOES: balsamic vinegar, basil, dill, oregano, parsley, rosemary

WINTER SQUASH: allspice, cloves, ginger, nutmeg, orange peel

(MUFAs). Follow the meal plan exactly; however, you can add herbs, spices, and other seasonings to each meal, as desired.

In Phase 1, we'll spell out exactly what to eat, how much, and when. Consider it a week at a spa—there's no need to figure out what to eat or when. We've done the work for you. Just take our handy Phase 1 Shopping List to the store ahead of time and stock up on the supplies you'll need, and you're ready to go. Your mission this week? Follow directions. To be more specific, be sure to:

▪ FOLLOW PHASE 1 MEALS EXACTLY. Try not to add, subtract, or substitute. For this week, stick to the set menu, which is carefully designed to give you balanced nutrition and the optimal amount of healthy MUFAs within the 1,600-calorie per day limit. This will help you get used to cooking and eating the Flat Belly Diet way. We want you to spend a week getting used to this healthy eating style and to the healthy mix of foods on your plate at every meal. When specific brands of foods are listed, try to buy and eat those. We've selected particular brands because of their taste, quality, availability, and nutritional value. Including these foods guarantees steady weight loss because their precise calorie counts and levels of carbohydrates and fiber have been incorporated into the plan. If you cannot find some of these items, replace them with comparable foods with as close to the same calorie, carbohydrate, and fiber level as possible.

The good news? You can spice things up a little, using our list of seasoning suggestions.

Of course, if you are allergic to any ingredient in any Flat Belly Diet Diabetes meal, skip it and substitute a similar item that's safe for you to eat.

▪ EAT FOUR MEALS A DAY. Phase 1 will introduce you to the pleasures of eating not three but four times a day. That's breakfast, lunch, dinner, plus a substantial snack. Our test panelists told us this schedule kept them from feeling hungry, tided them over when they knew there would be a long wait between meals, and added pleasure to every day. Yes, you may have less in your stomach after any one meal than you've been used to eating in the past, but the knowledge that there's another meal coming up in the next few hours is—we promise!—sure to help you stay on track.

■ MEASURE YOUR FOOD. For accuracy, we do request that you measure all of your food. Without measuring, it's very easy to accumulate extra calories. Use a kitchen measuring cup and kitchen measuring spoons—not regular silverware or the kind of cup you drink from—to do this. For these cup and spoon measurements (½ cup, 1 tablespoon, etc.), be sure to level the top, too.

■ DRINK WATER, TEA, OR COFFEE UNLESS OTHERWISE SPECIFIED. During Phase 1 and Phase 2, it is best to stick with plain water and unsweetened brewed hot and cold green, red, white, black, or herbal tea (or try refreshing Sassy Water). If possible, please limit alcohol consumption and go easy with sugar and milk or cream in your coffee, as both add extra calories to the diet. The calorie content of the meals has been carefully calculated, so added calories will change your results.

TRY SASSY WATER!

Developed by registered dietitian Cynthia Sass, MPH, RD, coauthor of the original *Flat Belly Diet!*, Sassy Water is a refreshing alternative to plain water or unsweetened iced tea. The perky flavor keeps you coming back for more—and that's great, because we recommend sipping one recipe's worth every day to meet your fluid needs.
Our recipe:

- 2 liters water (about 8½ cups)
- 1 teaspoon freshly grated ginger root
- 1 medium cucumber, peeled and thinly sliced
- 1 medium lemon, thinly sliced
- 12 mint leaves

Combine all ingredients in a large pitcher, chill in the refrigerator, and let flavors blend overnight.

Phase 1 Exercise

YOU'LL WALK 6 DAYS during Phase I. As we've already described in detail elsewhere in this book, exercise helps control blood sugar in several powerful ways—it makes cells more sensitive to insulin, it encourages muscle cells to pull more glucose from your bloodstream during and after you exercise, and it even helps you control your appetite. And, of course, exercise burns calories and helps you lose weight. That's a major payback for a small investment—just 15 minutes a day if you're new to exercise; 30 minutes a day if you're used to exercising.

If you have never exercised regularly before or haven't exercised in more than 6 months, start at the beginner level. If you do exercise regularly, start at the advanced level; if that's too challenging, you can always go back to the beginner level. At the advanced level, you'll be walking 30 minutes a day, which you can split into two, 15-minute walks instead of one long walk, if you prefer.

Since walking will also blast belly fat, we've named our basic Flat Belly Diet Diabetes exercise routine the Fat Blast Walk. To walk this way, simply warm up by walking at a slow pace for 3 minutes. Then walk briskly—10 minutes for beginners, 25 minutes for advanced exercisers. (A brisk pace is one at which you can hold a conversation with a walking partner, but you'd have trouble singing a song.) Then cool down with a slow walk for the last 2 minutes.

We recommend walking because you can do it virtually anytime, anyplace. As described in Chapter 11, if you cannot walk for at least 15 minutes due to diabetes-related foot problems (such as nerve damage or reduced circulation)—or for any other reason—consider investing in an economical "pedaler." Available online and in the sporting goods or exercise equipment section of many stores, these exercise machines are simply a set of pedals attached to a small base. (We love pedalers because they're small and easy to store!) Some allow you to adjust the resistance for a more challenging workout. To use, just place the pedaler in front of a kitchen chair, sit down, put your feet on the pedals, and begin pumping away.

If you already have an established exercise routine that you'd prefer to continue, go right ahead. Just be sure you're getting at least 15 to 30 minutes of activity 6 times a week for optimal calorie-burning, blood sugar–controlling results.

If you have knee or joint problems, heart disease, foot problems, or other health concerns, check with your doctor before starting this or any other exercise program.

Phase 1 Progressive Muscle Relaxation

IN PHASE 1, WE want you to set aside 10 minutes a day to practice the Progressive Muscle Relaxation exercise below. You can do it sitting in a chair or lying on your bed or even on the floor and at any time of day that's convenient for you. In Phase 2, we want you to continue setting aside 10 minutes of "me time" every day for a stress-busting activity of your choice.

PROGRESSIVE RELAXATION EXERCISE

In a quiet room, sit in a comfortable chair with both feet flat on the floor and your arms relaxed, hands in your lap. Or lie on the floor or in bed. Pick a time and place where you can be alone for 10 undisturbed minutes. Here we go:

RELAXATION EXERCISE	
FEET	Point or curl toes as you tighten foot muscles Tense for 5 seconds, then release and relax for 10 seconds. Repeat.
LOWER LEGS AND FEET	Clench big muscles in your calves. Tense for 5 seconds, then release and relax for 10 seconds. Repeat.
THIGHS	Tighten muscles in your upper legs from knees to hips. Tense for 5 seconds, then release and relax for 10 seconds. Repeat.
BUTTOCKS	Squeeze buttocks together. Tense for 5 seconds, then release and relax for 10 seconds. Repeat.
BACK	Squeeze shoulder blades together. Tense for 5 seconds, then release and relax for 10 seconds. Repeat.
ABDOMEN	Clench those tummy muscles. Tense for 5 seconds, then release and relax for 10 seconds. Repeat.
CHEST	Tense muscles of upper chest. Tense for 5 seconds, then release and relax for 10 seconds. Repeat.
HANDS	Clench fists. Tense for 5 seconds, then release and relax for 10 seconds. Repeat.
FOREARMS	Extend your arms with your elbows locked. Tense for 5 seconds, then release and relax for 10 seconds. Repeat.
UPPER ARMS	Bend your arms at the elbows and flex your biceps. Tense for 5 seconds, then release and relax for 10 seconds. Repeat.
NECK AND SHOULDERS	Clench muscles tightly. Tense for 5 seconds, then release and relax for 10 seconds. Repeat
JAW	Open your mouth wide and stick out your tongue. Tense for 5 seconds, then release and relax for 10 seconds. Repeat.
MOUTH	Press your lips together firmly. Tense for 5 seconds, then release and relax for 10 seconds. Repeat.
EYES	Close your eyes tightly. Tense for 5 seconds, then release and relax for 10 seconds. Repeat.
FOREHEAD	Wrinkle your forehead and eyebrows. Tense for 5 seconds, then release and relax for 10 seconds. Repeat

Introducing Mindful Eating

The first days of a new eating plan are never easy—new foods, new portion sizes, even whole new meals if you've been skipping breakfast or aren't used to fitting a substantial snack into your day. Of course, it's all going to be worth it. And we expect you'll begin seeing benefits by the end of Phase 1, as many of our test panelists did. "I felt wonderful," notes panelist Susan Hoar, who lost 1.8 pounds the first week.

To make it easier, we're including a mental tune-up on each day of Phase 1. These Mind Tricks are a way of giving a meal importance. They'll help you become mindful of what you're eating and why. Studies show that mindful eating can reduce binge eating. This practice harnesses all of your senses so that you're completely aware of what you're eating, how you're feeling, and how full you are. It's an important antidote to emotional and overeating. To help you further, we're asking you to register your sense of hunger and fullness before and after each meal. You'll learn how to stop as soon as you feel comfortably full—because it actually takes your stomach and brain about 20 minutes to register fullness.

I want you to have the experience of feeling really good at the end of every meal you eat—satisfied by the food you consumed and full enough. Not stuffed to the gills. Not still a little hungry. Simply good. If you haven't been taking good care of your body, or if you've been feeling guilty or downright bad about your weight or your health issues, you may bump up against the uncomfortable sense that you don't deserve to feel good. I'm here to tell you that you do! By eating mindfully, you can feel good emotionally and physically about the food you eat—secure in the knowledge that you're nourishing your body, giving yourself pleasure, and eating the right foods in the right amounts to support your journey toward an optimal body weight and blood sugar level.

For every meal in Phase 1 (and in Phase 2), assess your hunger or fullness status, using the following scale:

HOW HUNGRY ARE YOU?

For every meal in Phase 1 (and in Phase 2), we'll ask you to assess your hunger or fullness status, then circle the appropriate number on our Hunger Rating Chart. It uses the following scale:

RATING	HOW IT FEELS
1 = STARVING	You may feel shaky, like you're about to pass out, or like you want to devour the first thing you see and have a hard time slowing down.
3 = MILD TO MODERATE HUNGER	You have physical symptoms of hunger like a growling tummy and that "I need to eat soon" feeling, but you aren't starving or experiencing any unpleasant symptoms such as a headache, shaking, etc.
5 = JUST RIGHT	Just right. Your hunger is gone. You feel satisfied and full but not too full. Your mind is off food, and you're ready to take on the next task. You feel energized..
8 = OVERLY FULL	You think you overdid it. Your tummy feels stretched and uncomfortable. You may feel kind of sluggish, not energized at all.
10 = STUFFED!	The way you feel after a huge Thanksgiving dinner.

NOTE: Check in with yourself before, during, and after eating. Aim to eat when your hunger is at 3. Stop eating when your fullness and satisfaction level has reached about 5.

Track Your Progress

FOR PHASE 1, YOUR journal is incorporated into your meal and exercise plan. Each day you'll find an easy-to-follow page that spells it all out clearly and simply: what you'll eat, how much you'll exercise, a reminder to find time for relaxation, a Mind Trick, and some space for reflection and hunger ratings. Studies have continually shown that keeping a log of what you eat and how you feel while you're eating helps you stay on track with new lifestyle choices. There is now increasing evidence to support the concept that journaling has a positive impact on physical well-being. University of Texas at Austin researcher James W. Pennebaker, PhD, has scientifically shown that regular journaling strengthens immune cells called T lymphocytes.[1] Other research indicates that journaling may help decrease the symptoms of asthma and rheumatoid arthritis. Dr. Pennebaker believes that writing about stressful events helps you come to terms with them, thus reducing the impact of these stressors on your physical health. And in one recent study from Kaiser Permanente's Center for Health Research in Portland, Oregon, that tracked 1,685 men and women over 6 months while they followed a weight-loss program, those who kept a diary almost every day lost twice as much weight as those who didn't![2]

If you have diabetes, keeping a journal will also include recording some daily blood sugar readings taken with your blood glucose monitor. Test panelists checked their blood sugar 2 hours after each meal, in addition to monitoring at other times of the day as recommended by their doctors. The after-meal checks can help you assess how specific meals affect your blood sugar—you may find that some foods or combinations keep your blood sugar lower or nudge it up. These differences are very individual—what affects you might not affect someone else in the same way. We recommend doing checks 2 hours after most, if not all, meals at least during Phase 1 so that you can see for yourself how Flat Belly Diet Diabetes meals are affecting your blood sugar.

Later, when you complete Phase 1 and begin Phase 2 of the Flat Belly Diet Diabetes, we'll ask you to continue journaling about issues concerning food, health, and body image—the all-important Core Confidences that will help you gain important new tools for staying on track. For now, take these 7 days to get used to the format of the food journal—and start building the habit of sitting down and recording everything you've put into your mouth that day.

A few rules of the journaling journey:

1. Forget spelling and punctuation.
2. Write quickly to ward off your inner critic.
3. Speak from your heart.

Now it's time to get started!

Phase 1 Shopping List

PRODUCE

- ☐ Apples, 4 small (using 4)
- ☐ Avocado, 1; we like Hass avocados, but any type will work (using 1 cup, approximately 1 avocado)
- ☐ Baby carrots, 1-pound bag (using 2 cups)
- ☐ Bananas, 3 small (using 3)
- ☐ Blueberries, 1-pound bag frozen or 1 pint carton fresh (using 1 cup)
- ☐ Broccoli, 1 pound fresh or frozen (using 2 cups)
- ☐ Green beans, 10-ounce package frozen or 8 ounces fresh (using 1 cup)
- ☐ Lettuce, 2 (10-ounce) bags of romaine (using 2 bags)
- ☐ Mushrooms, 1 (8-ounce) package presliced baby portobellos (using 2 cups)
- ☐ Oranges, 2 medium (using 2)
- ☐ Red potatoes, about $\frac{1}{2}$ pound (using 6 ounces)
- ☐ Sugar snap peas, 1-pound bag frozen or 16 ounces fresh (using 2 cups)
- ☐ Sweet potato, 2 (4-ounce) potatoes (each about 5" long) (using 2)

DAIRY

- ☐ Eggs, $\frac{1}{2}$ dozen (using 2 eggs)
- ☐ Low-fat (1%) cottage cheese, 8-ounce tub (using $\frac{1}{2}$ cup)
- ☐ Low-fat/light Cheddar cheese slices, 1 (8-ounce) package (using 2 slices)
- ☐ Low-fat/light string cheese, 6 (using 6)
- ☐ Low-fat shredded Mexican blend cheese, 1 (6- to 8-ounce) package (using $\frac{1}{2}$ cup)
- ☐ Nonfat plain yogurt, 2 (6-ounce) containers (using 2 containers)

DRY GOODS

- ☐ Almonds, dry, unsalted, 1 (10-ounce) package (using $\frac{1}{2}$ cup)
- ☐ Balsamic vinegar, 1 (8-ounce) bottle (using 4 tablespoons)
- ☐ Black beans, 1 (15-ounce) can (using $\frac{1}{2}$ cup)
- ☐ Brown rice, 1 (14-ounce or smaller) box (using $\frac{1}{2}$ cup)
- ☐ Chicken and rice soup bowls, Campbell's or Healthy Choice, 2 (using 2)
- ☐ Dried cranberries, 1 (8-ounce) package (using 6 tablespoons)
- ☐ Oatmeal, 1 (18-ounce) carton or smaller (using $1\frac{1}{2}$ cups)
- ☐ Olive oil, 1 (8-ounce) bottle (using 11 tablespoons)
- ☐ Peanut butter, natural preferred, 1 (16-ounce or smaller) jar (using 6 tablespoons)
- ☐ Pineapple chunks canned in own juice, 1 (8-ounce) can (using 2 tablespoons)
- ☐ Pine nuts, 1 (4-ounce) package (using 4 tablespoons)

- Ranch dressing, light, 1 (16-ounce or smaller) bottle (using 4 tablespoons)
- Sunflower seeds, 1 (7-ounce) package (using 6 tablespoons)
- Tomato sauce, light, 1 (10- to 16-ounce) jar; look for a variety with about 50 to 60 calories per $\frac{1}{2}$ cup (using 1 cup)
- Walnuts, dried, unsalted, chopped, 1 (8-ounce) package (using 14 tablespoons)
- Wasa Rye Crispbread or ak-mak crackers, 1 box Wasa or 2 boxes ak-mak (using 15 Wasa or 21 ak-mak crackers)
- Whole wheat bread, 1 loaf (using 2 slices)
- Whole wheat English muffins, 1 package (using 4 muffins)
- Whole wheat pasta, 1 (13- to 16-ounce) box (using 1 cup)
- Whole wheat tortillas, 1 small package of 6" tortillas (approximately 75 calories per tortilla) (using 4)

MEAT/SEAFOOD
- Chicken breast, boneless, skinless, 4 ounces
- Cod, 10 ounces
- Deli turkey, 8 ounces
- Ground turkey breast (93% lean), 6 ounces
- Pork tenderloin (lean), 8 ounces

MISCELLANEOUS
- Hummus, 1 (8-ounce) tub (using $\frac{1}{2}$ cup)

ANY OF THESE APPROVED SALT-FREE SEASONINGS
- Fresh or dried (use only salt-free types): allspice, balsamic vinegar, basil, bay leaf, caraway seeds, cinnamon, chili powder, coriander, cumin, curry powder, dill, dry mustard, garlic, ginger, lemon or lime juice, marjoram, mint, nutmeg, dried onion powder or dried chopped onion, grated orange peel, oregano, paprika, parsley, pepper, poultry seasoning, red wine vinegar, rosemary, sage, tarragon, or thyme
- Original and Italian medley Mrs. Dash salt-free seasoning blends

PHASE 1, DAY 1

DATE:

BREAKFAST

- ☐ ½ cup dry oatmeal
- ☐ 1 medium banana (7"–8") cut into slices
- ☐ 2 tablespoons dried, unsalted, chopped walnuts

Cook oatmeal with desired amount of water. Add banana and walnuts to oatmeal and serve.

Calories=352, carb=56 g, fiber=7 g

LUNCH

- ☐ ½ cup 1% cottage cheese
- ☐ 2 tablespoons pineapple chunks canned in juice and drained
- ☐ 2 slices 100% whole wheat bread
- ☐ 2 tablespoons peanut butter

Mix pineapple into cottage cheese and serve with peanut butter sandwich.

Calories=423, carb=41 g, fiber=6 g

SNACK

- ☐ 5 Wasa Rye Crispbread crackers OR 7 ak-mak crackers
- ☐ 2 pieces low-fat string cheese
- ☐ 2 tablespoons sunflower seeds

Top crackers with light string cheese. Eat sunflower seeds on the side.

Calories=376, carb=40 g, fiber=8 g (Wasa)
Calories=376, carb=35 g, fiber=6 g (ak-mak)

DINNER

- ☐ 4 ounces raw boneless, skinless chicken breast
- ☐ 1 tablespoon olive oil
- ☐ 1 cup cooked green beans
- ☐ ½ cup cooked brown rice

Cut up chicken into strips. Heat oil in a skillet and add chicken. Sauté chicken until no longer pink. Add desired seasoning. Either steam fresh green beans or microwave frozen green beans. Cook brown rice according to package directions. Serve chicken with rice and green beans.

Calories=408, carb=34 g, fiber=6 g

☐ **MIND TRICK AT ONE MEAL TODAY:** Smile . . . at your plate. Research shows that 40 percent of us have "smile muscles"—using them sends a happy message to your brain. You may be one of them, so try it!

☐ **EXERCISE:** Walk or perform physical activity of your choice (swimming, biking, using a pedaler, exercise class, or video). Beginner: 15 minutes Advanced: 30 minutes (can be done in two 15-minute segments)

☐ **PROGRESSIVE MUSCLE RELAXATION**

JOURNAL, DAY 1

DATE:

BREAKFAST	
MOOD:	THOUGHTS

HUNGER BEFORE: 1   3   5   8   10 | HUNGER AFTER: 1   3   5   8   10

LUNCH	
MOOD:	THOUGHTS

HUNGER BEFORE: 1   3   5   8   10 | HUNGER AFTER: 1   3   5   8   10

SNACK	
MOOD:	THOUGHTS

HUNGER BEFORE: 1   3   5   8   10 | HUNGER AFTER: 1   3   5   8   10

DINNER	
MOOD:	THOUGHTS

HUNGER BEFORE: 1   3   5   8   10 | HUNGER AFTER: 1   3   5   8   10

☐ **BLOOD GLUCOSE LEVELS**
(Check as recommended by your doctor.)

Time:.....................

Reading: ....

Time:.....................

Reading: ....

Time:.....................

Reading: ....

Time:.....................

Reading: ....

Time:.....................

Reading: ....

Time:.....................

Reading: ....

PHASE 1, DAY 2

DATE:

BREAKFAST

- ☐ 1 whole wheat English muffin
- ☐ 2 tablespoons peanut butter
- ☐ 1 medium apple

Spread peanut butter on toasted English muffin and have apple on the side.

Calories=390, carb=51 g, fiber=9 g

LUNCH

- ☐ Campbell's Select Harvest Savory Chicken and Long Grain Rice Soup bowl OR 1 Healthy Choice Chicken with Rice Soup bowl
- ☐ ¼ cup dry, unsalted almonds

Calories=426, carb=43 g, fiber=6 g (Campbell's)
Calories=386, carb=33 g, fiber=8 g (Healthy Choice)

SNACK

- ☐ ½ cup blueberries, fresh or frozen (defrosted)
- ☐ 2 tablespoons walnuts
- ☐ 6 ounces nonfat plain yogurt
- ☐ 1 cup baby carrots
- ☐ 2 tablespoons light ranch dressing

Add blueberries and walnuts to yogurt and serve baby carrots with light ranch dressing on the side.

Calories=376, carb=39 g, fiber=6 g

DINNER

- ☐ 5 ounces raw cod fillet
- ☐ 1 tablespoon olive oil
- ☐ 3 ounces red potatoes
- ☐ 1 cup cooked sugar snap peas

Brush fish with 1 teaspoon oil and sprinkle desired seasoning on fish. Broil for 5 minutes. Carefully turn fish and brush with 1 teaspoon oil and broil for 4 to 6 minutes longer, or until fish flakes easily with a fork. Preheat oven to 350°F. Chop potatoes into small pieces, place in an ungreased glass baking dish, drizzle with remaining oil, and sprinkle with desired seasoning. Bake for 15 minutes, or until desired tenderness. Steam or microwave snap peas and serve with fish and potatoes.

Calories=379, carb=29 g, fiber=6 g

☐ **MIND TRICK AT ONE MEAL TODAY:** Cooking tonight? Use your food-prep time in the kitchen to immerse yourself in the aromas, textures, colors, and flavors of food. The creative act of chopping vegetables, cooking, adding pungent seasonings, and, finally, eating a great meal—is soul-satisfying.

☐ **EXERCISE:** Walk or perform physical activity of your choice (swimming, biking, using a pedaler, exercise class, or video).
Beginner: 15 minutes
Advanced: 30 minutes (can be done in two 15-minute segments)

☐ **PROGRESSIVE MUSCLE RELAXATION**

JOURNAL, DAY 2

DATE:

BREAKFAST	
MOOD:	THOUGHTS

HUNGER BEFORE: 1   3   5   8   10   HUNGER AFTER: 1   3   5   8   10

LUNCH	
MOOD:	THOUGHTS

HUNGER BEFORE: 1   3   5   8   10   HUNGER AFTER: 1   3   5   8   10

SNACK	
MOOD:	THOUGHTS

HUNGER BEFORE: 1   3   5   8   10   HUNGER AFTER: 1   3   5   8   10

DINNER	
MOOD:	THOUGHTS

HUNGER BEFORE: 1   3   5   8   10   HUNGER AFTER: 1   3   5   8   10

☐ **BLOOD GLUCOSE LEVELS** (Check as recommended by your doctor.)

Time:....................

Reading: ....

Time:....................

Reading: ....

Time:....................

Reading: ....

Time:....................

Reading: ....

Time:....................

Reading: ....

Time:....................

Reading: ....

PHASE 1, DAY 3

DATE:

BREAKFAST

- ☐ 1 whole wheat English muffin
- ☐ 1 cooked egg
- ☐ ¼ cup sliced avocado
- ☐ 1 slice reduced-fat Cheddar cheese
- ☐ 1 medium apple

Top toasted English muffin with egg, avocado, and cheese. Serve with apple on the side.

Calories=383, carb=49 g, fiber=10 g

LUNCH

- ☐ 3 cups romaine lettuce or other lettuce mix
- ☐ 2 tablespoons dried, unsalted, chopped walnuts
- ☐ 3 tablespoons dried cranberries
- ☐ 1 tablespoon olive oil
- ☐ 1 tablespoon balsamic vinegar
- ☐ 1 medium orange

Serve salad greens topped with walnuts, cranberries, and a mix of oil and vinegar. Serve orange on the side or on salad as desired.

Calories=393, carb=45 g, fiber=7 g

SNACK:

- ☐ 1 whole wheat tortilla
- ☐ 4 ounces deli turkey breast
- ☐ ¼ cup hummus
- ☐ 2 tablespoons pine nuts

Top tortilla with turkey, hummus, and pine nuts and roll up.

Calories=398, carb=35 g, fiber=6 g

DINNER:

- ☐ 4 ounces raw lean pork tenderloin
- ☐ 1 4-ounce sweet potato, about 5" long
- ☐ 1 tablespoon olive oil
- ☐ 1 cup cooked broccoli

Preheat oven to 425°F. Roast pork tenderloin for 15 to 20 minutes, or until internal temp is 160°F on meat thermometer. Bake sweet potato in the microwave oven for 10 minutes and drizzle with half the oil. Steam or microwave broccoli and drizzle with remaining oil. Serve pork with sweet potato and broccoli on the side.

Calories=428, carb=37 g, fiber=9 g

☐ **MIND TRICK AT ONE MEAL TODAY:** Avoid multitasking during at least one meal today. Turn off the radio or TV, shut the laptop, turn off the cell phone, and close the newspaper. When you avoid distractions and give food your complete attention, it's much more satisfying.

☐ **EXERCISE:** Walk or perform physical activity of your choice (swimming, biking, using a pedaler, exercise class, or video).
Beginner:
15 minutes
Advanced:
30 minutes (can be done in two 15-minute segments)

☐ **PROGRESSIVE MUSCLE RELAXATION**

JOURNAL, DAY 3

DATE:

BREAKFAST	
MOOD:	THOUGHTS

HUNGER BEFORE: 1   3   5   8   10   HUNGER AFTER: 1   3   5   8   10

LUNCH	
MOOD:	THOUGHTS

HUNGER BEFORE: 1   3   5   8   10   HUNGER AFTER: 1   3   5   8   10

SNACK	
MOOD:	THOUGHTS

HUNGER BEFORE: 1   3   5   8   10   HUNGER AFTER: 1   3   5   8   10

DINNER	
MOOD:	THOUGHTS

HUNGER BEFORE: 1   3   5   8   10   HUNGER AFTER: 1   3   5   8   10

❏ **BLOOD GLUCOSE LEVELS**
(Check as recommended by your doctor.)

Time:

Reading:

Time:

Reading:

Time:

Reading:

Time:

Reading:

Time:

Reading:

Time:

Reading:

PHASE 1, DAY 4

DATE:

BREAKFAST

- ☐ ½ cup dry oatmeal
- ☐ 1 medium banana (7"–8") cut into slices
- ☐ 2 tablespoons dried, unsalted, chopped walnuts

Cook oatmeal with desired amount of water. Add banana and walnuts to oatmeal and serve.

Calories=352, carb=56 g, fiber=7 g

LUNCH

- ☐ ¼ cup black beans
- ☐ ¼ cup sliced avocado
- ☐ ¼ cup shredded low-fat Mexican blend cheese
- ☐ 1 whole wheat tortilla
- ☐ 2 cups romaine lettuce or other lettuce blend
- ☐ 1 tablespoon olive oil
- ☐ 1 tablespoon balsamic vinegar

Place beans, avocado, and cheese in tortilla. Heat in the microwave oven to melt cheese, if desired. Serve with side salad of lettuce drizzled with oil and vinegar.

Calories=417, carb=38 g, fiber=9 g

SNACK

- ☐ 5 Wasa Rye Crispbread crackers OR 7 ak-mak crackers
- ☐ 2 pieces low-fat string cheese
- ☐ 2 tablespoons sunflower seeds

Top crackers with light string cheese. Eat sunflower seeds on the side.

Calories=376, carb=40 g, fiber=8 g (Wasa)
Calories=376, carb=35 g, fiber=6 g (ak-mak)

DINNER

- ☐ 1 tablespoon olive oil
- ☐ 3 ounces raw 93% lean ground turkey breast
- ☐ ½ cup cooked whole wheat pasta
- ☐ 1 cup cooked mushrooms
- ☐ ½ cup light tomato sauce

Heat oil in pan and add ground turkey. Cook until turkey is no longer pink. Cook pasta according to package directions. Add cooked or raw mushrooms to sauce, if desired, or serve on the side. Add cooked turkey to pasta and serve with sauce.

Calories=419, carb=37 g, fiber=9 g

☐ **MIND TRICK AT ONE MEAL TODAY:** Use dishes and silverware that you normally reserve for company or special occasions. Bring out the good china, the company silverware, the dinner-party glassware. Treating yourself like a special guest makes meals all the more special, and underlines the fact that you're treating your body to delicious, healthy food.

☐ **EXERCISE:** Walk or perform physical activity of your choice (swimming, biking, using a pedaler, exercise class, or video).
Beginner: 15 minutes
Advanced: 30 minutes (can be done in two 15-minute segments)

☐ **PROGRESSIVE MUSCLE RELAXATION**

JOURNAL, DAY 4

DATE:

BREAKFAST	
MOOD:	THOUGHTS

HUNGER BEFORE: 1   3   5   8   10   HUNGER AFTER: 1   3   5   8   10

LUNCH	
MOOD:	THOUGHTS

HUNGER BEFORE: 1   3   5   8   10   HUNGER AFTER: 1   3   5   8   10

SNACK	
MOOD:	THOUGHTS

HUNGER BEFORE: 1   3   5   8   10   HUNGER AFTER: 1   3   5   8   10

DINNER	
MOOD:	THOUGHTS

HUNGER BEFORE: 1   3   5   8   10   HUNGER AFTER: 1   3   5   8   10

❏ **BLOOD GLUCOSE LEVELS** (Check as recommended by your doctor.)

Time:.....................

Reading: ....

Time:.....................

Reading: ....

Time:.....................

Reading: ....

Time:.....................

Reading: ....

Time:.....................

Reading: ....

Time:.....................

Reading: ....

PHASE 1, DAY 5

DATE:

BREAKFAST

- ❑ 2 tablespoons peanut butter
- ❑ 1 whole wheat English muffin
- ❑ 1 medium apple

Spread peanut butter on toasted English muffin and have apple on the side.

Calories=390, carb=51 g, fiber=9 g

LUNCH

- ❑ 1 Campbell's Select Harvest Savory Chicken and Long Grain Rice Soup bowl OR 1 Healthy Choice Chicken with Rice Soup bowl
- ❑ ¼ cup dry, unsalted almonds

Calories=426, carb=43 g, fiber=6 g (Campbell's)
Calories=386, carb=33 g, fiber=8 g (Healthy Choice)

SNACK

- ❑ ½ cup blueberries, fresh or frozen (defrosted)
- ❑ 2 tablespoons walnuts
- ❑ 6 ounces nonfat plain yogurt
- ❑ 1 cup baby carrots
- ❑ 2 tablespoons light ranch dressing

Add blueberries and walnuts to yogurt. Serve baby carrots with light ranch dressing on the side.

Calories=376, carb=39 g, fiber=6 g

DINNER

- ❑ 5 ounces raw cod fillet
- ❑ 1 tablespoon olive oil
- ❑ 3 ounces red potatoes
- ❑ 1 cup cooked sugar snap peas

Brush fish with 1 teaspoon oil and sprinkle desired seasoning on fish. Broil for 5 minutes. Carefully turn fish and brush with 1 teaspoon oil and broil for 4 to 6 minutes longer, or until fish flakes easily with a fork. Preheat oven to 350°F. Chop potatoes into small pieces, place in an ungreased glass baking dish, drizzle with remaining oil, and sprinkle with desired seasoning. Bake for 15 minutes, or until desired tenderness. Steam or microwave snap peas and serve with fish and potatoes.

Calories=379, carb=29 g, fiber=6 g

❑ **MIND TRICK AT ONE MEAL TODAY:** Bite by bite, eat mindfully today. Notice the colors and textures of the food. Slowly savor your first bite. Put your silverware down between bites and ask yourself, "What am I tasting? What am I feeling?"

❑ **EXERCISE:** Walk or perform physical activity of your choice (swimming, biking, using a pedaler, exercise class, or video).
Beginner:
15 minutes
Advanced:
30 minutes (can be done in two 15-minute segments)

❑ **PROGRESSIVE MUSCLE RELAXATION**

JOURNAL, DAY 5

DATE: ....

BREAKFAST	
MOOD:	THOUGHTS

HUNGER BEFORE: 1   3   5   8   10   HUNGER AFTER: 1   3   5   8   10

LUNCH	
MOOD:	THOUGHTS

HUNGER BEFORE: 1   3   5   8   10   HUNGER AFTER: 1   3   5   8   10

SNACK	
MOOD:	THOUGHTS

HUNGER BEFORE: 1   3   5   8   10   HUNGER AFTER: 1   3   5   8   10

DINNER	
MOOD:	THOUGHTS

HUNGER BEFORE: 1   3   5   8   10   HUNGER AFTER: 1   3   5   8   10

☐ **BLOOD GLUCOSE LEVELS**
(Check as recommended by your doctor.)

Time:.....................

Reading: ....

Time:.....................

Reading: ....

Time:.....................

Reading: ....

Time:.....................

Reading: ....

Time:.....................

Reading: ....

Time:.....................

Reading: ....

PHASE 1, DAY 6

DATE:

BREAKFAST

- ❏ 1 whole wheat English muffin
- ❏ 1 cooked egg
- ❏ ¼ cup sliced avocado
- ❏ 1 slice reduced-fat Cheddar cheese
- ❏ 1 medium apple

Top toasted English muffin with egg, avocado, and cheese. Serve with apple on the side.

Calories=383, carb=49 g, fiber=10 g

LUNCH

- ❏ 3 cups romaine lettuce or other lettuce mix
- ❏ 2 tablespoons dried, unsalted, chopped walnuts
- ❏ 3 tablespoons dried cranberries
- ❏ 1 tablespoon olive oil
- ❏ 1 tablespoon balsamic vinegar
- ❏ 1 medium orange

Top salad greens with walnuts, cranberries, and a mix of oil and vinegar. Serve orange on the side or on the salad, as desired.

Calories=393, carb=45 g, fiber=7 g

SNACK

- ❏ 1 whole wheat tortilla
- ❏ 4 ounces deli turkey breast
- ❏ ¼ cup hummus
- ❏ 2 tablespoons pine nuts

Top tortilla with turkey, hummus, and pine nuts and roll up.

Calories=398, carb=35 g, fiber=6 g

DINNER

- ❏ 4 ounces raw lean pork tenderloin
- ❏ 1 (4-ounce) sweet potato, about 5" long
- ❏ 1 tablespoon olive oil
- ❏ 1 cup cooked broccoli

Preheat oven to 425°F. Roast pork tenderloin for 15 to 20 minutes, or until internal temp is 160°F on meat thermometer. Bake sweet potato in microwave oven for 10 minutes and drizzle with half the oil. Steam or microwave broccoli and drizzle with remaining oil. Serve pork with sweet potato and broccoli on the side.

Calories=428, carb=37 g, fiber=9 g

❏ **MIND TRICK AT ONE MEAL TODAY:** Choose a mantra for one meal today. It should be a calming word or phrase, such as, "I'm doing this meal plan for me." Repeat after each bite.

❏ **EXERCISE:** Walk or perform physical activity of your choice (swimming, biking, using a pedaler, exercise class, or video).
Beginner:
15 minutes
Advanced:
30 minutes (can be done in two 15-minute segments)

❏ **PROGRESSIVE MUSCLE RELAXATION**

JOURNAL, DAY 6

DATE:

BREAKFAST	
MOOD:	THOUGHTS

HUNGER BEFORE: 1   3   5   8   10   HUNGER AFTER: 1   3   5   8   10

LUNCH	
MOOD:	THOUGHTS

HUNGER BEFORE: 1   3   5   8   10   HUNGER AFTER: 1   3   5   8   10

SNACK	
MOOD:	THOUGHTS

HUNGER BEFORE: 1   3   5   8   10   HUNGER AFTER: 1   3   5   8   10

DINNER	
MOOD:	THOUGHTS

HUNGER BEFORE: 1   3   5   8   10   HUNGER AFTER: 1   3   5   8   10

☐ **BLOOD GLUCOSE LEVELS**
(Check as recommended by your doctor.)

Time:.....................

Reading: ....

Time:.....................

Reading: ....

Time:.....................

Reading: ....

Time:.....................

Reading: ....

Time:.....................

Reading: ....

Time:.....................

Reading: ....

PHASE 1, DAY 7

DATE:

BREAKFAST

- ☐ ½ cup dry oatmeal
- ☐ 1 medium banana (7"–8") cut into slices
- ☐ 2 tablespoons dried, unsalted, chopped walnuts

Cook oatmeal with desired amount of water. Add banana and walnuts to oatmeal and serve.

Calories=352, carb=56 g, fiber=7 g

LUNCH

- ☐ 1 whole wheat tortilla
- ☐ ¼ cup black beans
- ☐ ¼ cup sliced avocado
- ☐ ¼ cup shredded low-fat Mexican blend cheese
- ☐ 2 cups romaine lettuce or other lettuce blend
- ☐ 1 tablespoon olive oil
- ☐ 1 tablespoon balsamic vinegar

Top tortilla with beans, avocado, and cheese. Heat in the microwave oven to melt cheese, if desired. Serve with side salad of lettuce topped with oil and vinegar.

Calories=417, carb=38 g, fiber=9 g

SNACK

- ☐ 5 Wasa Rye Crispbread crackers or 7 ak-mak crackers
- ☐ 2 pieces low-fat string cheese
- ☐ 2 tablespoons sunflower seeds

Top crackers with string cheese. Eat sunflower seeds on the side.

Calories=376, carb=40 g, fiber=8 g (Wasa)
Calories=376, carb=35 g, fiber=6 g (ak-mak)

DINNER

- ☐ 1 tablespoon olive oil
- ☐ 3 ounces raw 93% lean ground turkey breast
- ☐ ½ cup cooked whole wheat pasta
- ☐ 1 cup cooked mushrooms
- ☐ ½ cup light tomato sauce

Heat oil in pan and add ground turkey. Cook until turkey is no longer pink. Cook pasta according to package directions. Add cooked or raw mushrooms to sauce, if desired, or serve on the side. Add cooked turkey to pasta and serve with sauce.

Calories=419, carb=37 g, fiber=9 g

☐ **MIND TRICK AT ONE MEAL TODAY:** Take some long, slow breaths that fill your lower lungs before you begin to eat this meal. This type of breathing soothes your parasympathetic nervous system, which remains "on alert" when we're stressed or anxious.

☐ **EXERCISE:** Walk or perform physical activity of your choice (swimming, biking, using a pedaler, exercise class, or video).
Beginner:
15 minutes
Advanced:
30 minutes (can be done in two 15-minute segments)

☐ **PROGRESSIVE MUSCLE RELAXATION**

JOURNAL, DAY 7

DATE: _____

BREAKFAST	
MOOD:	THOUGHTS

HUNGER BEFORE: 1   3   5   8   10   HUNGER AFTER: 1   3   5   8   10

LUNCH	
MOOD:	THOUGHTS

HUNGER BEFORE: 1   3   5   8   10   HUNGER AFTER: 1   3   5   8   10

SNACK	
MOOD:	THOUGHTS

HUNGER BEFORE: 1   3   5   8   10   HUNGER AFTER: 1   3   5   8   10

DINNER	
MOOD:	THOUGHTS

HUNGER BEFORE: 1   3   5   8   10   HUNGER AFTER: 1   3   5   8   10

☐ **BLOOD GLUCOSE LEVELS**
(Check as recommended by your doctor.)

Time:......................

Reading:...............

Time:......................

Reading:...............

Time:......................

Reading:...............

Time:......................

Reading:...............

Time:......................

Reading:...............

Time:......................

Reading:...............

READ A FLAT BELLY
SUCCESS
STORY

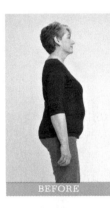

BEFORE

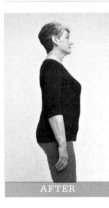

AFTER

Beth Gregory

AGE: 56

POUNDS LOST:

6.2

IN 35 DAYS

ALL-OVER
INCHES LOST:

4.25

**✳ BLOOD
SUGAR: A1C
WENT FROM
5.9 TO**

6.2

PERCENT

* The A1c is a check of long-term
blood sugar control; for most
people with diabetes, a reading
below 7 percent is considered ideal.

"CHOCOLATE WITHOUT GUILT!
I LOVED HAVING THE YOGURT
with fruit and chocolate chips in the
evening—to me it was dessert," Beth
says. "I never felt deprived or worried
that I was cheating. It's good knowing I
can fit in treats with confidence,
knowing my blood sugar won't go up,
and I don't have to feel guilty!"

Diagnosed with type 2 diabetes
4 years ago, Beth controls her blood
sugar with diet and exercise. "That
means every choice I make, at every
meal and snack, really counts," she
says. "I can't just take extra medication
if I eat too much of the wrong foods. So
it's wonderful finding a way of eating
that's filling and delicious and helps me
keep my blood sugar levels within a
healthy range—all at the same time."
Beth's A1c, a test of long-term blood
sugar control, rose slightly but stayed
within a healthy range. "I had surgery,
and my doctor thinks it was the stress,"
she says.

Discovering the many splendid
flavors and textures of MUFA-rich nuts
and seeds was a big *aha!* moment for
Beth. "When I started the Flat Belly Diet
Diabetes, I went out to the Whole

Foods grocery store and bought every nut and seed they had," she recalls. "It's a bit of an investment at first—every package was $6 or $7. But they last a long time, especially if you keep them in the refrigerator. I reorganized my fridge so that I could just reach in and grab a different one each time. I loved the lunch salad with cranberries and nuts—it's so easy with prewashed salad greens and dried cranberries. And you can really vary the taste by putting different nuts on top! Pistachios, almonds, sunflower seeds—I love them all now!"

Olive oil was new to her—and, she admits, it took some getting used to. "My salad dressing used to be all fat-free or low-fat. Now, it's olive oil and balsamic vinegar. That's a change that I think will be permanent."

Portability was another plus. "If I knew I would be out all day, I'd grab a meal bar, like an Odwalla bar, and make some trail mix. It was easy to carry and kept me from stopping at a fast-food drive-thru when I got hungry."

Flexibility made the plan a winner, too. "I'm Irish—and on St. Patrick's Day, I always have potato soup and a Guinness Stout beer. That didn't change on the plan. I enjoyed myself, and the next day I went right back to my Flat Belly Diet meals. Now that's something I can stick with for the rest of my life!"

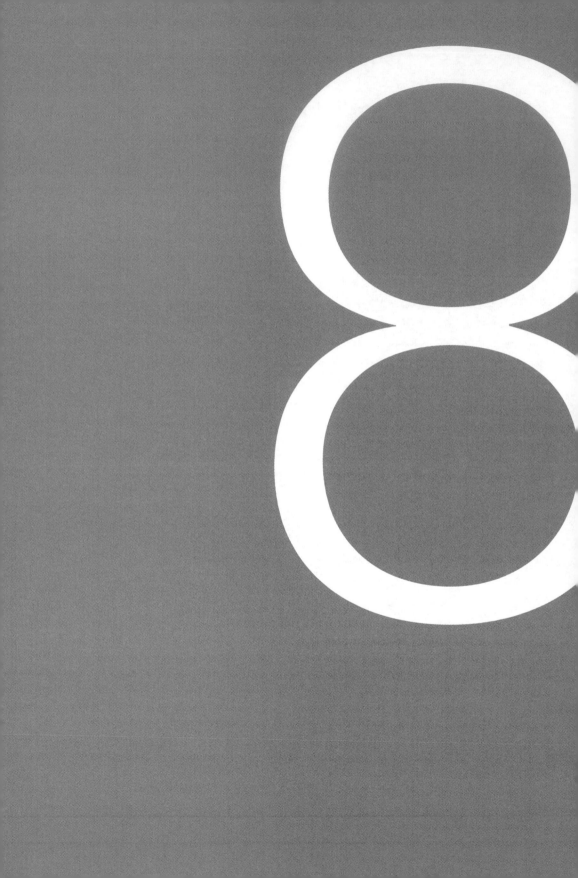

PHASE 2: THE 28-DAY
PLAN

WHAT A DIFFERENCE a week makes! In 7 short days, you've achieved a major Flat Belly Diet Diabetes milestone. Phase 1, our 7-Day Start-Up Plan, was all about changing the way you eat, the way you move, the way you relax—and perhaps most important of all, the way you think about your relationship with food. Now—*drumroll please*—you're on your way to mastering the elusive art of eating healthy meals four times a day *no matter what life throws at you.* (And we know that's no small feat!) You've fit in exercise and stress reduction. And if you completed each day's Mind Trick, you've accumulated lots of useful little strategies you can pull out of your pocket, so to speak, anytime, anyplace, to eat more mindfully—a practice proven to banish bingeing, emotional eating, and plain old overeating while it boosts eating pleasure and satisfaction.

By now, you may be seeing measurable improvements as you begin to lose pounds, trim inches from your waist (and hips . . . and thighs . . . and arms . . . and, well, all over!), and make changes aimed at keeping your blood sugar under better control. And you're ready for the next—and most life-changing—phase of the Flat Belly Diet Diabetes: You're ready to choose Flat Belly Diet meals and snacks that fit your tastes and your schedule.

For the next 28 days, you'll follow a more flexible version of the eating plan that sustained you throughout Phase 1. You'll have the freedom to choose virtually any meal you want—from home-cooked classics like Chicken Parmesan or Turkey Meat Loaf to a healthy grab-and-go meal bar or frozen entrée paired with a MUFA and other healthy items to turn the fastest fare into a healthy Flat Belly Diet Diabetes meal. You can dine out with confidence; just follow the tips on page 357 for a good time. How flexible is Phase 2? Let's put it this way: Our test panelists test-drove this meal plan by taking it everywhere their lives took them—including to a Caribbean island resort, out for a birthday dinner, to a St. Patrick's Day party, on business trips, and to family get-togethers. Every one was over the moon about their results—in terms of pounds and/or inches lost, blood sugar improvements, energy levels, and compliments from friends, family, and co-workers. Their verdict? This plan can go anywhere you go.

For the next 4 weeks, you'll also add variety and some new twists to your Flat Belly Diet Diabetes Workout as we introduce our Calorie Torch Walks, which use faster-paced intervals to burn more calories per step, and our body-toning, muscle-strengthening Metabolism Boost and Belly Routine workouts. These short, 10-minute routines help build sleek, toned muscle. You won't develop a bulging bodybuilder physique! You *will* improve muscle mass so that your body burns more calories round the clock. At the same time, these moves will improve your balance and your posture and give you a subtle feeling of power and confidence as everyday activities—from hauling groceries into the house to lifting toddlers, from doing yard work to walking all day during a terrific vacation—

become easier. There's even evidence that strength-training exercises like these improve insulin resistance, the core metabolic defect driving diabetes. So this 10-minutes-a-day investment can truly be life-changing!

The Heart of Phase 2

YOU KNOW THE RULES by now, but we want to reinforce that they remain at the heart of this revolutionary plan. As always, follow the Flat Belly Diet Diabetes rules and guidelines for best results in Phase 2:

- **RULE #1:** Stick to 400 calories per meal.
- **RULE #2:** Never go more than 4 hours without eating.
- **RULE #3:** Eat a MUFA at every meal.
- **RULE #4:** Exercise most days of the week.

Phase 2 Meals

IN THE CHAPTERS AHEAD—Chapter 9: The 28-Day Plan: Quick and Easy Meals and Chapter 10: The 28-Day Plan: Recipes—you'll find all of the secrets to satisfying, successful Flat Belly Diet Diabetes eating. Choose four 400-calorie meals per day from the list of Quick and Easy Meals in Chapter 9, from our delicious recipes (which come with easy ways to turn any recipe into a complete Flat Belly Diet Diabetes meal), or from our "Grab and Go" options. You can also repeat any of the meals from Phase 1, if you like. As we already revealed, here the key concept is flexibility. And we really mean flexibility! Take breakfast. Wake up on a lazy Saturday morning and you may want to make our sophisticated Asparagus Frittata (served with a toasted English muffin). But if it's an "I've got 5 minutes to munch something" Monday morning, choose an Apple Almond Butter Toast (sweetened with a dollop of orange marmalade). Uh-oh . . . it's an "I'm already 15 minutes late" kind of morning? No problem.

Grab a meal replacement bar (we have 21 options featuring five brands, in flavors ranging from cherry almond to gingersnap to chocolate pecan) plus a handful of nuts on your way out the door for a filling, 100 percent healthy Flat Belly Diet Diabetes breakfast. It's that easy.

Options for lunch, dinner, and your 400-calorie Flat Belly Diet Diabetes snack packs are equally diverse, allowing you to eat well and with confidence whether you bring your own lunch to work, find yourself in a restaurant, are cooking dinner in your own kitchen, or are grazing in a convenience store or hitting the drive-thru on your way to the kids' sports practice or other commitment. As you can see, this is the plan truly devised to fit your life.

Worried that 400 calories per meal for the next 28 days will leave you with a perpetually growling tummy? Our test panelists discovered that the meals in Phase 2 were even more satisfying than expected. But in case you need a little extra something, we've got it. Hungry? If you're a man of average or large build, or if you're extremely active and find yourself feeling extremely hungry on this meal plan, you can add an additional 200-calorie snack. Formulated to fill the nutritional and caloric needs of people who burn more calories than average every day, it's enough to keep you going without jeopardizing your weight loss or blood sugar goals. We recommend trying the 1,600-calorie daily plan first for a few days of Phase 2, and adding the snack only if you find that you need it. You'll find snack ideas on page 200.

Need more "bulk" at meal time? If you would like, you can add vegetables from the "Free Foods List" (on page 201) to one or two meals a day. This list includes a wide range of filling, low-calorie, high-fiber vegetables from green beans and asparagus to artichoke hearts and spinach. Use some to mix up a filling big salad or steam for a satisfying side dish. Buy them fresh or, if canned or bottled, packed in water—not oil! And don't slather with butter, margarine, or sauces. The idea of free foods is that you can fill up without adding significant extra calories to your daily total. A spritz of lemon on steamed "free foods" or a sprinkle of balsamic vinegar is a great, taste-boosting strategy.

Speaking of seasonings, keep on using the spice and seasoning suggestions found in Chapter 7, or experiment with some of your own as you prepare Flat Belly Diet Diabetes meals.

You can eat virtually any Flat Belly Diet Diabetes meal whenever you'd like (yes, you can have breakfast four times a day, or repeat *all* of the meals from Phase 1 if you'd like), if you follow a few important guidelines:

▪ Try not to choose more than one meal per day from the "Grab and Go" list. We know you're busy, but it's best to get your nutrition from whole foods—and as you know from Phase 1, it *is* possible to prepare healthy meals quickly and easily!

▪ Do not choose more than one meal per day that includes dark chocolate. We love that this decadent and delicious treat fits into our blood sugar–friendly meal plan, but the higher carbohydrate content (from the sugar in the chocolate) means it should be a once-a-day indulgence.

▪ Do not choose more than one meal per day that includes olives. Another fun food we're proud to feature in this eating plan, olives are high in sodium, but you can fit them into a healthy diet by limiting your olive consumption to once a day or less often.

YOU CAN EAT OUT IN PHASE 2! We have ordering ideas for national fast food and casual dining chains. For each selection, we include a recommended MUFA to pair it with—olives, nuts, or seeds. Keep these MUFA add-ons handy at home. Bag a portion in a zipper-lock bag before you head out the door for lunch or dinner. Plus, follow our tips for dining out anywhere on page 357, and you'll be able to enjoy your food without blowing your diet or your blood sugar levels.

Timing your meals is still vitally important for several reasons. It keeps energy levels high, protects against ravenous overeating, and helps supply your body with steady energy in the form of blood sugar, helping to avoid peaks and valleys. Space your meals about 4 hours apart. Your 400-calorie snack should be timed to help you do this. For example, if you have breakfast at 8:00 a.m.,

Partygoer's Guide

Who doesn't love a good party? The music! The conversation! The friends! And . . . uh-oh . . . the buffet table. From chips and dip to gourmet appetizers, decadent sweets, and indulgent drinks, festive food usually means calories—and a big challenge if you're following the Flat Belly Diet Diabetes. But we're here to help. Don't stay home or hide in the corner. Enjoy your next social gathering fully, with no guilt afterward, with these no-nonsense strategies:

Bring a beautiful platter . . . of Flat Belly Diet Diabetes "free foods." How about a sophisticated arrangement of lightly steamed, then chilled asparagus, green beans, and broccoli, served with lemon wedges? Or a refreshing summer tray of farm-stand bounty—cherry tomatoes, sliced peppers, sliced carrots, and cucumber? Or roasted, sliced beets or grilled eggplant? A filling, flavorful veggie platter is delicious and pretty, and no one need know it's filled with foods you can nibble to your heart's content.

Turn your Flat Belly Diet Diabetes snack into party food. Chocolate-Zucchini Snack Cake is too good to leave at home. Make one and bring it to your next book group, neighborhood picnic, or office party. Your strategy: Eat a slice as your daily, 400-calorie snack—at the party!

Chat more, eat less. Never stand by the chips and nosh while you talk with other party guests. Instead of letting conversation lead you into mindless eating, let socializing be the center-piece of your experience. When you arrive, grab a calorie-free drink (we love seltzer with a twist of lime) and scope out a great seat at a table or sofa filled with friends, family, or friendly strangers. This—and not the buffet—is your home base.

Make it a Flat Belly Diet Diabetes meal. If party food is taking the place of a meal, approach the buffet table or grill with a purpose: Grab a plate, add vegetables (zero in on types cooked without gobs of oil or butter or smothered in cheese or sauces), whole grains, lean protein (like lean beef or skinless chicken), and salad. Scope the selections for a MUFA—you may find an olive oil dressing, a bowl of nuts, homemade guacamole (it's made from avocado!), or olives. Help yourself to a Flat Belly Diet Diabetes portion of one of these MUFAs and you're set.

Dance, join the softball game, be part of the group going out Christmas caroling. Every party has its active participants and its kitchen denizens. Be part of the active crowd—you'll have fun, burn calories, and totally avoid the temptations lurking on kitchen counters.

Don't sweat the small stuff. You ended up splurging? No problem. Skip the morning-after guilt and get right back into the Flat Belly Diet Diabetes swing of things. That's what our test panelists did after special occasions that found them eating foods that weren't part of the plan.

lunch at noon, and dinner at 8:00 p.m., it would be best to eat the snack between lunch and dinner at around 4:00 p.m. But, if you have breakfast at 8:00 a.m., and your lunch will be delayed until 3:00 p.m., it would be best to have the snack around noon, and dinner at 7:00 or 8:00 p.m.

As in Phase 1, prepare the meals as directed. Always measure your ingredients and try to use the brands we recommend. You'll find more details in Chapter 9.

Phase 2 Exercise

IN PHASE 2, YOU'LL continue walking for 15 to 30 minutes a day, 6 days a week. But things will become much more varied and interesting. You'll begin our Metabolism Boost routine, a toning and strengthening routine for your arms, legs, and core. You'll begin alternating the Fat Blast Walk you learned in Phase 1 with faster-paced intervals of our Calorie Torch Walk. And you'll also begin to perform our Belly Routine, aimed at toning and tightening your midsection—without a single crunch, ever! (We promise!)

You'll find detailed instructions and photographs for all aspects of the Flat Belly Diet Diabetes Workout in Chapter 11. Here's a quick overview of how the two walks and two short exercise routines fit into Phase 2 (it may also help to take a look at the Flat Belly Diet Diabetes Exercise Program chart on page 166):

FAT BLAST WALK: Warm up by walking at a slow pace for 3 minutes. Then walk briskly—10 minutes for beginners, 25 minutes for advanced exercisers. Cool down with a slow walk for the last 2 minutes.

▮ HOW LONG: 15 minutes total for beginners, 30 minutes total for advanced exercisers in Weeks 2, 3, and 4. You'll increase that by 5 minutes in Week 5.

▮ HOW OFTEN: Six days in Week 2, and 3 days a week in Weeks 3, 4, and 5. (You'll be alternating with the Calorie Torch Walk in these weeks!)

CALORIE TORCH WALK: This walk features "intervals," in which you ramp up the speed for brief stretches, a strategy proven to burn more calories.

(Hence the name!) To perform it, first warm up for 3 minutes at a slow pace. Then do your first interval set like this: Walk briskly for 4 minutes, then walk a little faster (at a pace where you can talk in brief phrases, but you'd rather not) for 1 minute. That's one set. Beginners should do two sets. Advanced walkers should do five sets. Then cool down for 2 minutes.

■ HOW LONG: 15 minutes total for beginners, 30 minutes total for advanced exercisers. You'll increase that by 5 minutes in Week 5.

■ HOW OFTEN: Three days a week in Weeks 3, 4, and 5—you'll be alternating with the Fat Blast Walk.

METABOLISM BOOST ROUTINE: These four exercises use light dumbbells to build strength in your arms, legs, and core. Turn to Chapter 11 for complete instructions with photographs.

■ HOW MUCH WEIGHT: *Beginner*: Use 3- and 5-pound dumbbells; *Advanced*: Use 5- and 8-pound dumbbells.

■ HOW MANY REPS OF EACH EXERCISE: Do each move 10 times in Weeks 2, 3, and 4. You'll do each exercise 15 times in Week 5.

■ HOW OFTEN: Do the Metabolism Boost exercises 3 days a week in Weeks 2, 3, 4, and 5. You can schedule this strength-training routine for any days of the week as long as you don't do it 2 days in a row. Your muscles need a day off from strength training for recovery and repair.

■ ADJUSTING THE ROUTINE TO FIT YOUR FITNESS LEVEL: If you have never done any strength-training exercises (or haven't exercised in more than 6 months) or if you have any knee problems, start with the "Make it easier" option in each exercise description. Otherwise, start with the Main Move. If that's too challenging, perform the "Make it easier" option. If the Main Move is not challenging enough, perform the "Make it harder" option. Also, at the end of Week 4, if you find it's still challenging to complete 10 reps, stick with 10 reps rather than progressing to 15 reps in Week 5.

BELLY ROUTINE: These five moves further tighten, tone, and strengthen your core—working your abdominal and back muscles without a single crunch! For detailed instructions and photographs, turn to pages 306–315 in Chapter 11.

■ HOW MANY REPETITIONS OF EACH EXERCISE: Do each move 10 times in Week 4, 15 times in Week 5.

■ HOW OFTEN: Do the Belly Routine exercises 3 days a week in Weeks 4 and 5. You'll also be walking on these days. You can do the Belly Routine on any days of the week. We've suggested that you alternate with the Metabolism Boost, but you can combine them instead, if you prefer. Just start with the Metabolism Boost, then go right into the Belly Routine on those days; for the rest of the week, you won't do any strength or belly exercises at all. Remember that you shouldn't do the Metabolism Boost 2 days in a row.

■ ADJUSTING THE ROUTINE TO FIT YOUR FITNESS LEVEL: If you have never done any ab exercises (or haven't exercised in more than 6 months), start with the "Make it easier" option in the directions in Chapter 11. Otherwise, start with the Main Move. If that's too challenging, perform the "Make it easier" option. If the Main Move isn't challenging enough, perform the "Make it harder" option. Also, at the end of Week 4, if you find it's still challenging to complete 10 reps, stick with 10 reps rather than progressing to 15 reps in Week 5.

DAY BY DAY: THE FLAT BELLY DIET DIABETES EXERCISE PLAN IN ACTION

Here's our at-a-glance exercise calendar (page 166). Consult it any time you need to check what your physical activity "assignment" is for the day, or to see what's coming up tomorrow. You'll notice that you get a day off. You can move your free day anywhere in the week that you'd like or that fits your schedule— the plan is flexible. When you can, however, how about scheduling some fun physical activity? Go bowling or swimming, fly a kite or bike with the kids, or hop in a canoe at a local park. As the weeks go by, you'll notice that you have more strength, stamina, and flexibility, making everyday activity and fun stuff easier and more rewarding.

FLAT BELLY DIET DIABETES EXERCISE PROGRAM

WEEK	DAY 1	DAY 2	DAY 3	
1 7-Day Start-Up Plan	**Fat blast walk** beginners: 15 min advanced: 30 min	**Fat Blast Walk** beginners: 15 min advanced: 30 min	**Fat Blast Walk** beginners: 15 min advanced: 30 min	
2 Add Metabolism Boost	**Fat Blast Walk** beginners: 15 min advanced: 30 min **Metabolism Boost** 10 reps beginners: 3–5 lb advanced: 5–8 lb	**Fat Blast Walk** beginners: 15 min advanced: 30 min	**Fat Blast Walk** beginners: 15 min advanced: 30 min **Metabolism Boost** 10 reps beginners: 3–5 lb advanced: 5–8 lb	
3 Add Calorie Torch Walk	**Fat Blast Walk** beginners: 15 min advanced: 30 min **Metabolism Boost** 10 reps beginners: 3–5 lb advanced: 5–8 lb	**Calorie Torch Walk** beginners: 15 min advanced: 30 min	**Fat Blast Walk** beginners: 15 min advanced: 30 min **Metabolism Boost** 10 reps beginners: 3–5 lb advanced: 5–8 lb	
4 Add Belly Routine	**Fat Blast Walk** beginners: 15 min advanced: 30 min **Metabolism Boost** 10 reps beginners: 3–5 lb advanced: 5–8 lb	**Calorie Torch Walk** beginners: 15 min advanced: 30 min **Belly Routine** 10 reps	**Fat Blast Walk** beginners: 15 min advanced: 30 min **Metabolism Boost** 10 reps beginners: 3–5 lb advanced: 5–8 lb	
5 Add 5 minutes to walks; 5 reps to strength routines	**Fat Blast Walk** beginners: 20 min advanced: 35 min **Metabolism Boost** 10–15 reps beginners: 3–5 lb advanced: 5–8 lb	**Calorie Torch Walk** beginners: 20 min advanced: 35 min **Belly Routine** 10–15 reps	**Fat Blast Walk** beginners: 20 min advanced: 35 min **Metabolism Boost** 10–15 reps beginners: 3–5 lb advanced: 5–8 lb	

DAY 4	DAY 5	DAY 6	DAY 7
Fat Blast Walk beginners: 15 min advanced: 30 min	**Fat Blast Walk** beginners: 15 min advanced: 30 min	**Fat Blast Walk** beginners: 15 min advanced: 30 min	**Rest**
Fat Blast Walk beginners: 15 min advanced: 30 min	**Fat Blast Walk** beginners: 15 min advanced: 30 min	**Fat Blast Walk** beginners: 15 min advanced: 30 min	**Rest**
	Metabolism Boost 10 reps beginners: 3–5 lb advanced: 5–8 lb		
Calorie Torch Walk beginners: 15 min advanced: 30 min	**Fat Blast Walk** beginners: 15 min advanced: 30 min	**Calorie Torch Walk** beginners: 15 min advanced: 30 min	**Rest**
	Metabolism Boost 10 reps beginners: 3–5 lb advanced: 5–8 lb		
Calorie Torch Walk beginners: 15 min advanced: 30 min	**Fat Blast Walk** beginners: 15 min advanced: 30 min	**Calorie Torch Walk** beginners: 15 min advanced: 30 min	**Rest**
Belly Routine 10 reps	**Metabolism Boost** 10 reps beginners: 3–5 lb advanced: 5–8 lb	**Belly Routine** 10 reps	
Calorie Torch Walk beginners: 20 min advanced: 35 min	**Fat Blast Walk** beginners: 20 min advanced: 35 min	**Calorie Torch Walk** beginners: 20 min advanced: 35 min	**Rest**
Belly Routine 10–15 reps	**Metabolism Boost** 10–15 reps beginners: 3–5 lb advanced: 5–8 lb	**Belly Routine** 10–15 reps	

The Flat Belly Diet Diabetes Journal

As we've said before, a flat belly isn't just about food. It's about your attitude. That's why we're equipping you with an arsenal of tools that will help you reduce stress, become more mindful at every meal, and develop the confidence to give yourself the best care possible—emotionally and physically. That's why the Flat Belly Diet Diabetes Journal is so important. You'll find a page for each day of our 28-day Phase 2 program. Each one includes spaces for tracking food and exercise, your moods and reflections, your blood sugar and whether or not you found a few minutes just for you. Here's how all of these pieces fit together to help you develop the confidence and the awareness that will make your Flat Belly Diet Diabetes experience—and anything you do in the future that revolves around food, exercise, or your health—a resounding success:

■ **CORE CONFIDENCES: A FLAT BELLY DIET EXCLUSIVE.** In Phase 1, you worked every day on developing the art and science of mindful eat-

Flat Belly Diet, Family-Style

Husbands and wives, sons and daughters, sisters and brothers-in-law. Our test panelists regularly shared their Flat Belly Diet creations at the table with their nearest and dearest relations and got rave reviews. That's good news, because it means you can serve one meal to your entire family with confidence—no need to pick at an iceberg lettuce salad while everyone else digs into pasta or roast chicken! To make this way of eating truly family friendly, follow these suggested guidelines:

Don't put your spouse on a diet. Let your husband or wife decide for himself or herself how much of any food he or she will eat. It's just a good, relationship-friendly policy. If you have concerns about your spouse's weight or health, the loudest message you can send is via your actions—not your words.

Emphasize enjoying healthy, yummy food with kids. Kids simply shouldn't diet or attempt to lose weight, period. They need nutrients and calories for healthy growth and development and need to develop a healthy relationship with food.

ing, through our Mind Tricks. Continue to use them whenever you find yourself eating without realizing what's on your plate, on your fork, or even in your mouth! Mindfulness is a lifelong skill that disaster-proofs your meals and snacks against mindless overeating, against emotional eating, and against eating when you're already full. In Phase 2, we'll ask you to work on what we call a Core Confidence each day—a reflection related to your view of food, health, your body. Together, Core Confidences and Mind Tricks will help you get the most pleasure from the healthy foods you eat—and give you the tools you need to keep on making the right choices for your weight, your blood sugar, your health, and your energy levels—no matter what.

You'll find our Core Confidences in the Flat Belly Diet Diabetes Journal in Chapter 12.

■ **10 MINUTES OF "ME TIME."** We would also urge you to continue setting aside 10 minutes a day for some "me time." You can use it to de-stress with your Progressive Muscle Relaxation exercise, to write down your Core

You can serve Flat Belly Diet Diabetes foods with confidence because they're packed with nutrition and flavor and are satisfying and delicious. Sedentary to moderately active 4- to 8-year-olds need 400 to 470 calories per meal, those ages 9 to 13 need 530 to nearly 700, and teens need 600 to 730 if they're not very active, more if they're physically active, according to the Institute of Medicine.[1] So your brood may need larger portions than you're putting on your own plate. Childhood nutrition experts recommend keeping a lid on overeating via strategies such as serving a reasonable first helping of all foods, then allowing seconds on vegetables. (Of course, a hungry kid who's just spent 3 hours at soccer practice may legitimately need a little more of other foods as well, so be flexible!) You can also discourage overeating by putting food on plates in the kitchen, then carrying them to the table, rather than placing bowls of food on the table. In addition, we recommend pouring low-fat or fat-free milk for kids' beverages—they need plenty of bone-building calcium and vitamin D.

Confidence reflections, or to enjoy any activity that brings you back to yourself without distractions or anxiety.

■ **A DAILY FOOD AND EXERCISE LOG.** As we noted in Chapter 7, studies show that keeping a record of the food you eat can double your chances for weight-loss success. Test panelists told us, time and time again, that knowing they'd be writing down everything they ate motivated them to make healthy choices and to stick with healthy portion sizes. It's completely worth the few minutes it takes, they told us. Same goes for exercise. Writing it down makes you more accountable—to the most important person in this process: YOU!

■ **HUNGER RATINGS.** As in Phase 1, you'll note your hunger or fullness level before and after each meal. This helps you become more sensitive to physical signs of hunger and satisfaction—so that you can eat before you become ravenous and so that you can stop when comfortably full, not stuffed.

■ **BLOOD SUGAR LEVEL TRACKING.** If you have diabetes or prediabetes and monitor your blood sugar with a glucose meter, use the spaces in our journal to jot down your readings. (Of course, if you've been keeping a separate blood sugar log on paper or on your computer, continue to track your blood sugar there as well.) Test panelists checked their blood sugar 2 hours after each meal, in addition to monitoring at other times of the day as recommended by their doctors. The after-meal checks can help you assess how specific meals affect your blood sugar—you may find that some foods or combinations keep your blood sugar lower or nudge it up. These differences are very individual—what affects you might not affect someone else in the same way. We recommended performing these checks 2 hours after most, if not all, meals during Phase 1, and we suggest you continue doing so in Phase 2. That way, you will be able to see for yourself how Flat Belly Diet Diabetes meals are affecting your blood sugar.

Five Ways to Battle Belly Bloat

When is belly fat not really belly fat at all? When it's belly bloat, brought on by sluggish digestion, the wrong foods, or eating habits that encourage that overly full, button-popping feeling around your middle. You can flatten your belly significantly just by deploying these five anti-bloat strategies throughout the Flat Belly Diet Diabetes:

#1: Drink plenty of (noncarbonated) fluids. You've probably heard you need about eight glasses of water a day. Drinking water and even eating "watery" foods like melon, greens, and other fruits and vegetables has enormous health benefits, including warding off fatigue, maintaining your body's proper fluid balance, and guarding against water retention and constipation, which can cause bloating. Eight glasses is just a guideline; everyone's fluid needs vary according to activity level and body. But skip soda and fizzy water. Where do you think all those bubbles end up? In your belly!

#2: Avoid the salt shaker, salt-based seasonings, and highly processed foods. Water is attracted to sodium, so when you take in higher than usual amounts of sodium, you'll temporarily retain more fluid—which contributes to a sluggish feeling, a puffy appearance, and extra water weight. Cutting back on sodium and boosting your water intake will help bring your body back into balance. It'll also help reduce your risk of hypertension and osteoporosis. If you find your food lacks flavor without a few shakes of salt, use salt-free seasonings.

#3: Say no thanks to excess carbs. As a backup energy source, your muscles store a type of carbohydrate called glycogen. Every gram of glycogen is stored with about 3 grams of water. But unless you're running a marathon tomorrow, you don't need all this stockpiled fuel. Decreasing your intake, especially of refined carbs like white bread, as you will in Phases 1 and 2, will help you get rid of the excess energy and the excess stored fluid.

#4: Steer clear of sugar alcohols. These low-calorie sugar substitutes, which go by the names xylitol or maltitol, are often found in low-calorie, low-carb, and "diabetic" sweets such as cookies, candy, and some energy bars. But your GI tract can't absorb or completely digest them, leading to intestinal gas, abdominal distension, bloating, and diarrhea.

#5: Banish fried and spicy foods. Fatty foods, such as fried stuff, digest slowly, weighing you down. If you notice an extra-full feeling after downing a meal or snack containing foods seasoned with black pepper, nutmeg, cloves, chili powder, hot sauces, onions, garlic, mustard, chili, barbecue sauce, horseradish, ketchup, tomato sauce, or vinegar, try doing without them for a while. All can stimulate the release of excess stomach acid, which can cause irritation. Even alcohol, coffee, tea, and some fruit juices can be irritating because of their high acid content, so if you notice bloating after sipping one of these beverages, leave it off your menu to see if it makes a difference.

READ A FLAT BELLY
SUCCESS
STORY

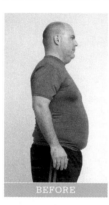

BEFORE

AFTER

Jay Hargis

AGE: 44

POUNDS LOST:

0

IN 35 DAYS

ALL-OVER
INCHES LOST:

1

✳ **BLOOD SUGAR: A1C FELL FROM 8.2 TO**

7.9
PERCENT

* The A1c is a test of long-term blood sugar control; levels below 7 percent are considered ideal for most people with diabetes.

"BREAKFAST WAS THE BEST PART! I TRAVEL A LOT IN MY JOB as a human resources consultant," says Jay. "Healthy meals away from home can be a real challenge, but it was easy on this plan. I could always find peanut butter or oatmeal at a hotel breakfast bar. Or go to Starbucks and order the Perfect Oatmeal. It really *is* perfect—you get the oats and the nuts. You just throw the nuts into the oatmeal and you're all set!"

Jay found that Flat Belly Diet Diabetes foods were good travel companions any time of day—whether he was waiting for a delayed flight in an airport far from home or dining out with a new client. "If the client says, 'Let's go to dinner,' you go. I would just have to make smart choices. And it was easy. You can always find grilled chicken and salad, and add some olives or avocado and top it with olive oil and vinegar or Italian dressing. Get the dressing on the side so you can control how much goes on the salad! It's always good. And it was so simple to throw meal bars and nuts into my bag so I'd have something to eat at the airport or on the plane.

"I definitely recommend measuring out servings so you can really visualize what they look like. Sometimes a serving is bigger than you expect; sometimes it's a little smaller. It's important to know what ⅔ cup of cereal really is when you pour it into a bowl. And I found out that 2 table-spoons of peanut butter—the amount I slathered on an English muffin at break-fast—was actually a lot more than I expected!"

Biggest lesson learned? "The impor-tance of combining foods—making sure I have a protein at every meal and that I have a MUFA along with grains or fruit or vegetables or even meat at a meal," he says. "It's a very Mediterranean way of eating that makes sense. It helps me control my blood sugar. And it's real food, not highly processed." Jay also developed some tricks of his own to boost meal flavors: "One lunch calls for a peanut butter sandwich and a side dish of cottage cheese and pineapple chunks. Well, if you put the pineapple on the sandwich, it tastes a lot like jelly—not bad!"

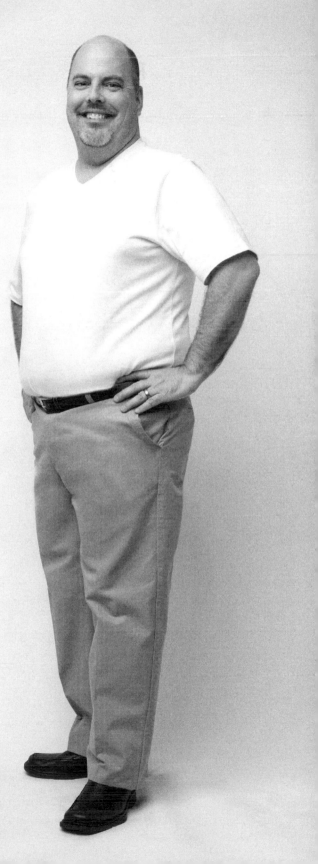

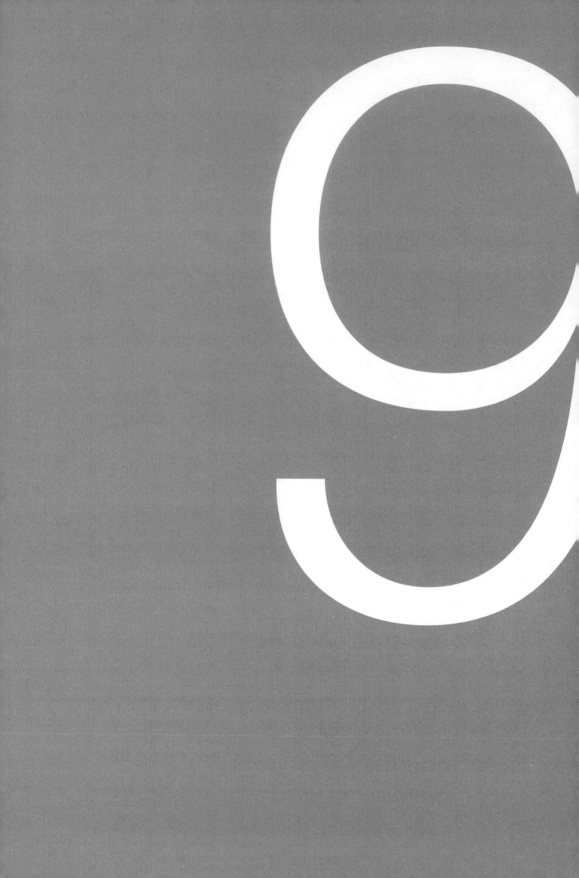

THE 28-DAY PLAN:
QUICK AND EASY
MEALS

PHASE 2 OF the Flat Belly Diet Diabetes won't trap you in a day-by-day, meal-by-meal, preset menu. (Big, loud cheer!) Instead, you will have a prescribed schedule of meals (four per day, including a snack—plus an additional, 200-calorie snack if you meet certain criteria). Meals and regular snacks have a predetermined calorie count—roughly 400. Each contains a MUFA, as part of our signature mix of blood sugar–friendly, belly-flattening food groups. Beyond that, we won't dictate what to eat when.

Instead, you get flexibility—by way of lots and lots of yummy suggestions. We offer everything from fast food and meal replacement bars to frozen entrées—all paired with MUFAs and other healthy fare to create a 100 percent healthy Flat Belly Diet Diabetes meal—to meals you can make quickly at home from a handful of basics. All of the meals are interchangeable, so you can mix and match all you want (with just a few exceptions, so read on). Our test panelists told us that this freedom of choice made it a pleasure to follow the plan faithfully, no matter where they went or what they were doing—well beyond the 5-week test period.

Some panelists stuck with the same breakfast, day in day out. Others ate something new every day. Some ate breakfasts for dinner sometimes. Others relied on meal replacement bars plus a MUFA while away on business; still others packed full meals to take to work. The possibilities are endless, as long as you follow the three basic food rules: Keep meals to 400 calories, include a MUFA at every meal, and eat every 4 hours. It's really that simple! Also, don't forget—no more than one meal a day with dark chocolate, and no more than one meal a day with olives.

You may be tempted to create your own meals right off the bat, but we caution you against this, at least for the first 28 days. It's important for you to get into the rhythm of the Flat Belly Diet Diabetes way of eating first. Once you are fully acquainted with the portion sizes, MUFA servings, and basic composition of the meals, feel free to create your own meals as often as you like. However, customiz-

Why so many calorie counts?

The numbers in the parentheses correspond to the calorie content of each ingredient. We provide them for a few reasons: First, to help you become familiar with the calorie levels of various ingredients—you may be surprised to find out just how many or few calories there are in certain foods. The second reason is to help you customize the plan. If you dislike a certain ingredient, don't have the same brand on hand, want to use up something you already have, or want to experiment with a different way of preparing a meal, you can. Just be sure the food you add provides about the same number of calories as the one you take away. Use the Nutrition Facts label information to check the calorie content of packaged foods; for fresh foods, you can check the foods database at www.prevention.com/healthtracker.

ing the meals to your taste is easy. The questions below will clarify the most important points for you to keep in mind when altering the meals in this chapter.

The Food Questions

Q: CAN I SWAP OUT INGREDIENTS IN A MEAL?

A: Yes and no. You should not move items from one meal to another—that is, you can't delete your MUFA from breakfast and add it to lunch. But you can swap out foods within a meal, as long as they're within the same food group, such as tomatoes and red peppers or turkey and chicken, and the food you added provides about the same number of calories as the food you took out. The calories for each ingredient appear in parentheses.

Q: DO I HAVE TO BUY THESE EXACT BRANDS?

A: We selected particular brands because of their taste, quality, availability, and, most importantly, nutritional value. The nutritional quality of foods in certain categories varies widely, so we scoured the supermarket aisles, read countless labels, and handpicked the high-quality brands that met our tough nutritional standards. Including these foods guarantees steady weight loss because their precise calorie level per serving has been incorporated into the plan. So, yes, I encourage you to use these brands. However, if you can't or prefer not to, simply replace them with comparable foods with as close to the same calorie levels.

Q: CAN I REALLY HAVE ANY MEAL OR 400-CALORIE SNACK—EVEN IF IT MEANS EATING THE SAME THING FOUR TIMES A DAY?

A: You could . . . but you might get bored! And we recommend having a meal or snack containing chocolate or olives no more often than once a day. These treats fit beautifully into this meal plan—testers said they *loved* not feeling guilty about having them—but the extra bit of sugar in the chocolate and the bit of excess sodium in our moderate portion of olives could become a little too big if repeated twice or three times in 1 day.

Flat Belly Breakfasts

What could be more filling than Banana Peanut Butter Oatmeal? MUFAs are in **boldface,** and ingredient calorie counts are in parentheses. Remember that you want to limit saturated fat to 10 percent of total calories—about 17 grams per day for most women or 21 grams for most men—and sodium intake to less than 2,300 milligrams. You'll see an asterisk on meals where the saturated fat or sodium levels are on the high side. If you choose those meals, just watch your saturated fat and sodium intake for the rest of the day.

Green Tea, Blueberry, and Banana Breakfast Drink: Microwave 3 tablespoons water (0) until hot, then add 1 green tea bag (0). Stir in 2 teaspoons honey (43). Combine 1½ cups frozen blueberries (119), ½ medium banana (53), ¾ cup calcium-fortified light vanilla soy milk (55), and 1 tablespoon **flaxseed oil** (120) in a blender. Add tea and blend 1 minute until smooth.
■ **Total Calories = 390**
5 g protein, 35 g carbohydrates, 17 g fat, 2 g saturated fat, 0 mg cholesterol, 95 mg sodium, 8 g fiber

Maple-Walnut Granola Parfait:
Arrange 1 cup strawberries (53), 6 ounces fat-free plain Greek yogurt (90), ½ cup maple-flavored granola (140), and 2 tablespoons toasted **walnuts** (82) in alternating layers in a tall glass.
■ **Total Calories = 365**
22 g protein, 41 g carbohydrates, 14 g fat, 1 g saturated fat, 0 mg cholesterol, 85 mg sodium, 7 g fiber

Macadamia Parfait: Arrange 1½ cups Kashi 7 Whole Grain Puffs (112), 6 ounces fat-free plain Greek yogurt (90), ½ banana, sliced (53), and 2 tablespoons **macadamia nuts** (120) in alternating layers in a tall glass.
■ **Total Calories = 375**
20 g protein, 46 g carbohydrates, 14 g fat, 2 g saturated fat, 0 mg cholesterol, 70 mg sodium, 5 g fiber

Blueberry Nut Cereal: Combine 2 tablespoons **cashews** (100), ¼ cup blueberries (21), and ¾ cup Kashi Good Friends Cereal (126). Top with ½ cup fat-free milk (42). Serve with 1 piece string cheese (80).
■ **Total Calories = 369**
17 g protein, 51 g carbohydrates, 14 g fat, 5 g saturated fat, 15 mg cholesterol, 350 mg sodium, 10 g fiber

Fruit and Nut Muesli: Combine 6 ounces Stonyfield Fat-Free French Vanilla

Yogurt (130) and 2 tablespoons old-fashioned oats (38). Stir well. Fold in 2 tablespoons chopped **pecans** (90) and ¼ cup raspberries (13). Serve with 2 ounces turkey breakfast sausage (130).

▦ **Total Calories = 401**

22 g protein, 35 g carbohydrates, 21 g fat, 5 g saturated fat, 50 mg cholesterol, 490 mg sodium, 4 g fiber

Banana Peanut Butter Oatmeal:
Cook ½ cup dry rolled oats (160) with water to consistency of your choice and mix in ½ banana, sliced (53), and 2 tablespoons **peanut butter** (188).

▦ **Total Calories = 401**

15 g protein, 49 g carbohydrates, 19 g fat, 3.5 g saturated fat*, 0 mg cholesterol, 150 mg sodium, 8 g fiber

Pumpkin Raisin Oatmeal:
Mix 2 tablespoons **pumpkin seeds** (148), ½ teaspoon pumpkin pie spice (3), and 2 tablespoons raisins (54) into ½ cup dry rolled oats (160). Add a pinch of ground ginger (0) and cook with water to consistency of your choice.

▦ **Total Calories = 365**

16 g protein, 48 g carbohydrates, 15 g fat, 2.5 g saturated fat, 0 mg cholesterol, 10 mg sodium, 6 g fiber

Strawberry Nut Butter Oatmeal:
Cook ½ cup dry rolled oats (160) with water to consistency of your choice and mix in ¾ cup organic frozen strawberries, warmed in the microwave oven for 1 minute and chopped (58), and 2 tablespoons **cashew butter** (190).

▦ **Total Calories = 408**

13 g protein, 51 g carbohydrates, 19 g fat, 3 g saturated fat, 0 mg cholesterol, 200 mg sodium, 8 g fiber

Apple Almond Butter Toast:
Spread 2 slices whole wheat bread, toasted (140), with 2 tablespoons **almond butter** (200) and top with 4 thin apple slices (13).

▦ **Total Calories = 351**

11 g protein, 38 g carbohydrates, 21 g fat, 2 g saturated fat, 0 mg cholesterol, 460 mg sodium, 6 g fiber

Cashew Crunch:
Spread 2 tablespoons **cashew butter** (190) on 2 slices toasted whole wheat bread (140), and sprinkle with 2 tablespoons raisins (54).

▦ **Total Calories = 384**

12 g protein, 51 g carbohydrates, 18 g fat, 3 g saturated fat, 0 mg cholesterol, 520 mg sodium, 5 g fiber

Cinnamon English Muffin with Almonds:
Split 1 whole wheat English muffin (135) in half and place on broiler pan. Spread ½ cup 1% dry-curd cottage cheese (62) on muffin halves. Sprinkle with pieces of 1 chopped apple (77), 2 tablespoons **almonds,** chopped (109), and dash of ground cinnamon (0). Broil for 2 minutes.

▦ **Total Calories = 383**

23 g protein, 52 g carbohydrates, 11 g fat, 1 g saturated fat, 5 mg cholesterol, 250 mg sodium, 10 g fiber

Tapenade Egg Sandwich: Toast 1 whole wheat English muffin (135) and spread 2 tablespoons **green olive tapenade** (54) on half. Cook 1 large egg (72) to desired style and place on other half with 1 slice reduced-fat Cheddar cheese (49). Serve with 1 cup cantaloupe (54) on side.

■ **Total Calories = 364**

21 g protein, 41 g carbohydrates, 14 g fat, 4 g saturated fat*, 215 mg cholesterol, 760 mg sodium*, 6 g fiber

English Muffin BLT: Spread 2 tablespoons **black olive tapenade** (88) on a whole wheat English muffin (135) and top with ½ fresh plum tomato, sliced (6), 3 large romaine lettuce leaves (3), 2 slices cooked turkey bacon (70), and 1 slice Muenster cheese (70).

■ **Total Calories = 372**

24 g protein, 28 g carbohydrates, 20 g fat, 5 g saturated fat*, 70 mg cholesterol, 480 mg sodium, 5 g fiber

Avocado and Egg Sandwich:

Spread 2 Laughing Cow Light Garlic & Herb Wedges (75) on 2 slices of toasted whole wheat bread (140). Fill the sandwich with ½ cup egg whites (60) cooked omelet-style and topped with ¼ cup sliced red onion (16), ½ fresh plum tomato, sliced (6), 3 large romaine lettuce leaves (3), and ¼ cup mashed **Hass avocado** (96).

■ **Total Calories = 396**

25 g protein, 43 g carbohydrates, 15 g fat, 3.5 g saturated fat*, 20 mg cholesterol, 1,040 mg sodium*, 8 g fiber

Avocado Breakfast Wrap: Warm 2 whole wheat wraps (212) and fill evenly with 4 scrambled egg whites (½ cup if using liquid substitute) (63), ½ cup fresh baby spinach leaves (5), 2 tablespoons low-fat shredded Cheddar cheese (40), 2 tablespoons salsa (10), and ¼ cup mashed **Hass avocado** (96).

■ **Total Calories = 426**

23 g protein, 45 g carbohydrates, 17 g fat, 3 g saturated fat, 10 mg cholesterol, 1050 mg sodium*, 10 g fiber

Scrambled Eggs and Potato Pancakes: Brown 2 frozen potato pancakes (118) in nonstick skillet with 1 tablespoon **high-oleic safflower oil** (120). Remove to plate and use same pan to scramble 4 egg whites (½ cup if using liquid substitute) (63). Top eggs with ¼ cup sliced red onion (16) and ½ fresh plum tomato, chopped (6). Serve with 1 orange (69).

■ **Total Calories = 392**

19 g protein, 35 g carbohydrates, 20 g fat, 2 g saturated fat, 40 mg cholesterol, 560 mg sodium, 5 g fiber

Country Breakfast: Brown 2 frozen potato pancakes (118) in a skillet with 1 tablespoon **high-oleic safflower oil** (120). Serve with 2 slices cooked organic turkey bacon (70) and 1 apple (72).

■ **Total Calories = 380**

15 g protein, 31 g carbohydrates, 23 g fat, 2 g saturated fat, 90 mg cholesterol, 340 mg sodium, 5 g fiber

Bacon and Avocado Omelet:

Whisk together 1 egg (71), 2 egg whites (32), 2 scallions, chopped (10), and a dash of hot-pepper sauce (0). Cook for about 3 minutes over medium heat in a nonstick skillet coated with cooking spray. Scatter 2 tablespoons shredded reduced-fat Cheddar cheese (40) on top and cook, covered, for 2 minutes. Chop and scatter 1 slice cooked lower-sodium natural turkey bacon (35) and ¼ cup mashed **Hass avocado** (96) on top. Fold in half. Let rest for 1 minute. Toast 1 whole wheat English muffin (135) to serve alongside.

■ **Total Calories = 419**

30 g protein, 35 g carbohydrates, 20 g fat, 5 g saturated fat*, 245 mg cholesterol, 620 mg sodium*, 9 g fiber

Cherry-Pecan Waffle: Toast 1 whole

wheat frozen waffle (90) and top with 1 cup frozen organic pitted sweet cherries, thawed (90). Sprinkle with a dash of nutmeg and 2 tablespoons **pecans** (90), chopped. Serve with 3 ounces maple-apple low-fat chicken sausage (161).

■ **Total Calories = 431**

19 g protein, 40 g carbohydrates, 25 g fat, 4.5 g saturated fat*, 75 mg cholesterol, 890 mg sodium*, 7 g fiber

Pineapple-Macadamia Waffles:

Toast 2 whole wheat frozen waffles (180) and top with ½ cup drained pineapple tidbits packed in juice (59). Sprinkle with cinnamon, nutmeg, and 2 tablespoons **macadamia nuts** (120), coarsely chopped.

■ **Total Calories = 359**

7 g protein, 46 g carbohydrates, 19 g fat, 3 g saturated fat, 0 mg cholesterol, 420 mg sodium, 6 g fiber

Breakfast—It's Always on the Flat Belly Diet Menu!

If you ever wondered whether skipping breakfast was a smart weight-control strategy or not, consider this statistic: An amazing 78 percent of successful dieters registered with the National Weight Control registry, a database of individuals who've lost 30 pounds or more and have kept it off for at least a year, eat a morning meal! What about the theory that skipping this meal is a natural way to eliminate calories? Studies show that breakfast skippers make up for those calories by unknowingly eating more later in the day. And there's emerging evidence that eating in the morning creates a feeling of satisfaction that helps guard against overeating later in the day, but skipping breakfast leads to cravings that later meals really don't fully satisfy.

Flat Belly Lunches

Our favorite lunch-bag treat? The Sunny Seeded Turkey Wrap. As always, MUFAs are in **boldface**, and ingredient calorie counts are in parentheses. Remember that you want to limit saturated fat to 10 percent of total calories—about 17 grams per day for most women or 21 grams for most men—and sodium intake to less than 2,300 milligrams. You'll see an asterisk on meals where the saturated fat or sodium levels are on the high side. If you choose those meals, just watch your saturated fat and sodium intake for the rest of the day.

Very Easy Veggie Burger: Cook 1 frozen vegan veggie burger (70) according to package instructions and serve on 1 whole wheat hamburger bun (114), dressed with 1 tablespoon ketchup (15), 3 large romaine lettuce leaves (3), 1/2 cup roasted red pepper strips (27), and 1/4 cup mashed **Hass avocado** (96). Serve with 1/2 ounce unsalted sweet potato chips (70).

■ **Total Calories = 395**

20 g protein, 51 g carbohydrates, 16 g fat, 2 g saturated fat, 0 mg cholesterol, 1,020 mg sodium*, 13 g fiber

Spicy Spinach Black Bean Pita:

Cook 1 frozen black bean veggie burger (110) according to package instructions and chop it up. Fill 1 whole wheat pita (140) with burger pieces, 1/2 cup fresh baby spinach leaves (3), 2 tablespoons chopped scallions (4), 1/4 cup mashed **Hass avocado** (96), and 3 tablespoons salsa (15).

■ **Total Calories = 368**

14 g protein, 54 g carbohydrates, 13 g fat, 2.5 g saturated fat, 20 mg cholesterol, 1,230 mg sodium*, 5 g fiber

Mediterranean Tomato Wrap:

Warm 1 whole grain tortilla (106) and spread with 2 tablespoons green olive **tapenade** (54). Sprinkle with 1/4 cup part-skim shredded mozzarella cheese (70) and 1/4 teaspoon dried oregano (1). Arrange 1 small thinly sliced tomato (16) and 1/4 cup slivered baby spinach leaves (3) on top. Fold burrito-style and serve with 6 ounces Stonyfield Fat-Free French Vanilla Yogurt (130) and 1/4 cup blueberries (21).

■ **Total Calories = 401**

19 g protein, 51 g carbohydrates, 14 g fat, 4 g saturated fat*, 20 mg cholesterol, 730 mg sodium*, 5 g fiber

Sunny Seeded Turkey Wrap:

Spread 1 tablespoon reduced-fat Neufchâtel (35) and 1 tablespoon honey mustard (30) on

1 whole wheat wrap (106) and sprinkle with 2 tablespoons **sunflower seeds** (90). Add 3 ounces honey maple turkey breast slices (75), 1/4 cup sliced red onion (16), 1 fresh plum tomato, sliced (11), and 3 large romaine lettuce leaves (3). Wrap up burrito-style.

■ **Total Calories = 366**

25 g protein, 33 g carbohydrates, 14 g fat, 3 g saturated fat, 45 mg cholesterol, 1,070 mg sodium*, 6 g fiber

Chicken Waldorf Pita: Combine 1/4

cup chopped celery (4), 1/4 chopped apple (24), 2 ounces grilled boneless skinless chicken breast (94), 2 tablespoons chopped **walnuts** (82), 2 tablespoons fat-free Greek yogurt (15), and 1 tablespoon raisins (27). Spoon into a multigrain pita (170).

■ **Total Calories = 416**

29 g protein, 53 g carbohydrates, 12 g fat, 1.5 g saturated fat, 50 mg cholesterol, 410 mg sodium, 7 g fiber

Roast Beef and Apricot Salad

Wraps: Combine 2 chopped apricots (34), 2 tablespoons toasted **pecans** (90), 1 tablespoon dried cranberries (23), 1 tablespoon crumbled blue cheese (30), and 1/2 cup arugula (3). Place apricot mixture on a whole wheat tortilla (106) along with 2 ounces lean roast beef (95) and fold up burrito-style.

■ **Total Calories = 381**

23 g protein, 34 g carbohydrates, 18 g fat, 3.5 g saturated fat*, 55 mg cholesterol, 820 mg sodium*, 6 g fiber

Salad Pita: Peel and chop 1/4 small seedless

cucumber (8), 10 **black olives** (50), and 1/4 small red onion (11) and toss together. Mix in 1/4 cup crumbled feta cheese (100). In another bowl, use a fork to mash 1/4 cup rinsed and drained canned chickpeas (65) with 1 tablespoon fat-free plain yogurt (6), 1/8 teaspoon dried oregano (1), and 1/8 teaspoon ground cumin (1). Place 2 medium romaine lettuce leaves (2) into 1 whole wheat pita (6" diameter) (170). Divide vegetables between pita halves and place the chickpea mixture on top.

■ **Total Calories = 414**

17 g protein, 57 g carbohydrates, 15 g fat, 7 g saturated fat*, 35 mg cholesterol, 1,170 mg sodium*, 10 g fiber

Sicilian Tuna Salad on Whole

Wheat: Combine 3 ounces solid white canned tuna (109) with 1 tablespoon finely chopped red onion (4), 1 tablespoon finely chopped parsley (1), 2 tablespoons chopped toasted **pine nuts** (113), and 1 tablespoon capers (1). Toss with 1 teaspoon olive oil (40) and 1/2 teaspoon lemon juice (1), and then season to taste with freshly ground black pepper. Serve between 2 slices whole wheat bread (140).

■ **Total Calories = 409**

29 g protein, 32 g carbohydrates, 21 g fat, 2 g saturated fat, 35 mg cholesterol, 730 mg sodium*, 5 g fiber

Pesto Ham & Cheese Sandwich:

Spread 1 tablespoon **pesto** (80) on 1 whole wheat English muffin (135). Fill the sandwich with 4 ounces thinly sliced ham (121), 1/2 fresh plum tomato, sliced (6), 3 large romaine leaves (3), and 1 slice provolone cheese (50). Serve with 1 cup grape tomatoes (27).

■ **Total Calories = 422**

37 g protein, 36 g carbohydrates, 15 g fat, 4.5 g saturated fat*, 65 mg cholesterol, 1,440 mg sodium*, 7 g fiber

Roast Beef and Creamy Horseradish Sandwich: Spread 1 tablespoon **canola oil mayonnaise** (100) and ½ teaspoon prepared horseradish (1) on 2 slices whole wheat bread, toasted (140). Fill the sandwich with 3 ounces thinly sliced lean roast beef (96) and 1 large red romaine lettuce leaf (3). Serve with 2 plums (61).

■ **Total Calories = 401**

24 g protein, 44 g carbohydrates, 16 g fat, 1.5 g saturated fat*, 50 mg cholesterol, 890 mg sodium*, 6 g fiber

Chicken-Cranberry Sandwich:

Toast 2 slices whole wheat bread (140) and spread 1 tablespoon reduced-fat Neufchâtel cheese (35) and ¼ cup mashed **Hass avocado** (96) onto one slice and 2 tablespoons cranberry sauce (50) onto the other slice. Fill the sandwich with 2 ounces thinly sliced cooked chicken breast (94) and ¼ cup baby spinach leaves (3).

■ **Total Calories = 418**

26 g protein, 47 g carbohydrates, 16 g fat, 4 g saturated fat*, 60 mg cholesterol, 440 mg sodium, 9 g fiber

Turkey Cranberry Muffin: Spread 1 Laughing Cow Light Garlic & Herb Wedge (35) on 1 whole wheat English muffin (135). Fill the muffin with 3 ounces sliced honey maple turkey (91), 1 tablespoon dried cranberries (23), and 2 tablespoons **walnuts** (82).

■ **Total Calories = 366**

13 g protein, 39 g carbohydrates, 13 g fat, 2 g saturated fat, 50 mg cholesterol, 570 mg sodium, 6 g fiber

Summer Couscous Salad: Cook ⅓ cup whole wheat couscous (140) according to package instructions. Add 1 tablespoon lemon juice (4), 1 teaspoon olive oil (40), ½ bell pepper, chopped (17), 2 tablespoons **pine nuts** (113), ⅓ cup canned chickpeas, rinsed and drained (67), and 2 tablespoons crumbled feta cheese (50). Toss until well combined. Garnish with basil, cilantro, or parsley.

■ **Total Calories = 431**

15 g protein, 49 g carbohydrates, 22 g fat, 4.5 g saturated fat*, 15 mg cholesterol, 440 mg sodium, 9 g fiber

Terrific Tuna Salad: Combine 2 cups organic mixed baby greens (18), 3 ounces chunk light water-packed tuna (109), 2 tablespoons **pumpkin seeds** (148), and 1 tablespoon crumbled blue cheese (30). Toss with 2 tablespoons Newman's Own Lighten Up Balsamic Vinaigrette Dressing (45) and serve with 1 apple (78).

■ **Total Calories = 428**

33 g protein, 31 g carbohydrates, 21 g fat, 4.5 g saturated fat*, 40 mg cholesterol, 790 mg sodium*, 7 g fiber

Niçoise Salad: Toss 2 cups organic mixed baby greens (18) with 2 tablespoons Annie's Naturals Organic Dijon Mustard (0). Top with 1 cup cooked, chopped skin-on red potatoes (101), 10 sliced large **black olives** (50), ½ cup chopped green beans (22), ¼ cup chopped

celery (4), ¹/₂ cup grape tomato halves (13), and 4 ounces chunk light water-packed tuna (145).

Total Calories = 353

34 g protein, 37 g carbohydrates, 9 g fat, 1.5 g saturated fat, 50 mg cholesterol, 1,270 mg sodium*, 9 g fiber

Spinach-Endive Salad: Chop 1 Belgian endive (14) and combine with 1 cup baby spinach (10) and ¹/₄ cup red seedless grapes (26). Toss with 2 tablespoons Newman's Own Lighten Up Balsamic Vinaigrette Dressing (20) and top with 2 tablespoons crumbled Gorgonzola or other blue cheese (60) and 2 tablespoons chopped, smoked, lightly salted **almonds** (99). Serve with 6 ounces Stonyfield Farm Fat-Free French Vanilla Yogurt (130) and ¹/₄ cup red seedless grapes (26) mixed together.

Total Calories = 385

16 g protein, 52 g carbohydrates, 17 g fat, 5 g saturated fat, 20 mg cholesterol, 900 mg sodium*, 6 g fiber

Sugar Snap Pea and Salmon Salad: Combine 3 ounces canned Alaskan wild salmon (116), ¹/₄ pound fresh sugar snap peas (53), ¹/₄ cup frozen peas, thawed (29), 1 tablespoon grated sweet onion (4), and ¹/₄ cup mango slices (27). Toss with 1 tablespoon Annie's Naturals Green Goddess Dressing (65) and top with 2 tablespoons **pumpkin seeds** (148).

Total Calories = 442

34 g protein, 27 g carbohydrates, 23 g fat, 4 g saturated fat*, 70 mg cholesterol, 530 mg sodium, 6 g fiber

Set a Lunch Date

A recent survey found that a whopping 74 percent of American office workers eat lunch at their desks. Eating while working can cause you to eat too fast, lose track of how much you've eaten, and distract you from the taste and enjoyment of your meal. Follow these lunchtime rules to help make your midday meal a priority:

- Set your cell phone or computer alarm to remind you to stop and eat. When it goes off, don't hit the snooze or dismiss it. You can pick up where you left off after your meal, and you will feel reenergized.

- Commit to eating lunch with a coworker. When you know a friend is waiting for you, you won't talk yourself into staying at your desk.

- Use real dishes and silverware. In Europe (where the average lunchtime is 50 percent longer but waistlines are smaller), people in France, Greece, Italy, Portugal, Spain, and other countries rely on this tradition to make each meal feel special. Store a set in your office kitchen—washing them will tack just a few seconds onto your meal.

- If you really have to eat at your desk, try not to work while you eat. Take a few deep breaths, and savor every bite—even if it's only for 10 minutes.

Chinese Chicken Salad with Toasted Almonds:
Combine 4 ounces boneless, skinless grilled chicken breast slices (187), 2 cups romaine lettuce, torn into bite-size pieces (15), ¼ cup shredded red cabbage (4), 1 scallion, sliced diagonally (5), ¼ cup pineapple tidbits packed in juice (29), and ½ cup mandarin oranges canned in water or own juice (18). Toss with 2 tablespoons reduced-fat sesame ginger dressing (60) and sprinkle with 2 tablespoons chopped toasted **almonds** (109).

■ **Total Calories = 427**

42 g protein, 28 g carbohydrates, 16 g fat, 2 g saturated fat, 95 mg cholesterol, 95 mg sodium, 5 g fiber

Green Salad with Ham, Feta, and Walnuts:
Combine 2 cups organic mixed baby greens (18), 1 chopped fresh plum tomato (11), 2 ounces chopped ham (61), 2 tablespoons crumbled reduced-fat feta (35), and 2 tablespoons **walnuts** (82). Toss with 1½ teaspoons olive oil (60) and 1½ teaspoons white wine vinegar (0). Serve with 1 medium pear (103).

■ **Total Calories = 370**

19 g protein, 36 g carbohydrates, 19 g fat, 3.5 g saturated fat*, 30 mg cholesterol, 870 mg sodium*, 10 g fiber

Dipping Trio:
Thaw ⅓ cup frozen **edamame** (81) and toss with 1 tablespoon Annie's Naturals Green Goddess Dressing (65). Serve with 2 dark rye crispbread crackers (73) and ½ cup organic baby carrots (27) with 2 tablespoons tahini sauce (178) for dipping.

■ **Total Calories = 424**

15 g protein, 36 g carbohydrates, 25 g fat, 3.5 g saturated fat*, 5 mg cholesterol, 210 mg sodium, 10 g fiber

Can I drink alcohol?

We suggest avoiding alcohol, along with all other calorie-containing beverages, during the Flat Belly Diet Diabetes. Even though alcohol can work within a healthy diet for people with diabetes, we want you to skip the extra calories—and sidestep the risk for overeating that can often become so tempting after a glass of wine or a cocktail!

There's also a health reason for our caution. Current dietary guidelines recommend that if you don't drink, you should not start. In moderation, alcohol has been shown to lower the risk of heart disease, but it also carries risks. Just one drink a day is linked to an increased risk of breast cancer in women, and more-than-moderate drinking is tied to liver cirrhosis, high blood pressure, cancers of the upper gastrointestinal tract, stroke, injuries, and violence. And some people are advised not to consume alcoholic beverages at all, including pregnant and lactating women and individuals taking medications that can interact with alcohol.

Flat Belly Dinners

These options pleased husbands, wives, kids, and extended family—and our testers loved whipping up extra portions to take for lunch, too. As with breakfasts and lunches, MUFAs are in **boldface** and ingredient calorie counts are in parentheses. Remember that you want to limit saturated fat to 10 percent of total calories—about 17 grams per day for most women or 21 grams for most men—and sodium intake to less than 2,300 milligrams. You'll see an asterisk on meals where the saturated fat or sodium levels are on the high side. If you choose those meals, just watch your saturated fat and sodium intake for the rest of the day.

Cheesy Veggies and Spaghetti:
Cook ½ cup chopped fresh red bell pepper (23), 1 cup broccoli florets (20), and 2 tablespoons sliced onions (6) in a nonstick skillet with 1 tablespoon **safflower oil** (120) until vegetables soften. Toss with ¾ cup cooked whole wheat spaghetti (130), ¼ cup nonfat ricotta cheese (45), and 2 tablespoons low-fat Italian blend shredded cheese (40).

◼ **Total Calories = 384**

18 g protein, 43 g carbohydrates, 17 g fat, 2.5 g saturated fat, 20 mg cholesterol, 200 mg sodium, 9 g fiber

Moo Shu Vegetable Wrap: Cook 1 cup shredded coleslaw mix (18), 1 shredded carrot (25), and ½ cup sliced mushrooms (8) in a large nonstick skillet with 1 teaspoon **canola oil** (41) until softened. Push vegetable mixture to the side and cook 1 lightly beaten egg (72) on the opposite side of the skillet. Add 1 chopped scallion (5) and 2 tablespoons chopped **peanuts** (110) and toss to combine. Warm a whole wheat tortilla (106), spread with 1 tablespoon hoisin sauce (35), and fill with the vegetable mixture.

◼ **Total Calories = 420**

16 g protein, 42 g carbohydrates, 22 g fat, 3.5 g saturated fat*, 210 mg cholesterol, 620 mg sodium*, 9 g fiber

Cashew-Chickpea Curry: Whisk 1 teaspoon cornstarch (10) in a bowl with ¼ cup reduced-sodium chicken broth (4) and set aside. Combine ½ teaspoon safflower oil (21), 2 tablespoons chopped onion (8), ½ teaspoon curry powder (3), and a pinch of salt and ground black pepper in a skillet and cook until fragrant. Add the cornstarch mixture, $\frac{1}{2}$ cup canned no-salt-added chickpeas (130) that have been rinsed and drained, and 2 tablespoons unsalted **cashews,** coarsely chopped (100), and simmer for 5 minutes, until thickened. Serve with $\frac{1}{3}$ cup brown rice (73) and top with 1 tablespoon chopped fresh cilantro (0) and 1 tablespoon fat-free Greek-style yogurt (8).

◼ **Total Calories = 357**

13 g protein, 50 g carbohydrates, 12 g fat, 2 g saturated fat, 0 mg cholesterol, 220 mg sodium, 8 g fiber

Pasta with Shrimp and Broccoli Rabe:
Cook 4 ounces broccoli rabe or broccolini (33) in a large pot of boiling water for 2 minutes, then remove with tongs. Cook $\frac{1}{2}$ cup whole wheat penne (106) in the same water according to package instructions. Cook 4 ounces raw shrimp (120) in 1 tablespoon **olive oil** (119) with $\frac{1}{2}$ teaspoon minced garlic (8) and a dash of red-pepper flakes until shrimp are opaque. Drain pasta and toss with broccoli rabe and shrimp mixture.

◼ **Total Calories = 386**

31 g protein, 28 g carbohydrates, 16 g fat, 2 g saturated fat, 170 mg cholesterol, 210 mg sodium, 3 g fiber

Sweet-and-Sour Shrimp Stir-Fry:
Cook 1$\frac{1}{2}$ cups frozen stir-fry bell pepper strips (38) in a large nonstick skillet with 1 teaspoon **canola oil** (40) until soft. Add 2 tablespoons apricot jam (97) and 1 teaspoon red wine vinegar (2), along with 4 ounces cooked, peeled, and deveined shrimp (112), and cook 2

minutes longer. Top with 2 tablespoons peanuts (110), chopped.

◼ **Total Calories = 399**

30 g protein, 38 g carbohydrates, 15 g fat, 2 g saturated fat, 220 mg cholesterol, 290 mg sodium, 3 g fiber

Chai Scallops with Bok Choy:
Steep 1 chai tea bag (0) in $\frac{1}{4}$ cup hot water (0) mixed with 2 tablespoons light coconut milk (24). Steam 1 small head baby bok choy, quartered lengthwise (11), in the microwave oven until softened. Cook 4 ounces sea scallops (100) in a nonstick skillet with $\frac{1}{2}$ teaspoon canola oil (21) for 2 minutes and then remove from pan. Add the tea mixture and $\frac{1}{2}$ teaspoon finely chopped fresh ginger (1) to the pan and cook for 1 to 2 minutes, until reduced by half. Toss with the bok choy, scallops, and 2 tablespoons **cashews** (100), chopped. Serve with $\frac{2}{3}$ cup steamed brown rice (146) and 1 lime wedge (0).

◼ **Total Calories = 403**

27 g protein, 47 g carbohydrates, 14 g fat, 3.5 g saturated fat*, 35 mg cholesterol, 830 mg sodium*, 4 g fiber

Asian Glazed Salmon with Greens:
Cook a 3-ounce skinless salmon fillet (156) in 1 tablespoon **canola oil** (124) over medium-high heat until fish flakes easily. Add 1 teaspoon reduced-sodium soy sauce (3) and 1 teaspoon honey (21) and turn to coat. Transfer salmon to plate and cook 1$\frac{1}{4}$ cups collard greens (14) and $\frac{1}{4}$ teaspoon fresh grated ginger (0) in same skillet until bright green and tender. Add 1 ounce cooked whole

wheat spaghetti (99), 2 tablespoons chopped scallions (4), and a pinch of red-pepper flakes (0). Toss to coat. Serve salmon on top of pasta and greens.

■ **Total Calories = 421**

23 g protein, 31 g carbohydrates, 24 g fat, 3 g saturated fat, 50 mg cholesterol, 270 mg sodium, 6 g fiber

Broiled Chicken Cutlets with Pesto:
Season a 5-ounce chicken breast cutlet (156) with salt-free spice mix of your choice and spread 1 tablespoon prepared **pesto** (80) on top. Broil for 5 minutes or until no longer pink in the thickest part. Slice a plum tomato (11) and arrange on top. Scatter 2 tablespoons shredded part-skim mozzarella cheese (36) and 2 teaspoons grated Parmesan cheese (14) over the tomato. Broil for 1 to 2 minutes longer, just until the cheese is melted and the tomato slices are heated. Serve with 1/2 cup cooked quinoa (111).

■ **Total Calories = 408**

45 g protein, 24 g carbohydrates, 14 g fat, 4.5 g saturated fat*, 100 mg cholesterol, 360 mg sodium, 4 g fiber

Chicken Pad Thai:
Cook 1 ounce flat rice noodles (99) according to package instructions and set aside. Cook 2 ounces thinly sliced boneless, skinless chicken breast strips (62) in a nonstick skillet with 1 teaspoon peanut oil (40). When the chicken is cooked through, push it to the side of the skillet and cook 1 egg (72), lightly beaten. Add 1 tablespoon lower-sodium ketchup (20), 1 teaspoon fish sauce (1), 1/4 teaspoon sugar (4), 1/4 teaspoon minced garlic (1),

and noodles. Cook for 1 minute, until heated through. Top with 1 chopped scallion (5), 1/2 cup bean sprouts (16), and 2 tablespoons unsalted **cashews,** finely chopped (100). Serve with lime wedges (0) if desired.

■ **Total Calories = 420**

26 g protein, 40 g carbohydrates, 18 g fat, 4 g saturated fat*, 245 mg cholesterol, 580 mg sodium, 3 g fiber

Chicken Zucchini Rotini:
Combine 3 ounces cooked chicken breast slices (140) with 1/2 cup cooked whole wheat rotini pasta (99), 1/4 cup 1% cottage cheese (41), 1/2 cup sliced zucchini (9), 2 chopped plum tomatoes (22), and 1 teaspoon salt-free Italian seasoning (0). Toss until coated and top with 2 tablespoons shredded reduced-fat mozzarella cheese (36). Microwave until heated through. Top with 10 medium **black olives,** sliced (50), just before serving.

■ **Total Calories = 397**

43 g protein, 33 g carbohydrates, 11 g fat, 3.5 g saturated fat*, 85 mg cholesterol, 780 mg sodium*, 6 g fiber

Super-Quick Chicken Fiesta:
Combine 1/2 cup cooked chicken breast chunks (116), 1/4 cup low-sodium black beans, rinsed and drained (50), 2 chopped plum tomatoes (22), and 1 teaspoon chili powder (8). Heat in a nonstick skillet and serve over 1/2 cup cooked brown rice (109) topped with 1/4 cup mashed **Hass avocado** (96) and 1 tablespoon fat-free sour cream (15).

■ **Total Calories = 416**

31 g protein, 44 g carbohydrates, 13 g fat, 2.5 g

saturated fat, 60 mg cholesterol, 110 mg sodium, 11 g fiber

Chicken with Banana Chutney Topping:
Chop ½ medium banana (53) and toss with 1 tablespoon mango chutney (55), 2 tablespoons chopped toasted **cashews** (100), and ½ teaspoon freshly squeezed lemon juice (1). Warm 4 ounces of boneless, skinless cooked chicken breast slices (187) and serve on a bed of 2 cups baby greens (18) topped with banana mixture.

◾ **Total Calories = 414**

40 g protein, 35 g carbohydrates, 12 g fat, 3 g saturated fat, 95 mg cholesterol, 220 mg sodium, 4 g fiber

Chicken Piccata:
Flatten 4 ounces boneless, skinless chicken tenders (125) and dredge lightly in 2 teaspoons flour (19). Cook for 2 minutes on each side in a nonstick skillet over high heat with 1 tablespoon **safflower oil** (120) until cooked through. Add 1 tablespoon chicken broth (3), 2 teaspoons freshly squeezed lemon juice (3), 1 teaspoon chopped fresh parsley (0), and ½ teaspoon capers (0), minced. Bring to a boil. Season with freshly ground black pepper (0). Serve with ¾ cup red potatoes (105) roasted with ½ teaspoon safflower oil (20).

◾ **Total Calories = 395**

30 g protein, 28 g carbohydrates, 17 g fat, 1.5 g saturated fat, 65 mg cholesterol, 130 mg sodium, 2 g fiber

Simple Sausage Pizza:
Brush 1 side of 1 whole wheat pita (170) with 1 tablespoon **extra-virgin olive oil** (119). Top with ¼ cup prepared marinara sauce (35), 1 ounce pre-cooked Italian-style low-fat chicken sausage, cut into pieces (50), and 2 tablespoons part-skim mozzarella cheese (40). Warm under the broiler or in a toaster oven to heat through.

◾ **Total Calories = 414**

17 g protein, 41 g carbohydrates, 21 g fat, 4.5 g saturated fat*, 35 mg cholesterol, 880 mg sodium*, 6 g fiber

Turkey Tacos with Avocado-Tomato Salsa:
Combine ¼ cup mashed **Hass avocado** (96), ½ cup cherry tomatoes, halved (13), and 1 teaspoon fresh lime juice (1). Warm 4 (6") corn tortillas (209) and place in 2 stacks. Divide 2 ounces cooked turkey breast strips (77), avocado mixture, and 2 tablespoons shredded low-fat Mexican blend cheese (40) between each stack and fold in half to serve.

◾ **Total Calories = 436**

28 g protein, 52 g carbohydrates, 15 g fat, 3.5 g saturated fat*, 55 mg cholesterol, 180 mg sodium, 11 g fiber

Pesto-Turkey Sliders:
Combine 4 ounces extra-lean ground turkey breast (120), 1 tablespoon finely chopped red onion (3), 2 teaspoons liquid egg white (5), 1 teaspoon minced fresh cilantro (0), ¼ teaspoon ground cumin (0), and ⅛ teaspoon salt (0). Shape into 2 burgers and cook on a skillet until centers register 165°F. Serve on 2 whole wheat dinner rolls (149), topped with 2 leaves lettuce (2), 1 sliced plum tomato (11), and 1 tablespoon **pesto** (80).

Total Calories = 370

37 g protein, 33 g carbohydrates, 11 g fat, 2.5 g saturated fat, 50 mg cholesterol, 760 mg sodium*, 6 g fiber

Island Pork Salad: Combine 3 ounces

grilled pork tenderloin slices (121), ½ cup pineapple tidbits (40), ¼ cup mango slices (27), ¼ cup fresh chopped red bell peppers (12), ¼ cup reduced-fat crumbled feta (70), 2 tablespoons balsamic vinegar (20), and 2 tablespoons chopped **macadamia nuts** (120). Toss to coat and serve on a bed of 2 cups organic mixed greens (18).

Total Calories = 428

33 g protein, 30 g carbohydrates, 21 g fat, 6 g saturated fat*, 23 mg cholesterol, 560 mg sodium, 7 g fiber

Steak Burger with Salad: Shape

3 ounces of 95% lean ground beef (117) into a patty. Slather with 2 teaspoons steak sauce (3) and season with salt-free seasoning mix (0). Grill until the temperature in the center registers 160°F. Serve on a whole grain hamburger bun (114) topped with ½-ounce slice reduced-fat Swiss cheese (41), 1 lettuce leaf (1), a tomato slice (5), and a thin red onion slice (3). Serve with 1 cup mixed greens (9) topped with 1 tablespoon **olive oil** (119) and 2 teaspoons balsamic vinegar (7).

Total Calories = 419

28 g protein, 28 g carbohydrates, 23 g fat, 6 g saturated fat*, 60 mg cholesterol, 440 mg sodium, 5 g fiber

Asian Beef and Rice Bowl: Cook 2

ounces thinly sliced top round steak (77) in a nonstick skillet with 2 teaspoons reduced-sodium soy sauce (7), 1 teaspoon canola oil (40), and 1 teaspoon finely chopped fresh ginger (2) until pink is gone. Add 1 cup frozen stir-fry or Asian vegetable mix (80) and cook until heated through. Serve over ½ cup brown rice (108) topped with 1 chopped scallion (4) and 2 tablespoons dry-roasted **peanuts** (110), coarsely chopped.

Total Calories = 428

24 g protein, 40 g carbohydrates, 19 g fat, 3 g saturated fat, 25 mg cholesterol, 680 mg sodium*, 6 g fiber

Dijon Pepper Steak and

Potatoes: Sprinkle 1½ teaspoons cracked

peppercorns (5) and ⅛ teaspoon salt (0) on both sides of a 5-ounce well-trimmed center-cut sirloin steak (191). Cook in a nonstick skillet with 1 tablespoon **olive oil** (119) over medium-high heat to desired doneness. Remove steak to a plate and add 1 tablespoon beef broth (1), 2 teaspoons balsamic vinegar (7), and ½ teaspoon Dijon mustard (3) to the pan along with ¾ cup cooked baby red potatoes (105). Spoon any remaining sauce over steak.

Total Calories = 431

33 g protein, 25 g carbohydrates, 20 g fat, 4.5 g saturated fat*, 65 mg cholesterol, 550 mg sodium, 2 g fiber

MEAL REPLACEMENT BARS

CHOOSE 1 OF THE FOLLOWING	CARBS	CALORIES	ADD YOUR MUFA
Clif Black Cherry Almond Bar	44 g	250	
Clif Crunchy Peanut Butter Bar	40 g	250	
Clif Chocolate Brownie bar	45 g	240	Add 1 light string cheese or 1 hard-boiled egg and a 100- to 150-calorie MUFA from the list on page 127, such as 2 tablespoons of (choose 1):
Nature's Path Optimum Pomegran Cherry energy bar	39 g	230	
Larabar Banana Bread	25 g	220	
Larabar Chocolate Coconut	28 g	220	
Larabar Ginger Snap	24 g	220	■ almonds (109)
Odwalla Banana Nut bar	41 g	220	■ Brazil nuts (110)
Larabar Cinnamon Roll	27 g	210	■ peanuts (110)
Larabar Pecan Pie	22 g	200	■ macadamia nuts (120)
Luna Chocolate Pecan Pie bar	25 g	200	OR
Nature's Path Optimum Blueberry Flax & Soy energy bar	37 g	200	Add a 150- to 200-calorie MUFA from the list on page 127, such as 2 tablespoons of (choose 1):
Larabar Chai Tea bar	25 g	190	
Larabar Cherry Pie	28 g	190	
Luna LemonZest bar	26 g	180	■ natural peanut butter (188)
Luna Nutz Over Chocolate bar	25 g	180	■ almond butter (200)
Luna Peanut Butter Cookie bar	23 g	180	
Luna S'mores bar	27 g	180	

FROZEN MEALS

CHOOSE 1 OF THE FOLLOWING MEALS	CARBS	CALORIES	ADD YOUR MUFA
Amy's Black Bean Enchilada Whole Meal	53 g	330	Add a 50- to 100-calorie MUFA from the list on page 127, such as: ▪ 10 large green or black olives (or 5 of each) (50)
Amy's Indian Mattar Paneer	54 g	320	
Seeds of Change Fettuccine Alfredo di Roma	45 g	320	
Amy's Indian Vegetable Korma	41 g	310	
Seeds of Change Hanalei Vegetarian Chicken Teriyaki	47 g	300	
Kashi Lemongrass Coconut Curry	38 g	300	
Kashi Red Chicken Curry	40 g	300	
Amy's Organic Brown Rice, Black-Eyed Peas & Veggies Bowl	38 g	290	
Amy's Organic Teriyaki Bowl	52 g	290	Add a 100- to 150-calorie MUFA from the list on page 127, such as 2 tablespoons of (choose 1): ▪ almonds (109) ▪ peanuts (110) ▪ pumpkin seeds (148)
Amy's Veggie Loaf Whole Meal	47 g	290	
Boca Lasagna with Chunky Tomato and Herb Sauce	42 g	290	
Kashi Chicken Florentine	31 g	290	
Kashi Chicken Pasta Pomodoro	38 g	280	
Seeds of Change Lasagna Calabrese with Eggplant and Portobello Mushrooms	42 g	270	
Amy's Indian Mattar Tofu	40 g	260	
Kashi Southwest Style Chicken	32 g	240	
Cedarlane Low Fat Veggie Pizza Wrap	32 g	220	Add a 150- to 200-calorie MUFA from the list on page 127, such as: ▪ ¼ cup chocolate chips (207)
Yves Veggie Penne	36 g	210	
Amy's Light in Sodium Shepherd's Pie	27 g	160	
Boca Meatless Chili	25 g	150	

FAST FOOD

MENU ITEM(S)	CARBS	CALORIES	ADD YOUR MUFA
McDonald's Premium Southwest Salad with Grilled Chicken and Newman's Own Ligthen Up Italian Dressing	38 g	380	Add a 50- to 100- calorie MUFA from the list on page 127, such as:
Jack in the Box Asian Grilled Chicken Salad with Roasted Slivered Almonds and Low-Fat Balsamic Dressing	27 g	325	◼ 10 large green or black olives (or 5 of each) (50)
Baja Fresh Baja Ensalada with Charbroiled Chicken with Fat-Free Salsa Verde	29 g	310	◼ 2 tablespoons walnuts (82) ◼ 2 tablespoons pistachios (89)
Pizza Hut Fit n' Delicious Pizza (2 slices) with Green Pepper, Red Onion & Diced Tomato (12″)	48 g	300	◼ 2 tablespoons sunflower seeds (90)
Panda Express String Bean Chicken Breast with Mixed Vegetables	26 g	290	
Wendy's Large Chili	29 g	280	Add a 100- to 150- calorie MUFA from the list on page 127, such as:
Arby's Junior Roast Beef Sandwich	37 g	270	
Chick-fil-A Chargrilled Chicken Sandwich	33 g	260	◼ 2 tablespoons pumpkin seeds (148)
Panera Low-Fat Vegetarian Garden Vegetable Soup with a Whole Grain Loaf	51 g	260	
Subway Oven Roasted Chicken Salad with Fat-Free Italian Dressing and Roasted Chicken Noodle Soup	22 g	245	Add a 150- to 200- calorie MUFA from the list on page 127, such as 2 tablespoons of (choose 1):
Taco Bell Burrito Supreme Chicken (Fresco Style)	49 g	180	◼ natural peanut butter (188) ◼ almond butter (200)

400-Calorie MUFA Snack Packs

Like the breakfasts, lunches, and dinners, your MUFA Snack Packs are all about 400 calories each and contain a MUFA. As such, they can be used interchangeably with your other meals. We've provided a variety of savory, sweet, and grab-and-go options for you. MUFAs are in **boldface**, and calorie counts are in parentheses. Remember that you want to limit saturated fat to 10 percent of total calories—about 17 grams per day for most women or 21 grams for most men—and sodium intake to less than 2,300 milligrams. You'll see an asterisk on meals where the saturated fat or sodium levels are on the high side. If you choose those meals, just watch your saturated fat and sodium intake for the rest of the day.

Zesty Citrus Mustard Dip: Combine 2 tablespoons Dijon mustard (30), 2 teaspoons frozen orange juice concentrate, thawed (19), 2 tablespoons plain yogurt (19), 2 tablespoons reduced-fat sour cream (41), and 1 teaspoon white wine vinegar (0). Serve as a dip for 1 ounce thin pretzels (111), 1 cup baby carrots (53), and 1 cup broccoli florets (20). Have 2 tablespoons **peanuts** (110) on the side.

◾ **Total Calories = 403**

12 g protein, 56 g carbohydrates, 15 g fat, 4 g saturated fat*, 15 mg cholesterol, 1,390 mg sodium*, 7 g fiber

Hummus Dip: Sprinkle 2 tablespoons **pine nuts** (113) onto ¾ cup hummus (300). Serve with 1 cup broccoli florets (20).

◾ **Total Calories = 433**

9 g protein, 42 g carbohydrates, 24 g fat, 0.5 g saturated fat, 0 mg cholesterol, 1,030 mg sodium*, 15 g fiber

Black Bean Dip 'n' Tomatoes: Mix ½ cup canned black beans, rinsed, drained, and mashed (100), with 1 cup halved grape tomatoes (27). Top with ¼ cup mashed **Hass avocado** (96) and 1 chopped low-fat string cheese (70). Serve with 3 RyKrisp crackers (110).

◾ **Total Calories = 403**

20 g protein, 54 g carbohydrates, 16 g fat, 5 g saturated fat*, 15 mg cholesterol, 350 mg sodium, 17 g fiber

Decadent Deli Wrap: Top 4 ounces reduced-sodium deli turkey slices (118) with

2 teaspoons pesto (50), then sprinkle with 2 tablespoons **pumpkin seeds** (148) and 1 cup cherry tomatoes, chopped (27). Roll up and serve with 1 medium orange (69).

■ **Total Calories = 412**

37 g protein, 28 g carbohydrates, 18 g fat, 3 g saturated fat*, 45 mg cholesterol, 790 mg sodium*, 6 g fiber

Open-Faced Tomato-Olive Sandwich: Spread ½ cup part-skim
ricotta cheese (171) on a 100% whole wheat English muffin (135) and top with 1 cup halved grape tomatoes (27) and 10 **black olives,** chopped (50).

■ **Total Calories = 383**

22 g protein, 41 g carbohydrates, 16 g fat, 7 g saturated fat*, 40 mg cholesterol, 790 mg sodium*, 7 g fiber

Italian-Style Ham Roll-Ups:

Spread 2 tablespoons garlic and herb Boursin cheese (120) evenly between 2 slices (2 ounces) reduced-sodium deli-baked ham (61) and sprinkle with 2 tablespoons **sunflower seeds** (90) and 1 teaspoon chopped fresh parsley (0). Cut ham slices in half and roll pieces around 4 grissini or Italian breadsticks (99). Stir together 1 tablespoon reduced-fat sour cream (20) and 1 teaspoon grainy deli-style mustard (5) to use as a dip.

■ **Total Calories = 395**

19 g protein, 24 g carbohydrates, 26 g fat, 11 g saturated fat*, 65 mg cholesterol, 860 mg sodium*, 3 g fiber

Barbecued Edamame: Cook 1 cup
fresh or frozen **edamame** (244) in boiling water for 5 minutes. Heat 1 teaspoon olive oil (40) in a skillet and add ¼ teaspoon chili powder (0), ⅛ teaspoon ground cumin (0), and a dash of ground red pepper (0). Cook for 30 seconds until fragrant. Toss edamame in seasoning mix to coat and sprinkle ⅛ teaspoon salt (0) on top. Serve with 8 (8") celery sticks (51) and 2 tablespoons hummus (50).

■ **Total Calories = 385**

26 g protein, 35 g carbohydrates, 20 g fat, 2 g saturated fat, 0 mg cholesterol, 730 mg sodium*, 13 g fiber

Pineapple "Sundae": Combine 1 cup
canned pineapple (109) with 1 cup nonfat cottage cheese (123). Sprinkle with 2 tablespoons **pumpkin seeds** (148).

■ **Total Calories = 380**

35 g protein, 35 g carbohydrates, 13 g fat, 2.5 g saturated fat, 10 mg cholesterol, 25 mg sodium, 3 g fiber

Strawberry-Chocolate "Sundae": Mix 1 cup sliced strawberries
(53) and ¼ cup **semisweet chocolate chips** (207) into ¾ cup cottage cheese (135).

■ **Total Calories = 395**

21 g protein, 51 g carbohydrates, 13 g fat, 7 g saturated fat*, 15 mg cholesterol, 680 mg sodium*, 6 g fiber

Glazed Pineapple Rings: Cook
2 pineapple rings (56), fresh or canned packed in juice and drained, for 2 minutes over medium-high heat. Add 1 tablespoon

water (0), 1 teaspoon brown sugar (12), and $\frac{1}{2}$ teaspoon trans-free margarine (14) and toss to coat. Serve slices drizzled with the pan juices and top with 1 teaspoon sour cream (10) and 2 tablespoons finely chopped **macadamia nuts** (120). Mix 2 tablespoons dried cranberries (47) and 1 tablespoon semisweet chocolate chips (104) to serve on side as trail mix.

▨ **Total Calories = 363**

3 g protein, 46 g carbohydrates, 22 g fat, 7 g saturated fat*, 5 mg cholesterol, 20 mg sodium, 5 g fiber

Apple Snack:
Serve 1 medium apple (77) cut into wedges with 2 tablespoons **peanut butter** (188) as a dip. Serve with 4 cups light microwaved popcorn (137).

▨ **Total Calories = 402**

12 g protein, 50 g carbohydrates, 19 g fat, 4 g saturated fat*, 0 mg cholesterol, 310 mg sodium, 10 g fiber

Apple Cashew Butter Snack:
Spread 2 tablespoons **cashew butter** (190) on 1 apple (77) and stir 1 teaspoon maple syrup (17) into 6 ounces non-fat plain yogurt (80).

▨ **Total Calories = 364**

16 g protein, 49 g carbohydrates, 13 g fat, 3 g saturated fat, 5 mg cholesterol, 300 mg sodium, 4 g fiber

Grab and Go Option 1:
1 piece low-fat string cheese (70), 1 medium banana (105), 1 cup baby carrots (53), and 2 tablespoons **almonds** (109).

▨ **Total Calories = 337**

14 g protein, 43 g carbohydrates, 16 g fat, 4.5 g

saturated fat*, 15 mg cholesterol, 300 mg sodium, 8 g fiber

Grab and Go Option 2:
1 piece low-fat string cheese (70), 5 cups popped light microwave popcorn (172), 1 teaspoon grated Parmesan (7), and 2 tablespoons **macadamia nuts** (120).

▨ **Total Calories: 369**

15 g protein, 33 g carbohydrates, 23 g fat, 6 g saturated fat*, 15 mg cholesterol, 460 mg sodium, 7 g fiber

Grab and Go Option 3:
2 pieces low-fat string cheese (140), 5 Wasa crackers (124), and 2 tablespoons **pumpkin seeds** (148).

▨ **Total Calories = 412**

28 g protein, 34 g carbohydrates, 24 g fat, 9 g saturated fat*, 30 mg cholesterol, 570 mg sodium, 7 g fiber

Grab and Go Option 4:
Stir 2 tablespoons **walnuts** (82) and $\frac{1}{2}$ cup raspberries (32) into 6 ounces Stonyfield Fat-Free French Vanilla Yogurt (130). Serve with 1 cup baby carrots (53) and 2 tablespoons light ranch dressing (77) for dipping.

▨ **Total Calories = 374**

11 g protein, 49 g carbohydrates, 17 g fat, 2.5 g saturated fat, 15 mg cholesterol, 470 mg sodium, 8 g fiber

Blueberry Smoothie:
Blend 1 cup fat-free or soy milk (83), 6 ounces nonfat plain yogurt (80), and 1 cup frozen blueberries (79) for 1 minute. Transfer to a glass, and

stir in 1 tablespoon organic cold-pressed **flaxseed oil** (120).

■ **Total Calories = 362**

16 g protein, 45 g carbohydrates, 15 g fat, 1.5 g saturated fat, 10 mg cholesterol, 210 mg sodium, 4 g fiber

Chocolate Malted Milkshake:

Combine ½ cup vanilla frozen yogurt (95), 1 tablespoon malted milk powder (52), 2 teaspoons cocoa powder (8), ¼ teaspoon instant espresso coffee powder (0), 1 cup fat-free or soy milk (83), and ½ teaspoon vanilla extract (6). Process until smooth and stir in 1 tablespoon **flaxseed oil** (120).

■ **Total Calories = 364**

15 g protein, 45 g carbohydrates, 15 g fat, 2 g saturated fat, 5 mg cholesterol, 200 mg sodium, 1 g fiber

Chocolate-Strawberry Smoothie:

Blend 1 cup fat-free milk (83), ¼ cup **semisweet chocolate chips** (207), 1 scoop protein powder (100), and ½ cup frozen strawberries (26) for 1 minute. Transfer to a glass and enjoy.

■ **Total Calories = 416**

35 g protein, 47 g carbohydrates, 12.5 g fat, 7.5 g saturated fat*, 8 mg cholesterol, 196 mg sodium, 4 g fiber

Apple Pie Smoothie:

Blend 6 ounces Stonyfield Fat-Free French Vanilla Yogurt (130), ½ cup fat-free or soy milk (42), 1 teaspoon apple pie spice (6), ½ medium apple, peeled, cored, and chopped (32), 2 tablespoons **cashew butter** (190), and a handful of ice for 1 minute. Transfer to a glass and eat with a spoon.

■ **Total Calories = 400**

17 g protein, 47 g carbohydrates, 18 g fat, 4 g saturated fat*, 5 mg cholesterol, 360 mg sodium, 3 g fiber

DID YOU KNOW?

Eating at the drive-thru? Stick with our Flat Belly Diet Diabetes fast-food suggestions. A recent Cornell University study has found that people consistently underestimated the calories in fast-food entrées, fries, and sodas by as much as 22 to 30 percent! The bigger the meal, the more off-base their estimates. Bottom line: Unless you know the calorie count, chances are you're eating way more than you think![1]

Create Your Own Snack Pack

Keep the total calorie count around 400, include a selection from the MUFA list on page 127, and pair with foods such as the ones on this list. Keep your total carb counts between 25 and 45 grams. Have one snack pack per day.

GRAINS

Corn tortillas (2), 105 calories, 21 g carbs

Food For Life Ezekiel 4:9 Organic Sesame Sprouted Grain Bread (1 slice), 80 calories, 14 g carbs

Nature's Path Organic Flax Plus Frozen Waffle (1), 90 calories, 12 g carbs

Oatmeal, instant, plain, (1 packet, 1 ounce) 100 calories, 17 g carbs

Popcorn; Smart Balance Light or Newman's Own 94% fat-free (4 cups popped) 100 calories, 15 g carbs

DAIRY

Cottage cheese, fat-free (½ cup), 81 calories, 3 g carbs

Kraft Natural Mexican Style Four Cheese (¼ cup), 100 calories, 0 g carbs

Milk, fat-free (1 cup) 83 calories, 13 g carbs

String cheese, low-fat (1 ounce), 80 calories, 0 g carbs

Yogurt, fat-free plain (6 ounces), 80 calories, 12 g carbs

FRUITS

Apple, any variety, medium (size of a tennis ball), 77 calories, 15 g carbs

Banana, medium, 105 calories, 27 g carbs

Blueberries (1 cup), 84 calories, 11 g carbs

Grapes (1 cup), 104 calories, 27 g carbs

Orange, medium, 69 calories, 6 g carbs

Peach, medium, 59 calories, 15 g carbs

Pineapple, canned in pineapple juice (4 ounces or ½ cup), 59 calories, 18 g carbs

Raisins, unsweetened (¼ cup), 123 calories, 33 g carbs

VEGETABLES

Baby carrots (1 cup), 53 calories, 5 g carbs

Broccoli florets, raw (2 cups), 40 calories, 10 g carbs

Grape tomatoes (1 cup), 30 calories, 5 g carbs

Mixed baby field greens (2 cups), 18 calories, 10 g carbs

Red bell pepper, sliced (1 cup), 28 calories, 5 g carbs

PROTEINS

Black beans, canned, drained (½ cup), 100 calories, 15 g carbs

Chicken breast, pre-cooked (3 ounces), 122 calories, 0 g carbs

Chunk light tuna in water (3 ounces), 105 calories, 0 g carbs

Deli turkey slices (4 ounces), 122 calories, 0 g carbs

Egg, large (1), 78 calories, 0 g carbs

Optional 200-Calorie Snacks

If you're a man of medium to large build or are a man or woman who's extremely active, you may find that you're a bit too hungry on our 1,600-calorie meal plan. Just for you, we've added an additional 200-calorie snack. These 200-calorie snacks don't necessarily contain MUFAs or don't use MUFAs in the same serving sizes we use in the meals. So you can't use two of these snacks to replace one of your meals. These snacks are only to be used as an addition to the meals if you find you're still hungry.

- ¼ cup almonds (low-carb choice)
- 10 walnut halves and ⅔ cup red grapes
- 2 tablespoons peanuts and 100-calorie bag microwave popcorn (4 cups popped)
- 2 tablespoons walnuts, 5 (8") celery stalks, and 2 tablespoons light cream cheese (low-carb choice)
- 2 tablespoons peanuts and 4 ounces Stonyfield Farm nonfat vanilla yogurt
- 1 tablespoon cashews and 1 Kashi TLC Chewy Trail Mix bar
- 2 tablespoons almonds, 2 tablespoons dried cranberries, and 1 tablespoon semisweet chocolate chips
- 2 tablespoons chopped walnuts, 6 ounces nonfat plain yogurt, and ¼ cup blueberries
- 1 large apple with 1 tablespoon peanut butter

- 8 (8") celery stalks with 1½ tablespoons almond butter (low-carb choice)
- 1 medium banana with 1 tablespoon cashew butter
- ⅓ cup dry rolled oats cooked with water; 1 tablespoon cashew butter mixed in
- ⅓ cup pineapple with 1 cup low-fat cottage cheese
- 4 ak-mak or 3 Wasa rye crispbread crackers with 3 wedges Laughing Cow Light Garlic & Herb cheese
- Kashi TLC Chewy Cherry Dark Chocolate bar and 1 low-fat string cheese
- 1 ounce whole wheat pita (½ Thomas's whole wheat pita) with ⅓ cup hummus
- 1 cup baby carrots with ⅓ cup hummus
- 15 Kashi TLC Honey Sesame crackers with 1 hard-boiled egg

Free Foods List

Looking for another alternative if you still feel a bit hungry after your four MUFA meals? Munch on some veggies from the list below. This list includes a wide range of filling, low-calorie, high-fiber vegetables that you can add to one of your meals or eat on their own. As we noted earlier, be careful of how you prepare your vegetables. Buy them fresh or frozen, if you can, and avoid cooking with butter, margarine, or oily or sugary sauces. Instead, eat them raw or steamed with low-calorie seasonings, such as the ones listed on page 130 in Chapter 7.

- Artichoke hearts
- Asparagus
- Beets
- Bell peppers
- Broccoli
- Brussels sprouts
- Cabbage
- Carrots
- Cauliflower
- Celery
- Collard greens
- Cucumbers
- Eggplant
- Kale
- Lettuce
- Mushrooms
- Onions
- Radishes
- Spinach
- String/green beans
- Summer squash
- Tomatoes
- Water chestnuts
- Zucchini

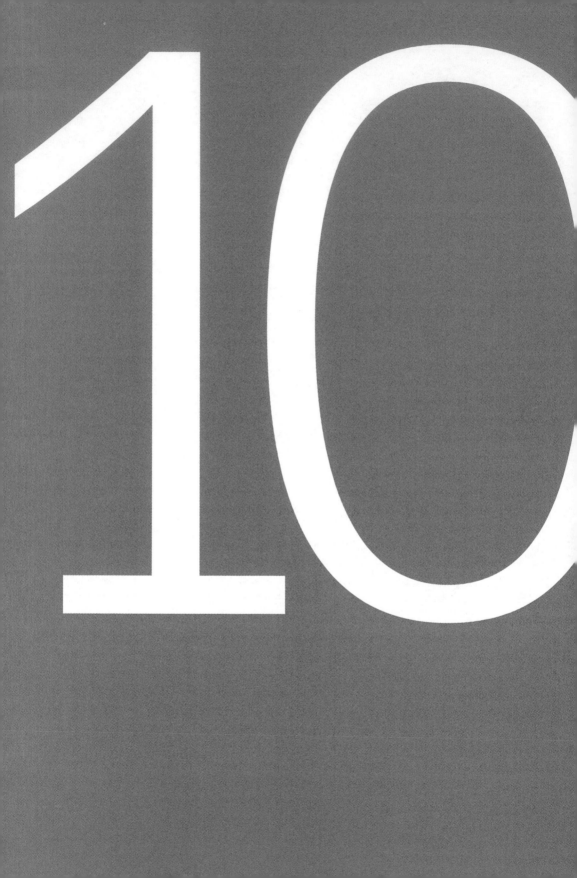

THE 28-DAY PLAN:
RECIPES

WHEN WE TURNED our Flat Belly Diet Diabetes test panelists loose
with these recipes, we knew that several things would happen. And they
did. The cooks in the group got busy, thrilling themselves and their families with everything from roast pork tenderloin to stuffed French toast
to zucchini and chocolate chip cake. A few confirmed non-cooks stuck
with the quick and easy options you discovered in Chapter 9. As for the
"I don't mind cooking if it's really, really easy" middle group, they made
a big discovery: Flat Belly Diet Diabetes cooking is easy and delicious.

As test panelist Phil Hernandez told us later, "If I make a recipe, it
can't have more than a handful of ingredients, and they have to be
things I can remember off the top of my head when I'm shopping in
the grocery store. This plan fulfilled those requirements, and as a
result, I ate very, very well!"

Formulated to be healthy and to meet the specific needs of people with diabetes and prediabetes, these recipes were a complete success. And when panelists went on to tell us they were still cooking their favorites months after the plan was over—and serving them to guests and passing the recipes around at work—we knew we really had something special.

Now it's your turn to give 'em a try. The recipes you'll find here are sufficiently gourmet to make your mouth water and get your creative chef juices flowing. But they're also extremely simple. Take the Tortellini Pasta Salad on page 222. It takes 15 minutes! Or the Strawberry-Almond Topped French Toast on page 212—a mere 10 minutes start to finish. And believe me, the flavors will astound you.

But what really makes these recipes extraordinary is not how easy or fast they are to prepare but how well they fit into the Flat Belly Diet Diabetes. Each serving contains several diabetes-fighting ingredients—a fruit or vegetable, whole grains, and lean protein, as well as a MUFA, for starters. As you know, MUFAs are the only foods that can specifically help reduce belly fat. You can spot them in the ingredient lists; they're in boldface.

In addition, beside most recipes is a very important component titled "Make It a Flat Belly Diet Meal." This box tells you what to add to one serving of that recipe to turn it into a meal that you can slot right into your menu plan. Let's say you decide to start your day with a serving of the delicious Asparagus Frittata on page 211. Your MUFA is included (in this case, it's sunflower oil) in the recipe. But remember that every meal on the Flat Belly Diet Diabetes should equal roughly 400 calories. When you sit down to your delicious 221-calorie slice of Asparagus Frittata, you should also add a toasted whole wheat English muffin (135 calories) and 2 teaspoons of margarine (53 calories) to round out the meal and raise it to the appropriate calorie level healthfully. Remember, the numbers in parentheses refer to the calorie counts of specific ingredients.

Confused? Don't be. All you have to do is follow the instructions in the "Make It a Flat Belly Diet Meal" box at the end of each recipe, and you'll stay within the Flat Belly Diet Diabetes rules. Now let's get cookin'.

RECIPE INDEX

Garden Breakfast Wraps

Cooking time: 8 minutes / Makes 4 servings

- 4 spinach-flavored flour tortillas (12" diameter)
- 2 teaspoons trans-free margarine
- 4 eggs + 4 egg whites, beaten
- 1/4 cup grated Parmesan cheese
- 4 cups baby arugula or baby spinach

MUFA: 1 Hass avocado, sliced

Hot-pepper sauce (optional)

1. Preheat a grill pan over medium-high heat. Lightly toast 1 tortilla in the pan about 20 seconds, flip, and cook 10 seconds longer. Set aside on a plate and cover with a slightly damp paper towel. Repeat with the remaining tortillas.

2. Melt the margarine in a large nonstick skillet over medium heat. Pour in the eggs, egg whites, and cheese. Cook, stirring, for 2 minutes. Add the greens. Continue cooking, stirring, for about 1 minute longer, or until the eggs are set and the greens are wilted.

3. Mound one-quarter of the mixture on the bottom half of 1 tortilla, add one-quarter of the sliced avocado, flap up the 2 sides, and roll into a tube. Repeat with remaining tortillas and filling. Cut the wraps diagonally in half and serve with hot-pepper sauce, if desired.

■ Eat One Serving:

344

calories, 22 g protein, 36 g carbohydrates, 17 g fat, 4.5 g saturated fat*, 220 mg cholesterol, 620 mg sodium*, 4 g fiber

MAKE IT A FLAT BELLY DIET MEAL: Serve with 1/2 medium orange (35).

■ Total Meal:

379

calories, 22 g protein, 44 g carbohydrates, 17 g fat, 4.5 g saturated fat*, 220 mg cholesterol, 620 mg sodium*, 4 g fiber

* Limit saturated fat to no more than 10 percent of total calories—about 17 grams per day for most women or 21 grams for most men—and sodium intake to no more than 2,300 milligrams.

Breakfast Tacos

Cooking time: 30 minutes / Makes 4 servings

1 teaspoon ground cumin
1 (15-ounce) can no-salt-added pink beans, rinsed and drained
4 scallions, sliced
1 small red bell pepper, cut into thin strips
½ cup reduced-sodium chicken broth
2 cloves garlic, minced
4 eggs

MUFA: 40 black olives (1⅓ cups), chopped

4 tablespoons fat-free Greek-style yogurt
4 tablespoons salsa
8 (6") corn tortillas, toasted Hot-pepper sauce (optional)

1. Heat a 10" nonstick skillet over medium-high heat. Add the cumin and cook, stirring occasionally, for about 30 seconds, or until fragrant. Add the beans, scallions, bell pepper, broth, and garlic. Bring to a boil, then reduce the heat so the mixture simmers. Cook for 8 minutes, or until the vegetables are tender and most of the broth is evaporated. With the back of a large silicone or wooden spoon, smash the beans until they are lumpy.

2. Use the back of the spoon to make four indentations in the beans. Working one at a time, break each egg into a custard cup and pour in each indentation. Cover and cook for about 8 minutes, or until the eggs are cooked to the desired doneness.

3. Scoop each portion of egg-topped bean mixture onto a plate. Sprinkle the olives over and around the beans. Top each serving with 1 tablespoon of the yogurt and 1 tablespoon of the salsa. Serve with the tortillas and hot-pepper sauce, if desired.

■ Eat One Serving:

315

calories, 15 g protein, 41 g carbohydrates, 11 g fat, 3 g saturated fat, 210 mg cholesterol, 660 mg sodium*, 9 g fiber

MAKE IT A FLAT BELLY DIET MEAL: Serve with 1 medium orange (69).

■ Total Meal:

384

calories, 17 g protein, 51 g carbohydrates, 11 g fat, 3 g saturated fat, 210 mg cholesterol, 800 mg sodium*, 10 g fiber

* Limit saturated fat to no more than 10 percent of total calories—about 17 grams per day for most women or 21 grams for most men—and sodium intake to no more than 2,300 milligrams.

Barbecue Hash

Cooking time: 25 minutes / Makes 4 servings

MUFA: ¼ cup olive oil

3 sweet potatoes, peeled and chopped
1 (8-ounce) package tempeh, chopped
1 onion, finely chopped
1 red bell pepper, finely chopped
1 tablespoon store-bought barbecue sauce
1 teaspoon Cajun seasoning
¼ cup chopped fresh parsley
4 eggs
Hot-pepper sauce (optional)

1. Heat 3 tablespoons of the oil in a large nonstick skillet over medium-high heat. Add the sweet potatoes and tempeh and cook, stirring occasionally, for 5 minutes, or until the mixture begins to brown. Reduce the heat to medium.

2. Add the onion and bell pepper and cook for 12 minutes longer, stirring more frequently at the end of the cooking time, until the tempeh is browned and the potatoes are tender.

3. Add the barbecue sauce, Cajun seasoning, and parsley. Toss to combine, then divide among 4 serving plates.

4. Wipe out the skillet with a paper towel. Reduce the heat to medium-low and add the remaining 1 tablespoon oil. Break the eggs into the skillet and cook to the desired doneness.

5. Slide an egg on top of each portion of the hash and serve at once. Pass hot-pepper sauce, if desired, at the table.

■ Eat One Serving:

388

calories, 15 g protein, 36 g carbohydrates, 21 g fat, 4 g saturated fat*, 210 mg cholesterol, 190 mg sodium, 7 g fiber

A SINGLE SERVING OF THIS RECIPE COUNTS as a Flat Belly Diet Meal without any add-ons!

* Limit saturated fat to no more than 10 percent of total calories—about 17 grams per day for most women or 21 grams for most men—and sodium intake to no more than 2,300 milligrams.

Olive and Herb Frittata

Cooking time: 45 minutes / Makes 4 servings

1 teaspoon olive oil, preferably extra-virgin
¾ cup chopped red bell pepper
¾ cup chopped green bell pepper
¾ cup (3 ounces) shredded reduced-fat Monterey Jack cheese
2 tablespoons chopped fresh basil
5 eggs + 2 egg whites, lightly beaten

MUFA: 40 black olives (1⅓ cups), chopped

¼ teaspoon salt
Ground black pepper

1. Preheat the oven to 375°F. Coat a 9″ ovenproof skillet with vegetable oil spray. Place over medium-high heat. Add the oil. Heat for 30 seconds. Add the bell peppers. Cook, stirring occasionally, for about 5 minutes, or until just soft. Sprinkle the cheese and basil into the pan. Add the eggs, egg whites, olives, salt, and pepper.

2. Bake for about 30 minutes, or until the eggs are set. Let stand to cool slightly. Cut into wedges.

■ **Eat One Serving:**

232

calories, 16 g protein, 8 g carbohydrates, 16 g fat, 5 g saturated fat*, 285 mg cholesterol, 820 mg sodium*, 1 g fiber

MAKE IT A FLAT BELLY DIET MEAL:

Serve with 1 whole wheat English muffin (135) and 2 teaspoons trans-free margarine (53).

■ **Total Meal:**

420

calories, 21 g protein, 35 g carbohydrates, 23 g fat, 6 g saturated fat*, 285 mg cholesterol, 1,300 mg sodium*, 7 g fiber

* Limit saturated fat to no more than 10 percent of total calories—about 17 grams per day for most women or 21 grams for most men—and sodium intake to no more than 2,300 milligrams.

Asparagus Frittata

Cooking time: 25 minutes / Makes 4 servings

MUFA: ¼ cup sunflower oil

½ pound asparagus, cut into 1" pieces
¼ onion, finely chopped
4 eggs
2 egg whites
2 tablespoons cold water
2 teaspoons freshly grated orange zest
¼ teaspoon salt
Freshly ground black pepper

1. Preheat the oven to 350°F. Heat a 10" nonstick ovenproof skillet over medium heat for 1 minute. Add the oil and heat for 30 seconds. Add the asparagus and onion. Cook, stirring, for about 2 minutes, or until the asparagus is bright green.

2. Meanwhile, whisk the eggs, egg whites, water, orange zest, and salt. Pour into the pan and cook for 2 minutes, or until starting to set on the bottom. Use a silicone spatula to lift up the set edges and allow the uncooked mixture to run underneath. Season well with the pepper.

3. Transfer to the oven and bake for 6 minutes. Use the spatula to lift the edge of the egg mixture, and tip the pan to allow any uncooked egg and oil to run underneath. Bake for about 6 minutes longer, or until puffed and golden.

■ Eat One Serving:

221

calories, 9 g protein, 4 g carbohydrates, 19 g fat, 3 g saturated fat, 215 mg cholesterol, 240 mg sodium, 1 g fiber

MAKE IT A FLAT BELLY DIET MEAL:

Serve with 1 whole wheat English muffin (135) and 2 teaspoons trans-free margarine (53).

■ Total Meal:

409

calories, 15 g protein, 31 g carbohydrates, 26 g fat, 4 g saturated fat*, 215 mg cholesterol, 720 mg sodium*, 6 g fiber

* Limit saturated fat to no more than 10 percent of total calories—about 17 grams per day for most women or 21 grams for most men—and sodium intake to no more than 2,300 milligrams.

Strawberry-Almond Topped French Toast

Cooking time: 10 minutes / Makes 1 serving

1 egg
¼ cup fat-free milk
¼ teaspoon ground cinnamon
1 slice whole grain bread
1 teaspoon trans-free margarine
½ cup sliced strawberries

MUFA: 2 tablespoons sliced almonds, toasted

1. Beat the egg in a shallow bowl with the milk and cinnamon. Dip both sides of the bread in the egg mixture.

2. Melt the margarine in a nonstick skillet over medium heat. Cook the bread for about 2 to 3 minutes per side, or until golden. Cut in half diagonally. Place half on a plate. Top with half of the strawberries and almonds. Cover with the other toast half and the remaining strawberries and almonds.

■ **Eat One Serving**

304

calories, 16 g protein, 26 g carbohydrates, 16 g fat, 3 g saturated fat, 210 mg cholesterol, 270 mg sodium, 5 g fiber

MAKE IT A FLAT BELLY DIET MEAL: Serve with 3 slices Applegate Farms Organic Turkey Bacon (105).

■ **Total Meal:**

409

calories, 34 g protein, 26 g carbohydrates, 20 g fat, 3 g saturated fat, 285 mg cholesterol, 270 mg sodium, 5 g fiber

Chocolate Chip Pancakes

Cooking time: 25 minutes / Makes 12 servings

²/₃ cup whole
  wheat flour
²/₃ cup unbleached
  all-purpose
  flour
¹/₃ cup cornmeal
  1 tablespoon
  baking powder
¹/₂ teaspoon
  baking soda
  2 cups nonfat
  vanilla yogurt
³/₄ cup fat-free egg
  substitute

**MUFA: 3 cups
semisweet mini
chocolate chips**

  2 tablespoons
  canola oil
³/₄ cup nondairy
  whipped
  topping

1. Combine the flours, cornmeal, baking powder, and baking soda in a large bowl. Stir in the yogurt, egg substitute, chocolate chips, and oil.

2. Coat a large nonstick skillet with cooking spray and heat over medium heat.

3. For each pancake, spoon 2 tablespoons of the batter into the skillet. Cook pancakes for 2 minutes, or until bubbles appear on the surface and edges set. Flip and cook until lightly browned, about 2 minutes longer. Repeat with the remaining batter.

4. Top each pancake with 1 teaspoon whipped topping.

**■ Eat One Serving
(4 pancakes per
serving):**

344

calories, 7 g protein, 48 g carbohydrates, 17 g fat, 9 g saturated fat*, 0 mg cholesterol, 220 mg sodium, 4 g fiber

**MAKE IT A FLAT
BELLY DIET MEAL:**

Serve with 2 slices Applegate Farms Organic Turkey Bacon (70).

■ Total Meal:

414

calories, 19 g protein, 48 g carbohydrates, 20 g fat, 9 g saturated fat*, 50 mg cholesterol, 220 mg sodium, 4 g fiber

* Limit saturated fat to no more than 10 percent of total calories—about 17 grams per day for most women or 21 grams for most men—and sodium intake to no more than 2,300 milligrams.

Chocolate Walnut Waffles

Cooking time: 35 minutes / Makes 6 servings

1½ cups whole grain pastry flour
½ cup unsweetened cocoa powder
2 teaspoons baking powder
¼ teaspoon baking soda
1 cup 1% milk
½ cup packed brown sugar
2 teaspoons espresso powder
3 tablespoons light olive oil
3 egg whites
⅛ teaspoon salt
3 tablespoons maple syrup

MUFA: ¾ cup walnuts, toasted and chopped

1. Whisk together the flour, cocoa powder, baking powder, and baking soda in a large bowl until combined. Make a well in the center of the flour mixture and add the milk, sugar, espresso powder, and oil. Whisk the ingredients together until blended.

2. Preheat a waffle iron for 4 minutes, or according to the manufacturer's instructions. (A drop of water should sizzle and bounce when dropped on the iron.) Meanwhile, beat the egg whites and salt with an electric mixer at high speed just until they form soft peaks. Fold the whites into the chocolate batter in 3 additions, folding just until the mixture is combined.

3. Coat the heated waffle grids with cooking spray right before using. Add enough batter to almost cover the waffle grids (⅔ cup) and cook for 3 to 4 minutes. Repeat with the remaining batter. (To keep warm, place a single layer of waffles on a foil-lined baking sheet in a preheated 250°F oven.) Serve each waffle topped with ½ tablespoon maple syrup and 2 tablespoons walnuts.

■ **Eat One Serving (1 waffle per serving):**

379

calories, 10 g protein, 50 g carbohydrates, 18 g fat, 2.5 g saturated fat, 0 mg cholesterol, 290 mg sodium, 7 g fiber

A SINGLE SERVING OF THIS RECIPE COUNTS as a Flat Belly Diet Meal without any add-ons!

Chilled Summer Soup

Cooking time: 45 minutes + chilling time / Makes 4 servings

4 large carrots, coarsely chopped

2 cans (14½ ounces each) reduced-sodium chicken broth

1 large yellow summer squash, chopped

½ small red onion, chopped

1 clove garlic

¾ teaspoon ground cumin

½ teaspoon salt

¼ teaspoon ground coriander

¼ teaspoon ground black pepper

¾ cup low-fat plain yogurt

MUFA: 1 Hass avocado, pitted and sliced

Fresh chives, cut in ¼" lengths (optional)

1. Combine the carrots and broth in a large covered saucepan and bring to a boil. Reduce the heat to medium and simmer about 7 minutes, or until the carrots begin to soften.

2. Add the squash, onion, garlic, cumin, salt, coriander, and pepper. Cover and raise heat to high. As soon as the mixture begins to boil, reduce the heat to low and simmer for 15 to 20 minutes, or until the vegetables are very tender and the flavors are blended.

3. In the bowl of a food processor fitted with a metal blade, in a blender, or with an immersion blender, puree the soup until smooth. Pour into a bowl, cover, and refrigerate for 1 hour.

4. Stir the yogurt into the soup until combined. Garnish each serving with ¼ of the avocado slices and chives, if desired.

■ **Eat One Serving (1½ cups per serving):**

146

calories, 7 g protein, 18 g carbohydrates, 7 g fat, 1.5 g saturated fat, 5 mg cholesterol, 470 mg sodium, 6 g fiber

MAKE IT A FLAT BELLY DIET MEAL:

Top 2 slices of whole grain bread (140) with 2 tablespoons light mayonnaise (33), 2 ounces deli turkey (53), and 1 ounce low-fat Cheddar cheese (50).

■ **Total Meal:**

422

calories, 29 g protein, 50 g carbohydrates, 15 g fat, 3 g saturated fat, 37 mg cholesterol, 1,712 mg sodium*, 10g fiber

* Limit saturated fat to no more than 10 percent of total calories—about 17 grams per day for most women or 21 grams for most men—and sodium intake to no more than 2,300 milligrams.

Tomato Avocado Soup

Cooking time: 1 hour 15 minutes/ Makes 4 servings

1 can (28 ounces) whole tomatoes
½ sweet onion, sliced
1 cup reduced-sodium vegetable broth
1 cup water
½ teaspoon ground pepper
1 cup buttermilk
¼ cup fat-free Greek-style yogurt

MUFA: 1 Hass avocado, sliced

1. Preheat the oven to 350°F.

2. Pour the tomatoes (with juice) into an 11″ x 17″ baking dish. Scatter the onion on top and bake for 1 hour, or until the mixture is thick and the onion begins to brown.

3. Transfer the mixture to a blender. Add the broth, water, and pepper and puree until smooth.

4. Heat the soup mixture in a pot over medium-low heat for 5 minutes, or until heated through. Add the buttermilk and stir to combine.

5. Garnish each serving with 1 tablespoon of the yogurt and ¼ of the avocado slices.

■ Eat One Serving (1¼ cups per serving):

155

calories, 6 g protein, 19 g carbohydrates, 6 g fat, 1 g saturated fat, 0 mg cholesterol, 500 mg sodium, 5 g fiber

MAKE IT A FLAT BELLY DIET MEAL:

Serve with a grilled cheese sandwich made from 2 slices of whole grain bread (140) and a slice of reduced-fat provolone (75) cooked in 2 teaspoons of trans-free margarine (52).

■ Total Meal:

422

calories, 19 g protein, 42 g carbohydrates, 19 g fat, 6 g saturated fat*, 20 mg cholesterol, 1,010 mg sodium*, 9 g fiber

* Limit saturated fat to no more than 10 percent of total calories—about 17 grams per day for most women or 21 grams for most men—and sodium intake to no more than 2,300 milligrams.

African Peanut Soup

Cooking time: 1 hour / Makes 4 servings

1 tablespoon canola oil
1 onion, chopped
2 ribs celery, chopped
2 carrots, chopped
1 clove garlic, minced
1 tablespoon grated ginger
3 cups reduced-sodium vegetable broth

MUFA: ½ cup creamy natural unsalted peanut butter

2 tablespoons freshly squeezed lemon juice
2 tablespoons chopped unsalted peanuts
2 tablespoons chopped fresh cilantro

1. Heat the oil in a large pot or Dutch oven over medium-high heat. Add the onion, celery, and carrots. Cook, stirring occasionally, for 5 minutes, or until the onion softens.

2. Add the garlic, ginger, and 2 cups of the broth. Reduce the heat to low, cover, and simmer for 30 minutes, or until the vegetables are very tender.

3. Transfer the soup to a food processor fitted with a metal blade or a blender (in batches, if necessary). Process until smooth.

4. Return the soup to the pot and stir in the peanut butter, lemon juice, and remaining 1 cup broth. Cook for 5 minutes, or until the peanut butter melts and the flavors blend.

5. Garnish each serving with the chopped nuts and cilantro.

■ Eat One Serving (1¼ cups per serving):

300

calories, 9 g protein, 18 g carbohydrates, 22 g fat, 2.5 g saturated fat, 0 mg cholesterol, 160 mg sodium, 5 g fiber

MAKE IT A FLAT BELLY DIET MEAL:

Serve with a baked sweet potato (103) and ½ cup cooked greens (25).

■ Total Meal:

428

calories, 13 g protein, 45 g carbohydrates, 22 g fat, 2.5 g saturated fat, 0 mg cholesterol, 500 mg sodium, 11 g fiber

Lentil Soup

Cooking time: 45 minutes / Makes 4 servings

1 tablespoon olive oil

1½ teaspoons whole cumin seeds

1 large onion, chopped

4 cloves garlic, minced

½ teaspoon ground coriander

½ teaspoon freshly ground black pepper

1 teaspoon paprika

1⅓ cups (½ pound) lentils, sorted and rinsed

5 cups water

1 can (14½ ounces) diced tomatoes

2 cups packed shredded fresh spinach

MUFA: ½ cup unsalted peanuts, chopped

½ teaspoon salt

½ cup fat-free Greek-style yogurt

1. Place the oil and cumin seeds in a Dutch oven or heavy large saucepan over medium heat.

2. Cook, stirring, for 2 to 3 minutes, or until fragrant. Stir in the onion, garlic, coriander, and pepper and cook, stirring often, for 4 to 6 minutes, or until the onion and garlic are tender. Stir in the paprika.

3. Add the lentils and water. Cover and bring to a boil. Reduce the heat to low and simmer, covered, for 30 to 35 minutes, or until the lentils are very tender.

4. Stir in the tomatoes, spinach, peanuts, and salt. Increase the heat and simmer, uncovered, for 5 minutes longer.

5. Garnish each serving with 2 tablespoons of yogurt.

▪ Eat One Serving (2 cups per serving):

402

calories, 24 g protein, 48 g carbohydrates, 13 g fat, 2 g saturated fat, 0 mg cholesterol, 370 mg sodium, 21 g fiber

A SINGLE SERVING OF THIS RECIPE COUNTS as a Flat Belly Diet Meal without any add-ons!

Italian Greens and Bean Soup

Cooking time: 45 minutes / Makes 8 servings

1 tablespoon olive oil
1 large onion, chopped
4 carrots, chopped
1 can (14½ ounces) diced tomatoes with roasted garlic (juice reserved)
2 cans (14½ ounces each) reduced-sodium chicken broth
3 cans (15 ounces each) no-salt-added cannellini beans, rinsed and drained
1 tablespoon chopped dried rosemary
3 cups water
½ pound escarole, coarsely chopped
½ teaspoon salt
½ cup grated Romano cheese

MUFA: ½ cup pesto

1. Heat the olive oil in a large pot over medium-high heat. Cook the onion and carrots for 10 minutes, or until vegetables soften.

2. Add the tomatoes and their juice, broth, beans, rosemary, and 3 cups water. Cover and cook about 10 minutes, or until the mixture begins to simmer.

3. Reduce heat and add the escarole and salt. Cook, uncovered, 15 minutes longer, or until flavors combine. Stir in the cheese.

4. Spoon 1 tablespoon of pesto into the center of each serving.

■ **Eat One Serving (1 cup per serving):**

266

calories, 14 g protein, 26 g carbohydrates, 12 g fat, 3.5 g saturated fat, 10 mg cholesterol, 660 mg sodium*, 8 g fiber

MAKE IT A FLAT BELLY DIET MEAL: Serve with 3 ounces lean Italian turkey sausage (140).

■ **Total Meal:**

406

calories, 37 g protein, 26 g carbohydrates, 18 g fat, 5 g saturated fat*, 45 mg cholesterol, 660 mg sodium*, 8 g fiber

* Limit saturated fat to no more than 10 percent of total calories—about 17 grams per day for most women or 21 grams for most men—and sodium intake to no more than 2,300 milligrams.

Cheese-Free Beef Onion Soup

Cooking time: 1 hour 20 minutes / Makes 4 servings

MUFA: 4 tablespoons safflower oil

- 8 ounces beef tenderloin, trimmed
- 3 large onions, thinly sliced
- 2 teaspoons sugar
- 2 cloves garlic, minced
- 2 tablespoons balsamic vinegar
- 4 cups reduced-sodium beef broth
- 1 teaspoon Worcestershire sauce
- 1 slice day-old whole wheat bread
  Chives (optional)

1. Heat 1 tablespoon of the oil in a large pot over medium-high heat. Add the beef and cook for about 2 to 3 minutes per side for medium rare. Transfer to a cutting board and let stand for 5 minutes. Slice across the grain into thin strips.

2. Add the remaining 3 tablespoons oil to the pot and reduce the heat to medium. Add the onions and sugar and cook, stirring occasionally, about 25 minutes, or until golden.

3. Add the garlic and cook for 2 minutes.

4. Increase heat to medium-high, pour in the vinegar, and bring to a boil. Cook, stirring constantly, for about 1 minute, or until the vinegar is almost completely evaporated.

5. Add the broth and Worcestershire sauce. Bring to a boil, reduce to a simmer, and cook, covered, for 15 minutes.

6. Tear the bread into chunks and whirl in the food processor to form crumbs. Stir the crumbs into the soup and cook for 2 to 3 minutes, or until slightly thickened.

7. Top each serving with an equal portion of the reserved beef slices and garnish with chives, if desired.

■ **Eat One Serving (1¼ cups per serving):**

314

calories, 18 g protein, 20 g carbohydrates, 18 g fat, 2 g saturated fat, 33 mg cholesterol, 528 mg sodium, 2 g fiber

MAKE IT A FLAT BELLY DIET MEAL: Serve with 1 slice whole grain French bread, toasted and rubbed with garlic (93).

■ **Total Meal:**

407

calories, 22 g protein, 38 g carbohydrates, 19 g fat, 2.5 g saturated fat, 40 mg cholesterol, 740 mg sodium*, 3 g fiber

* Limit saturated fat to no more than 10 percent of total calories—about 17 grams per day for most women or 21 grams for most men—and sodium intake to no more than 2,300 milligrams.

Broccoli-Pecan Salad

Cooking time: 15 minutes/ Makes 4 servings

3 tablespoons canola oil mayonnaise

1 tablespoon red or white wine vinegar

⅛ teaspoon salt

2 cups broccoli florets

MUFA: ½ cup pecans, toasted

¼ cup slivered red onion

¼ teaspoon red-pepper flakes

1. Combine the mayonnaise, vinegar, and salt in a large serving bowl. Whisk until smooth.

2. Add the broccoli, pecans, onion, and red-pepper flakes. Toss to coat. Refrigerate until ready to serve.

■ **Eat One Serving:**

191

calories, 3 g protein, 5 g carbohydrates, 19 g fat, 1.5 g saturated fat, 5 mg cholesterol, 150 mg sodium, 3 g fiber

MAKE IT A FLAT BELLY DIET MEAL: Serve with the Turkey Panini with Avocado, Tomato, and Dijon on page 234, but omit the avocado (190).

■ **Total Meal:**

381

calories, 19 g protein, 26 g carbohydrates, 23 g fat, 1.5 g saturated fat, 25 mg cholesterol, 810 mg sodium*, 5 g fiber

* Limit saturated fat to no more than 10 percent of total calories—about 17 grams per day for most women or 21 grams for most men—and sodium intake to no more than 2,300 milligrams.

Tortellini Pasta Salad

Cooking time: 15 minutes / Makes 4 servings

1 package
(9 ounces)
refrigerated
tricolor cheese
tortellini
2 cups trimmed
sugar snap peas
2 cups baby
carrots
2 cups broccoli
florets
2 tablespoons
pesto
1 cup cherry
tomatoes,
halved

MUFA: 40 chopped black olives

¼ teaspoon
ground black
pepper
Fresh basil
(optional)

1. Place the tortellini into a large pot of boiling water. Cook according to package directions, stirring occasionally. Add the sugar snap peas, carrots, and broccoli and cook for the last 3 minutes, or until tender but still crisp.

2. Drain the pasta and vegetables, and rinse with cold water. Place into a large bowl and toss with the pesto. Gently fold in the tomatoes, olives, and pepper. Garnish with basil, if using.

■ **Eat One Serving:**

367

calories, 15 g protein, 50 g carbohydrates, 13 g fat, 4 g saturated fat*, 30 mg cholesterol, 780 mg sodium*, 8 g fiber

A SINGLE SERVING OF THIS RECIPE COUNTS as a Flat Belly Diet Meal without any add-ons!

* Limit saturated fat to no more than 10 percent of total calories—about 17 grams per day for most women or 21 grams for most men—and sodium intake to no more than 2,300 milligrams.

Barley and Bean Salad

Cooking time: 55 minutes / Makes 6 servings

1 cup barley
3 tablespoons olive oil
1 leek, white and light green parts only, thinly sliced
½ butternut squash, peeled and chopped (about 2 cups)
¼ cup water
3 tablespoons chopped fresh parsley
1 can (15 ounces) no-salt-added black beans, rinsed and drained
½ teaspoon salt

MUFA: ¾ cup pine nuts, toasted

2 tablespoons lemon juice
¼ teaspoon ground black pepper
Grated lemon peel (optional)

1. Cook the barley according to the package directions. Drain, if necessary, and set aside.

2. Meanwhile, heat 2 tablespoons of the oil in a large nonstick skillet over medium-high heat. Add the leek and squash and cook, tossing or stirring, until slightly softened and lightly browned, about 10 minutes. Add the water and half of the parsley and cook 2 to 3 minutes longer. Transfer the vegetables to a large bowl.

3. Add the barley, black beans, salt, and the remaining 1 tablespoon oil and remaining parsley. Stir to combine. Add in pine nuts. Season with lemon juice and pepper. Garnish with lemon peel, if desired.

■ **Eat One Serving:**

348

calories, 10 g protein, 38 g carbohydrates, 19 g fat, 2 g saturated fat, 0 mg cholesterol, 210 mg sodium, 10 g fiber

MAKE IT A FLAT BELLY DIET MEAL:
Serve with 1 tangerine (47).

■ **Total Meal:**

395

calories, 10 g protein, 50 g carbohydrates, 19 g fat, 2 g saturated fat, 0 mg cholesterol, 210 mg sodium, 10 g fiber

Spinach Salad with Avocado, Fresh Mozzarella, and Strawberry Dressing

Cooking time: 25 minutes / Makes 4 servings

- 2 cups hulled and sliced strawberries
- 2 tablespoons extra-virgin olive oil
- 2 tablespoons honey
- 1 tablespoon + 1 teaspoon balsamic vinegar
- $\frac{1}{2}$ teaspoon salt
- $\frac{1}{8}$ teaspoon freshly ground black pepper
- 1 bag (6 ounces) baby spinach
- 1 ripe medium mango, peeled and cut in small chunks
- 5 ounces fresh mozzarella, cut in small chunks

MUFA: 1 Hass avocado, peeled and cut in small chunks

- 3 tablespoons chopped almonds, toasted

1. Put $\frac{1}{2}$ cup of the strawberries, the oil, honey, and balsamic vinegar in a food processor. Process until smooth. Scrape into a salad bowl and stir in the salt and pepper.

2. Add the spinach, mango, and remaining 1$\frac{1}{2}$ cups strawberries to the dressing and toss to mix well. Sprinkle the mozzarella, avocado, and almonds over the top.

■ **Eat One Serving:**

370

calories, 11 g protein, 40 g carbohydrates, 25 g fat, 7 g saturated fat*, 25 mg cholesterol, 470 mg sodium, 8 g fiber

A SINGLE SERVING OF THIS RECIPE COUNTS as a Flat Belly Diet Meal without any add-ons!

French Lentil Salad with Goat Cheese

Cooking time: 40 minutes / Makes 4 servings

1 cup French or
brown lentils
3 cups reduced-
sodium
vegetable broth
2 bay leaves
2 whole cloves
garlic, peeled

**MUFA: 1/4 cup
walnut oil**

2 tablespoons red
wine vinegar
1/4 teaspoon salt
1/4 teaspoon
freshly ground
black pepper
1 carrot,
shredded
2 tablespoons
chopped
parsley
1 log (4 ounces)
herbed goat
cheese
Ground
coriander

1. Combine the lentils, broth, bay leaves, and garlic in a medium pot and bring to a boil over medium-high heat. As soon as the lentils reach the boiling point, reduce the heat so the mixture simmers. Cover and simmer for 25 to 30 minutes, or until the lentils are tender. Drain any excess broth. Set aside the garlic cloves. Discard the bay leaves. Spread the lentils on a tray to cool.

2. Combine the oil, vinegar, salt, pepper, and reserved garlic cloves in a salad bowl. Whisk, smashing the garlic, until smooth. Add the lentils, carrot, and parsley. Toss to coat. Spoon the mixture onto 4 plates.

3. Cut the cheese into 4 slices. Lay flat. Dust both sides lightly with coriander. Place on a microwaveable dish. Microwave on medium for about 30 seconds, or just until the cheese is warm. Set a piece of cheese on each salad.

■ Eat One Serving:

394

calories, 17 g protein, 32 g carbohydrates, 22 g fat, 7 g saturated fat*, 22 mg cholesterol, 422 mg sodium, 8 g fiber

A SINGLE SERVING OF THIS RECIPE COUNTS as a Flat Belly Diet Meal without any add-ons!

* Limit saturated fat to no more than 10 percent of total calories—about 17 grams per day for most women or 21 grams for most men—and sodium intake to no more than 2,300 milligrams.

Easy Egg Salad Platter

Cooking time: 20 minutes / Makes 4 servings

6 large eggs, hard-boiled and peeled (discard 3 yolks)

3 ribs celery, chopped

½ cup peeled, chopped hothouse cucumber

3 radishes, chopped

2 scallions, thinly sliced, or ¼ cup chopped sweet white onion

MUFA: ¼ cup canola oil mayonnaise

2 tablespoons snipped fresh dill

½ teaspoon grainy mustard

½ teaspoon freshly ground black pepper

⅛ teaspoon salt Leaf lettuce, for serving

2 large tomatoes, cut into wedges

8 Wasa crispbreads, for serving

1. Coarsely chop the eggs and egg whites and place in a medium bowl. Add the celery, cucumber, radishes, scallions, mayonnaise, dill, mustard, pepper, and salt and mix well.

2. Arrange the lettuce leaves on a platter or plates. Mound the salad on top and surround with the tomato wedges. Serve with the crispbreads.

■ Eat One Serving:

277

calories, 13 g protein, 22 g carbohydrates, 16 g fat, 2 g saturated fat, 165 mg cholesterol, 400 mg sodium, 5 g fiber

MAKE IT A FLAT BELLY DIET MEAL:
Serve with 4 ounces broiled shrimp (112) and 1 medium plum (33).

■ Total Meal:

422

calories, 37 g protein, 30 g carbohydrates, 16 g fat, 4.5 g saturated fat, 120 mg cholesterol, 325 mg sodium*, 6 g fiber

* Limit saturated fat to no more than 10 percent of total calories—about 17 grams per day for most women or 21 grams for most men—and sodium intake to no more than 2,300 milligrams.

Classic Greek Shrimp Salad

Cooking time: 20 minutes + standing time / Makes 4 servings

- 2 tablespoons olive oil
- 1 tablespoon lemon juice
- 1 tablespoon red wine vinegar
- ½ teaspoon dried oregano, crumbled
- ½ teaspoon freshly ground black pepper
- 2 large red tomatoes, cut into chunks
- 1 can (15 ounces) chickpeas, rinsed and drained
- 2 cups peeled, chopped cucumber
- ½ cup thinly sliced red onion
- ½ cup coarsely chopped fresh flat-leaf parsley

MUFA: 40 kalamata olives (1⅓ cups), pitted and sliced

- ¾ pound peeled cooked shrimp, thawed if frozen
- 4 cups torn mixed greens, such as escarole and romaine lettuce
- 2 ounces feta cheese, chopped

1. Combine the oil, lemon juice, vinegar, oregano, and pepper in a large salad bowl and mix with a fork until blended.

2. Add the tomatoes, chickpeas, cucumber, red onion, parsley, olives, and shrimp. Toss to mix well. Let salad sit for 15 minutes to allow time for flavors to combine.

3. Add the greens and feta and toss again.

■ **Eat One Serving:**

416

calories, 30 g protein, 25 g carbohydrates, 23 g fat, 4.5 g saturated fat*, 185 mg cholesterol, 1,120 mg sodium*, 7 g fiber

A SINGLE SERVING OF THIS RECIPE COUNTS as a Flat Belly Diet Meal without any add-ons!

* Limit saturated fat to no more than 10 percent of total calories—about 17 grams per day for most women or 21 grams for most men—and sodium intake to no more than 2,300 milligrams.

Curried Barley and Shrimp Salad

Cooking time: 1 hour / Makes 6 servings

1 cup barley
1 teaspoon curry powder
½ teaspoon turmeric
Juice of 4 limes
1 tablespoon vegetable oil
½ jalapeño chile pepper, seeded and finely chopped
1 clove garlic, minced
¼ teaspoon salt
1 pound cooked shrimp, peeled and deveined
2 tomatoes, seeded and chopped (about 1½ cups)
1 green bell pepper, seeded and chopped
1 cucumber, peeled, seeded and chopped
12 cups baby greens
¼ cup chopped fresh basil

MUFA: ¾ cup macadamia nuts, toasted

2 ounces semisoft goat cheese, crumbled

1. Bring 3 cups of water to a boil in a large saucepan. Stir in the barley, curry, and turmeric. Cover and reduce the heat to low. Cook for about 45 minutes, or until the water is absorbed and the barley is tender. Remove from the heat and let sit uncovered to cool slightly.

2. Meanwhile, whisk together the lime juice, oil, chile pepper, garlic, and salt in a large bowl. Add the shrimp, tomatoes, bell pepper, cucumber, and barley. Toss to coat.

2. Place 2 cups of baby greens on each of 6 plates. Divide the salad evenly on top of the greens and sprinkle with the basil, macadamia nuts, and goat cheese.

■ **Eat One Serving:**

402

calories, 25 g protein, 37 g carbohydrates, 20 g fat, 4.5 g saturated fat*, 120 mg cholesterol, 280 mg sodium, 10 g fiber

A SINGLE SERVING OF THIS RECIPE COUNTS as a Flat Belly Diet Meal without any add-ons!

* Limit saturated fat to no more than 10 percent of total calories—about 17 grams per day for most women or 21 grams for most men—and sodium intake to no more than 2,300 milligrams.

Mushroom, Zucchini, and Avocado Sandwich with Artichoke Tapenade

Cooking time: 40 minutes / Makes 2 servings

ARTICHOKE TAPENADE

1 cup canned artichoke
Juice of ½ lemon
1 tablespoon olive oil
1 teaspoon minced garlic
1 teaspoon white vinegar
¼ teaspoon salt
Ground black pepper, to taste

MUSHROOM, ZUCCHINI, AND AVOCADO SANDWICH

2 portobello mushroom caps
1 zucchini, cut in 3" segments, then sliced lengthwise
2 tablespoons olive oil
1 medium tomato, sliced
2 multigrain rolls, insides scooped out

MUFA: ¼ Florida avocado, sliced

2 ounces fresh goat cheese

1. To prepare the tapenade: Combine all tapenade ingredients in the bowl of a food processor fitted with a metal blade. Pulse about 8 times, scraping down the sides of the bowl as needed, or until the mixture is spreadable. Season to taste with additional pepper. Set aside 2 tablespoons. Refrigerate remainder in an airtight container for use in other recipes for up to 3 days.

2. To prepare the sandwich: Preheat the oven to 400°F. Arrange the mushrooms and zucchini on a nonstick baking sheet. Drizzle with 1 tablespoon olive oil. Roast for 10 minutes. Arrange the tomato slices on the same baking sheet, drizzle with the remaining tablespoon of olive oil, and continue roasting, flipping the vegetables halfway through cooking, for 20 minutes, or until sizzling and any liquid is cooked away.

3. Divide the sandwich fillings between the rolls or bread, layering the mushrooms, then zucchini, avocado, cheese, tomato, and tapenade. Serve with an orange on the side.

■ **Eat One Serving:**

400

calories, 16 g protein, 50 g carbohydrates, 19 g fat, 7.5 g saturated fat*, 22 mg cholesterol, 403 mg sodium, 16 g fiber

A SINGLE SERVING OF THIS RECIPE COUNTS as a Flat Belly Diet Meal without any add-ons!

* Limit saturated fat to no more than 10 percent of total calories—about 17 grams per day for most women or 21 grams for most men—and sodium intake to no more than 2,300 milligrams.

Grilled Mushroom Burgers

Cooking time: 10 minutes / Makes 2 servings

2 large portobello mushroom caps (8 ounces total), stems removed

4 teaspoons balsamic vinegar

½ cup roasted red bell pepper strips

2 100% whole wheat buns

MUFA: 2 tablespoons pesto

2 slices (¾ ounce each) Provolone

4 leaves frisée lettuce

1. Preheat a grill pan over medium heat.

2. Grill the mushrooms for 8 minutes, turning halfway during cooking and brushing with the vinegar. Warm the pepper strips and buns on the grill pan.

3. Spread 1 tablespoon pesto on each bun bottom, then place a mushroom topped with 1 slice of cheese and half the pepper slices. Place 2 frisée leaves on top of each burger, drizzle with additional vinegar, if desired, and cap with bun top.

■ **Eat One Serving:**

318

calories, 16 g protein, 33 g carbohydrates, 15 g fat, 6 g saturated fat*, 20 mg cholesterol, 670 mg sodium*, 6 g fiber

MAKE IT A FLAT BELLY DIET MEAL: Serve with ½ cup 1% low-fat cottage cheese (81) and ¼ cup pineapple chunks canned in their own juice (27).

■ **Total Meal:**

426

calories, 30 g protein, 43 g carbohydrates, 16 g fat, 7 g saturated fat*, 25 mg cholesterol, 1,130 mg sodium*, 7 g fiber

* Limit saturated fat to no more than 10 percent of total calories—about 17 grams per day for most women or 21 grams for most men—and sodium intake to no more than 2,300 milligrams.

Olive–Cream Cheese Sandwiches

Cooking time: 10 minutes / Makes 4 servings

1 package
(8 ounces)
Neufchâtel
cheese,
softened

**MUFA: 40
pimiento-stuffed
green olives,
chopped (about 1⅓
cups)**

4 scallions,
minced
¼ teaspoon hot-
pepper sauce
(optional)
12 lower-sodium
wheat crackers
2 plum tomatoes,
thinly sliced

1. Combine the cheese, olives, scallions, and hot-pepper sauce, if desired, in a small bowl.

2. Spread on the crackers. Top with the tomatoes.

■ **Eat One Serving:**

373

calories, 10 g protein, 38 g carbohydrates, 21 g fat, 9 g saturated fat*, 40 mg cholesterol, 1,290 mg sodium*, 4 g fiber

MAKE IT A FLAT BELLY DIET MEAL:
Serve with ½ cup seedless green grapes (52).

■ **Total Meal:**

425

calories, 11 g protein, 52 g carbohydrates, 21 g fat, 9 g saturated fat*, 40 mg cholesterol, 1,290 mg sodium*, 5 g fiber

* Limit saturated fat to no more than 10 percent of total calories—about 17 grams per day for most women or 21 grams for most men—and sodium intake to no more than 2,300 milligrams.

Salmon Sandwiches with Wasabi and Pickled Ginger

Cooking time: 8 minutes / Makes 4 servings

MUFA: ¼ cup canola oil mayonnaise

¼–½ teaspoon wasabi paste
2 cups (14.75-ounce can) canned Alaskan wild salmon, drained
8 thin slices 100% whole wheat bread, toasted
4 thin slices red onion
4 thin rings red bell pepper
4 teaspoons sliced pickled ginger
1 cup arugula

1. Combine the mayonnaise and ¼ teaspoon of the wasabi paste and stir until smooth. Add more wasabi, if desired, to suit your taste. Gently fold in the salmon.

2. Place 4 slices of the bread on a work surface and top each with ½ cup of the salmon mixture, 1 onion slice separated into rings, 1 pepper ring, 1 teaspoon ginger, and ¼ cup arugula. Top with the remaining 4 slices of bread.

■ **Eat One Serving:**

350

calories, 17 g protein, 28 g carbohydrates, 18 g fat, 1.5 g saturated fat, 40 mg cholesterol, 390 mg sodium, 5 g fiber

MAKE IT A FLAT BELLY DIET MEAL:

Serve with ¼ cup frozen, thawed shelled edamame (61).

■ **Total Meal:**

411

calories, 21 g protein, 32 g carbohydrates, 20 g fat, 1.5 g saturated fat, 40 mg cholesterol, 390 mg sodium, 7 g fiber

Cheesy Chicken Sandwich

Cooking time: 10 minutes / Makes 1 serving

MUFA: 1 tablespoon canola oil

- 2 corn tortillas (6" diameter)
- 1 slice (¾ ounce) reduced-fat Cheddar cheese
- 1 ounce thinly sliced cooked boneless, skinless chicken breast
- 1 leaf lettuce, cut into shreds
- 2 teaspoons salsa
- 2 teaspoons minced fresh cilantro

1. Heat the oil in a nonstick skillet over medium-high heat. Cook the tortillas for about 1 minute on each side, or until lightly browned (they will become crisp as they cool). Transfer the tortillas to a work surface. Lay the cheese on top of 1 tortilla.

2. Place the chicken in the skillet (do not wipe it out first) and cook for 30 seconds, or until warm.

3. Top the cheese-covered tortilla with the chicken, lettuce, salsa, cilantro, and finally the remaining tortilla. With a serrated knife, cut into 2 half-moons.

■ **Eat One Serving:**

315

calories, 17 g protein, 23 g carbohydrates, 18 g fat, 2.5 g saturated fat, 30 mg cholesterol, 240 mg sodium, 3 g fiber

MAKE IT A FLAT BELLY DIET MEAL:

Serve with the Tomato Avocado Soup on page 216, but omit the avocado (98).

■ **Total Meal:**

413

calories, 22 g protein, 38 g carbohydrates, 18 g fat, 3 g saturated fat, 30 mg cholesterol, 730 mg sodium*, 6 g fiber

* Limit saturated fat to no more than 10 percent of total calories—about 17 grams per day for most women or 21 grams for most men—and sodium intake to no more than 2,300 milligrams.

Turkey Panini with Avocado, Tomato, and Dijon

Cooking time: 10 minutes / Makes 2 servings

4 slices whole wheat bread
¼ pound deli-sliced reduced-sodium turkey breast
4 beefsteak tomato slices

MUFA: ½ Hass avocado, sliced

¼ cup baby arugula
2 teaspoons Dijon mustard
1 teaspoon extra-virgin olive oil

1. Place 1 slice of the bread on a work surface. Top with half the turkey, tomato slices, avocado slices, and arugula. Spread another slice of bread with half the mustard and set, mustard side down, on the arugula. Repeat with the remaining ingredients.

2. Heat a ridged nonstick grill pan over medium heat until hot. Working with one sandwich at a time, lightly brush the outsides of each sandwich with ¼ teaspoon oil and place on the pan. Set a heavy-bottomed skillet on top of the sandwich and cook for 1 to 2 minutes per side, or until toasted and warm in the center.

■ Eat One Serving:

247

calories, 17 g protein, 24 g carbohydrates, 9 g fat, 1 g saturated fat, 20 mg cholesterol, 660 mg sodium*, 4 g fiber

MAKE IT A FLAT BELLY DIET MEAL:

Serve with 1 medium pear (65) and 1 cup baby carrots (53).

■ Total Meal:

365

calories, 20 g protein, 51 g carbohydrates, 9 g fat, 1 g saturated fat, 20 mg cholesterol, 730 mg sodium*, 8 g fiber

* Limit saturated fat to no more than 10 percent of total calories—about 17 grams per day for most women or 21 grams for most men—and sodium intake to no more than 2,300 milligrams.

Grilled Ham, Pear, and Blue Cheese Sandwiches

Cooking time: 15 minutes / Makes 4 servings

8 slices multigrain bread, toasted
2 tablespoons canola oil mayonnaise
1 cup baby arugula or watercress sprigs
¼ pound thinly sliced lean, low-sodium baked ham
1 ripe red Bartlett pear, quartered, cored, and cut into thin wedges
¼ cup crumbled Gorgonzola cheese

MUFA: ½ cup sliced almonds

1. Preheat the broiler. Arrange the bread on a baking sheet. Spread 4 slices with the mayonnaise and mound the arugula or watercress on top, dividing evenly. Cover the same slices with equal portions of ham and arrange the pear wedges on top. Sprinkle the cheese and sliced almonds over the pear.

2. Place under the broiler for 1 to 2 minutes, or until the cheese is melted. Top with the remaining bread. Cut on the diagonal and serve warm.

■ **Eat One Serving:**

375

calories, 19 g protein, 38 g carbohydrates, 17 g fat, 3 g saturated fat, 25 mg cholesterol, 690 mg sodium*, 11 g fiber

A SINGLE SERVING OF THIS RECIPE COUNTS as a Flat Belly Diet Meal without any add-ons!

* Limit saturated fat to no more than 10 percent of total calories—about 17 grams per day for most women or 21 grams for most men—and sodium intake to no more than 2,300 milligrams.

Chicken with Avocado-Orange Salsa

Cooking time: 25 minutes / Makes 4 servings

4 boneless, skinless chicken breast halves (1½ pounds)

4 cups water

½ teaspoon + ⅛ teaspoon salt

1 cup mandarin oranges packed in water or own juice

MUFA: 1 cup diced Hass avocado

4 radishes, thinly sliced

¼ cup chopped fresh basil + additional for garnish

1. In a large saucepan, combine the chicken, water, and ½ teaspoon salt. Cover and bring to a gentle boil over high heat. Lower the heat and let simmer for 15 minutes, or until a thermometer inserted in the thickest portion registers 165°F.

2. Place mandarin orange segments into a bowl. Add the avocado, radishes, basil, and the remaining ⅛ teaspoon salt. Gently toss to mix.

3. Drain the chicken breasts, discarding the liquid. Let cool for 5 minutes, then cut crosswise into ½" slices. Divide the orange mixture among 4 plates and add one-quarter of the chicken slices to each, drizzling the chicken with juice from the orange mixture. Garnish with basil leaves, if using.

■ **Eat One Serving:**

272

calories, 40 g protein, 10 g carbohydrates, 8 g fat, 1.5 g saturated fat, 100 mg cholesterol, 490 mg sodium, 3 g fiber

MAKE IT A FLAT BELLY DIET MEAL: Serve with ½ cup steamed brown rice (109).

■ **Total Meal:**

381

calories, 43 g protein, 33 g carbohydrates, 8 g fat, 1.5 g saturated fat, 100 mg cholesterol, 490 mg sodium, 5 g fiber

Chicken and Summer Vegetable Sauté

Cooking time: 45 minutes / Makes 4 servings

1 egg
1 tablespoon water
¼ cup ground flaxseed
¼ cup all-purpose flour
½ teaspoon salt
4 boneless, skinless chicken breast halves (1 pound)

MUFA: ¼ cup sunflower oil

1 onion, cut into ½" wedges
1 zucchini, halved lengthwise and sliced
2 cups grape tomatoes, halved
1 teaspoon dried basil
½ lemon
2 cups cooked whole wheat couscous

1. Preheat the oven to 425°F. Coat a baking sheet with cooking spray.

2. Place the egg and water in a shallow dish and whisk to combine. Combine the flaxseed, flour, and salt in another shallow dish. Dip the chicken into the egg mixture and then into the flaxseed mixture. Place the chicken on the prepared sheet. Bake, turning once, for 15 minutes, or until a thermometer inserted in the center reaches 160°F.

3. Meanwhile, coat a large nonstick skillet with cooking spray and heat the oil over medium-high heat. Add the onion and zucchini and cook, stirring, for 5 minutes, or until well browned. Add the tomatoes and basil and cook for 3 minutes, or until tender. Remove from the heat. Squeeze the lemon over the tomato mixture and toss to coat.

4. Place the chicken on 4 plates. Arrange one-quarter of the tomato mixture around each piece. Serve with hot couscous.

■ **Eat One Serving:**

432

calories, 34 g protein, 31 g carbohydrates, 20 g fat, 2 g saturated fat, 120 mg cholesterol, 400 mg sodium, 6 g fiber

A SINGLE SERVING OF THIS RECIPE COUNTS as a Flat Belly Diet Meal without any add-ons!

Orange Chicken and Broccoli Stir-Fry

Cooking time: 30 minutes / Makes 4 servings

2 bunches broccoli (about 2 pounds)
½ cup orange juice
2 tablespoons reduced-sodium soy sauce
2 teaspoons cornstarch
2 tablespoons orange marmalade

MUFA: ¼ cup canola oil

1¼ pounds chicken tenders, trimmed and cut into 1" pieces
3 scallions, sliced
3 large cloves garlic, minced
1 tablespoon minced fresh ginger
Pinch of red-pepper flakes
⅓ cup reduced-sodium chicken broth
1 red bell pepper, thinly sliced

1. Cut the broccoli into small florets. Trim and discard about 2" of the tough broccoli stems. Thinly slice the remaining stems.

2. Combine the orange juice, soy sauce, cornstarch, and orange marmalade in a small bowl. Stir until blended. Set the sauce aside.

3. In a wok or large nonstick skillet, heat the oil over medium-high heat. Add the chicken and cook, stirring frequently, for 2 to 3 minutes, or until cooked through. Add the scallions, garlic, ginger, and red-pepper flakes and stir to combine. With a slotted spoon, remove the chicken to a plate.

4. Add the broth and broccoli to the mixture in the wok and reduce the heat to medium. Cover and cook for 2 minutes. Increase the heat to high and add the bell pepper. Cook, stirring frequently, for 2 minutes, or until the broth evaporates and the vegetables are crisp-tender. Stir the sauce and add to the wok along with the chicken. Cook, stirring constantly, for 1 to 2 minutes, or until the sauce thickens and the chicken is hot.

■ **Eat One Serving:**

401

calories, 40 g protein, 31 g carbohydrates, 16 g fat, 1 g saturated fat, 85 mg cholesterol, 420 mg sodium, 7 g fiber

A SINGLE SERVING OF THIS RECIPE COUNTS as a Flat Belly Diet Meal without any add-ons!

Szechuan Chicken and Rice

Cooking time: 20 minutes / Makes 4 servings

1 teaspoon
minced garlic
1 teaspoon
grated fresh
ginger
½ teaspoon salt-
free lemon-
pepper
seasoning
½ teaspoon
crushed fennel
seeds
Pinch of ground
cloves
1 pound chicken
tenders, cut
into ½"-thick
crosswise slices

**MUFA: ¼ cup
canola oil**

12 ounces bok
choy, cut into
½"-thick
crosswise slices
¼ cup chicken
broth
1 tablespoon
reduced-
sodium soy
sauce
2⅔ cups cooked
brown rice
Red-pepper
flakes (optional)

1. Combine the garlic, ginger, lemon-pepper seasoning, fennel seeds, and cloves in a large bowl. Add the chicken. With your hands or a fork, toss well to coat all the pieces with seasoning.

2. Set a wok or large skillet over medium-high heat until very hot. Add the oil and swirl to coat the pan. Place the chicken pieces in the pan so they are separated. Cook for 1 to 2 minutes, or until the chicken begins to brown on the bottom. Turn and cook for 1 minute longer, until browned. Reduce the heat to medium. Add the bok choy. Cook, tossing, for about 2 minutes, or until the bok choy leaves are wilting. Add the broth and soy sauce. Bring almost to a boil. Reduce the heat and simmer for 2 minutes, or until the chicken is cooked through.

3. Serve with ⅔ cup cooked brown rice per serving and garnish with red-pepper flakes, if desired.

■ **Eat One Serving:**

395

calories, 31 g protein, 33 g carbohydrates, 16 g fat, 1.5 g saturated fat, 65 mg cholesterol, 240 mg sodium, 3 g fiber

A SINGLE SERVING OF THIS RECIPE COUNTS as a Flat Belly Diet Meal without any add-ons!

Chicken with Pears and Walnuts

Cooking time: 50 minutes / Makes 4 servings

2 tablespoons all-purpose flour
½ teaspoon salt
¼ teaspoon freshly ground black pepper
2 large boneless, skinless chicken breast halves (6–8 ounces each), halved widthwise, or 4 chicken cutlets (3–4 ounces each)
2 tablespoons canola oil
1 large onion, cut into wedges
2 medium pears, halved, cored, and sliced
1 bag (6 ounces) baby spinach
½ cup apple cider or apple juice
1½ teaspoons fresh thyme leaves or ½ teaspoon dried
½ cup crumbled reduced-fat blue cheese

MUFA: ½ cup walnuts, toasted and chopped

1. Combine the flour, salt, and pepper in a shallow dish. Dredge the chicken in the mixture and set aside.

2. Heat 1 tablespoon of the oil in a large nonstick skillet over medium heat. Add the onion and cook for 5 minutes, or until lightly browned. Add the pears and cook for 3 minutes, or until lightly browned. Add the spinach and cook for 1 minute, or until wilted. Place the mixture on a serving plate.

3. Heat the remaining 1 tablespoon oil in the same skillet. Cook the chicken, turning once, for 6 to 8 minutes, or until browned. Add the cider and thyme and bring to a boil. Reduce the heat to low and simmer for 5 minutes, or until the sauce is reduced by half.

4. Place the chicken on the spinach mixture, drizzle with the cider mixture, and sprinkle with the cheese and walnuts.

■ **Eat One Serving:**

397

calories, 28 g protein, 31 g carbohydrates, 20 g fat, 3 g saturated fat, 55 mg cholesterol, 650 mg sodium*, 7 g fiber

A SINGLE SERVING OF THIS RECIPE COUNTS as a Flat Belly Diet Meal without any add-ons!

* Limit saturated fat to no more than 10 percent of total calories—about 17 grams per day for most women or 21 grams for most men—and sodium intake to no more than 2,300 milligrams.

Mexican Chicken with Pumpkin Seeds

Cooking time: 25 minutes / Makes 4 servings

2 teaspoons canola oil
½ onion, chopped
½ red bell pepper, chopped
1 teaspoon ground cumin
1 teaspoon chopped fresh oregano
¼ teaspoon salt
1 tablespoon flour
¼ teaspoon freshly ground black pepper
1 cup reduced-sodium chicken broth
1 pound chicken tenders

MUFA: ½ cup pumpkin seeds

3 cups cooked wild rice
Fresh cilantro for garnish (optional)

1. Heat the oil in a large nonstick skillet over medium-high heat. Add the onion, bell pepper, cumin, oregano, and salt. Stir to mix. Cover and cook over medium heat, stirring occasionally, for 3 minutes, or until the vegetables have softened.

2. Add the flour and black pepper. Stir so the flour thoroughly coats the vegetables. Add the broth and cook, stirring constantly, for 2 minutes, or until thickened. Add the chicken. Cover and simmer for 10 minutes, or until the chicken is cooked through. Add the pumpkin seeds and stir into the sauce.

3. Serve each portion on top of ¾ cup cooked wild rice, garnished with cilantro if desired.

■ Eat One Serving:

394

calories, 37 g protein, 34 g carbohydrates, 13 g fat, 2 g saturated fat, 65 mg cholesterol, 250 mg sodium, 4 g fiber

A SINGLE SERVING OF THIS RECIPE COUNTS as a Flat Belly Diet Meal without any add-ons!

Baked Lemon Chicken

Cooking time: 1 hour / Makes 4 servings

1 tablespoon extra-virgin olive oil
  Grated peel and juice of 1 lemon
1 tablespoon minced garlic
1 teaspoon dried oregano
¼ teaspoon salt
¾ teaspoon ground black pepper
¾ teaspoon paprika
4 skinless chicken legs or thighs, trimmed of fat (1 pound total)
1 medium red bell pepper, cut into 8 wedges
1 medium orange bell pepper, cut into 8 wedges
2 medium Yukon gold potatoes, each cut into 8 wedges
1 medium red onion, cut into 8 wedges

MUFA: 40 kalamata olives, pitted

Chopped fresh mint or parsley, grated lemon peel, and lemon wedges (optional)

1. Preheat the oven to 400°F. Coat a 17" x 12" rimmed baking pan with cooking spray. Add the oil, lemon peel, lemon juice, garlic, oregano, salt, black pepper, and paprika.

2. Place the chicken on one side of the pan and the bell peppers, potatoes, and onion on the other. Toss to coat with seasonings.

3. Roast for 20 minutes. Turn the chicken and stir the vegetables. Roast for another 20 to 25 minutes, or until a thermometer inserted in the thickest part of the chicken registers 165°F and the vegetables are lightly browned and tender. Arrange the chicken and vegetables on serving plates and scatter 10 olives over each portion. Garnish with the mint or parsley, lemon peel, and lemon wedges, if using.

■ **Eat One Serving:**

399

calories, 27 g protein, 30 g carbohydrates, 18 g fat, 3 g saturated fat, 90 mg cholesterol, 870 mg sodium*, 6 g fiber

A SINGLE SERVING OF THIS RECIPE COUNTS as a Flat Belly Diet Meal without any add-ons!

* Limit saturated fat to no more than 10 percent of total calories—about 17 grams per day for most women or 21 grams for most men—and sodium intake to no more than 2,300 milligrams.

Chicken Parmesan

Cooking time: 30 minutes / Makes 4 servings

1 egg
1 tablespoon water

MUFA: ½ cup pine nuts, finely chopped

¼ cup whole wheat bread crumbs
½ teaspoon Italian seasoning
4 chicken cutlets (about 3 ounces each)
2 cups prepared marinara sauce
¼ cup shredded part-skim mozzarella cheese (about 2 ounces)

1. Preheat the oven to 425°F. Coat a baking sheet with cooking spray.

2. Whisk the egg with the water in a shallow dish. Combine the pine nuts, bread crumbs, and seasoning in another shallow dish. Dip the chicken into the egg and then the nut mixture. Place the chicken on the prepared baking sheet.

3. Bake for 10 minutes. Turn the chicken over and top each with ½ cup of the marinara sauce and some of the cheese. Bake for 5 to 10 minutes longer, or until the cheese has melted and the chicken is cooked through.

■ **Eat One Serving:**

327

calories, 29 g protein, 14 g carbohydrates, 18 g fat, 3 g saturated fat, 110 mg cholesterol, 670 mg sodium*, 3 g fiber

MAKE IT A FLAT BELLY DIET MEAL:
Serve with 2 cups steamed spaghetti squash (84).

■ **Total Meal:**

411

calories, 31 g protein, 34 g carbohydrates, 19 g fat, 3 g saturated fat, 110 mg cholesterol, 730 mg sodium*, 7 g fiber

* Limit saturated fat to no more than 10 percent of total calories—about 17 grams per day for most women or 21 grams for most men—and sodium intake to no more than 2,300 milligrams.

Stuffed Chicken Roulade with Pasta and Pistachios

Cooking time: 35 minutes / Makes 4 servings

4 ounces multigrain spaghetti
¼ cup finely chopped onion
1 clove garlic, minced
¼ teaspoon red-pepper flakes (or to taste)
2 teaspoons olive oil
¼ cup grated Parmesan cheese
1 package (10 ounces) frozen chopped spinach, thawed and squeezed dry
4 chicken breast cutlets (about 1 pound)
2 tablespoons minced dry packed sun-dried tomatoes
½ cup low-sodium chicken broth

MUFA: ½ cup pistachios, coarsely chopped

1. Cook spaghetti according to package directions. Drain and keep warm.

2. In a medium nonstick skillet over medium heat, cook the onion, garlic, and pepper flakes in 1 teaspoon oil for 30 seconds. Reduce the heat to low, cover, and cook, stirring once, for about 3 minutes, or until softened. Combine the onion mixture, Parmesan, and spinach in a small bowl.

3. Pound the chicken gently with a meat mallet to an even thickness. Spread equal amounts of the tomatoes and spinach mixture over the cutlets. Carefully roll up each cutlet, ending with the narrow tip, and secure with wooden picks.

4. Add the remaining oil to the skillet and set over medium heat. Add the chicken and cook about 10 minutes. Add the broth. Cover and cook over low heat for about 7 minutes. Transfer the roulades to a serving platter. Cover to keep warm.

5. Boil the remaining juices in the skillet for about 5 minutes, or until reduced by half. Toss pasta and nuts in pan juices. Cut the roulades into diagonal slices and serve on top of pasta.

■ Eat One Serving:

400

calories, 39 g protein, 29 g carbohydrates, 13 g fat, 2.5 g saturated fat, 70 mg cholesterol, 320 mg sodium, 5 g fiber

A SINGLE SERVING OF THIS RECIPE COUNTS as a Flat Belly Diet Meal without any add-ons!

Santa Fe Turkey Pizzas

Cooking time: 30 minutes / Makes 4 servings

4 whole wheat tortillas (8″ diameter)
6 ounces ground turkey breast
1 small red bell pepper, chopped
1 small zucchini, thinly sliced
¼ cup chopped red onion
1 cup corn
1 cup canned no-salt added black beans, rinsed and drained

MUFA: 40 chopped black olives

1 tablespoon chili powder
1½ cups mild chunky salsa
2 tablespoons chopped cilantro
⅓ cup reduced-fat shredded Mexican cheese blend
2 tablespoons chopped jalapeño chile pepper (optional)
2 cups shredded escarole
¼ cup reduced-fat sour cream (optional)

1. Preheat the oven to 450°F. Arrange the oven racks to divide the oven into thirds. Place the tortillas on 2 baking sheets.

2. In a large nonstick skillet over medium-high heat, cook the turkey, bell pepper, zucchini, and onion, stirring frequently to break up the turkey, for 5 minutes, or until the turkey is no longer pink. Stir in the corn, beans, olives, and chili powder, and ¾ cup of the salsa. Cook for 2 minutes, stirring, until heated through. Stir in the cilantro.

3. Top the tortillas with the turkey mixture, spreading to ½″ from the edges. Bake for 8 minutes, rotating the cookie sheets halfway through, or until the tortillas are crisp and browned at the edges. Sprinkle with the cheese and bake for 1 to 2 minutes, or until melted. Sprinkle with the jalapeño (if using) and the escarole. Serve with the sour cream, if desired, and the remaining ¾ cup salsa on the side.

■ **Eat One Serving:**

403

calories, 25 g protein, 55 g carbohydrates, 11 g fat, 2 g saturated fat, 25 mg cholesterol, 1,260 mg sodium*, 11 g fiber

A SINGLE SERVING OF THIS RECIPE COUNTS as a Flat Belly Diet Meal without any add-ons!

* Limit saturated fat to no more than 10 percent of total calories—about 17 grams per day for most women or 21 grams for most men—and sodium intake to no more than 2,300 milligrams.

Turkey Meat Loaf

Cooking time: 1 hour 30 minutes / Makes 4 servings

2 teaspoons olive oil
1 large carrot, grated
4 scallions, thinly sliced
1 clove garlic, minced

MUFA: ½ cup walnuts, chopped

2 slices whole wheat bread
¼ cup fat-free milk
2 egg whites, lightly beaten
1 pound extra-lean ground turkey breast (99% fat-free)
¼ cup chopped fresh flat-leaf parsley
¼ cup grated Parmesan cheese
1 teaspoon dried sage
½ teaspoon salt
½ teaspoon freshly ground black pepper

1. Preheat the oven to 350°F. Line a rimmed baking sheet with foil and coat the foil with olive oil spray.

2. Heat the oil in a small nonstick skillet over medium heat. Add the carrot, scallions, and garlic and cook, stirring often, for about 3 minutes, or until tender. Remove from the heat.

3. Meanwhile, chop the walnuts in a food processor fitted with a metal blade. Break up the bread and add to the walnuts. Pulse until both are ground to fine crumbs. Transfer to a large bowl. With a fork, stir in the milk and egg whites. Add the turkey, parsley, cheese, sage, salt, pepper, and carrot mixture. Mix gently just until blended.

4. Shape into a free-form loaf about 7" long and 4½" wide on the prepared baking sheet. Bake for 50 to 60 minutes, or until a thermometer inserted in the center of the loaf registers 165°F. Let stand a few minutes before slicing.

■ **Eat One Serving:**

322

calories, 37 g protein, 14 g carbohydrates, 15 g fat, 2 g saturated fat, 50 mg cholesterol, 570 mg sodium, 3 g fiber

MAKE IT A FLAT BELLY DIET MEAL: Serve with 1 cup steamed broccoli (44) sprinkled with 1 tablespoon grated Parmesan cheese (21).

■ **Total Meal:**

387

calories, 43 g protein, 22 g carbohydrates, 17 g fat, 3 g saturated fat, 55 mg cholesterol, 680 mg sodium*, 8 g fiber

* Limit saturated fat to no more than 10 percent of total calories—about 17 grams per day for most women or 21 grams for most men—and sodium intake to no more than 2,300 milligrams.

Zesty Turkey Chili

Cooking time: 1 hour 30 minutes / Makes 8 servings

MUFA: ½ cup olive oil

- 2 pounds extra-lean ground turkey breast
- 1 large onion, chopped
- 2 red or yellow bell peppers, chopped
- 4 large cloves garlic, minced
- 3 tablespoons tomato paste
- 2 tablespoons chili powder
- 1 tablespoon ground cumin
- 1 teaspoon dried oregano
- 1 teaspoon salt
- 1 large sweet potato, peeled and cut into ½" cubes
- 1 can (28 ounces) diced tomatoes
- 1 can (14 ounces) chicken broth
- 1 chipotle chile pepper in adobo sauce, minced (optional)
- 2 cans (15–16 ounces each) mixed beans for chili, rinsed and drained
- 1 zucchini, chopped

1. Warm the oil in a large soup pot or Dutch oven over medium-high heat. Cook the turkey, onion, and bell peppers, stirring frequently, for 8 minutes, or until the turkey is cooked through. Add the garlic, tomato paste, chili powder, cumin, oregano, and salt. Cook, stirring constantly, for 1 minute.

2. Add the sweet potato, diced tomatoes (with juice), chicken broth, and chile peppers, if using. Bring to a boil. Reduce the heat to low and simmer, covered, stirring occasionally, for 30 minutes.

3. Stir in the beans and zucchini. Return to a simmer. Cover and simmer for 30 minutes longer, stirring occasionally, or until the flavors are well blended and the vegetables are tender.

■ Eat One Serving:

388

calories, 36 g protein, 28 g carbohydrates, 16 g fat, 2 g saturated fat, 45 mg cholesterol, 1,000 mg sodium*, 7 g fiber

A SINGLE SERVING OF THIS RECIPE COUNTS as a Flat Belly Diet Meal without any add-ons!

* Limit saturated fat to no more than 10 percent of total calories—about 17 grams per day for most women or 21 grams for most men—and sodium intake to no more than 2,300 milligrams.

Lemon Aioli Tuna Burger

Preparation time: 5 minutes / Cooking time: 4 minutes / Makes 4 servings

**MUFA: ¼ cup
canola oil
mayonnaise**

1 tablespoon
lemon juice
½ clove garlic,
minced
½ green onion,
thinly sliced
4 (4-ounce)
yellowfin tuna
steaks
2 teaspoons
canola oil
¼ teaspoon salt
4 hamburger
buns
1 cup fresh
arugula leaves
¼ cucumber, cut
into 12 slices

1. Coat a grill rack with cooking spray. Prepare the grill for medium-high heat.

2. Combine the mayonnaise, lemon juice, garlic, and onion in a bowl and mix well.

3. Brush the tuna steaks with the oil and sprinkle with the salt. Grill for 2 minutes per side, or until well marked and cooked to desired doneness.

4. Arrange the bun bottoms on each of 4 plates. Top each with ¼ cup arugula, 3 cucumber slices, and 1 tuna steak. Spread the top half of each bun with the mayonnaise mixture and set each on the tuna steak. Serve immediately.

■ **Eat One Serving:**

369

calories, 32 g protein, 22 g carbohydrates, 17 g fat, 2.1 g saturated fat, 56 mg cholesterol, 498 mg sodium, 1 g fiber

MAKE IT A FLAT BELLY DIET MEAL:
Serve with ½ cup red grapes (52).

■ **Total Meal:**

421

calories, 32 g protein, 36 g carbohydrates, 17 g fat, 2.1 g saturated fat, 56 mg cholesterol, 498 mg sodium, 1 g fiber

range Frappé
ith Strawberries
age 285

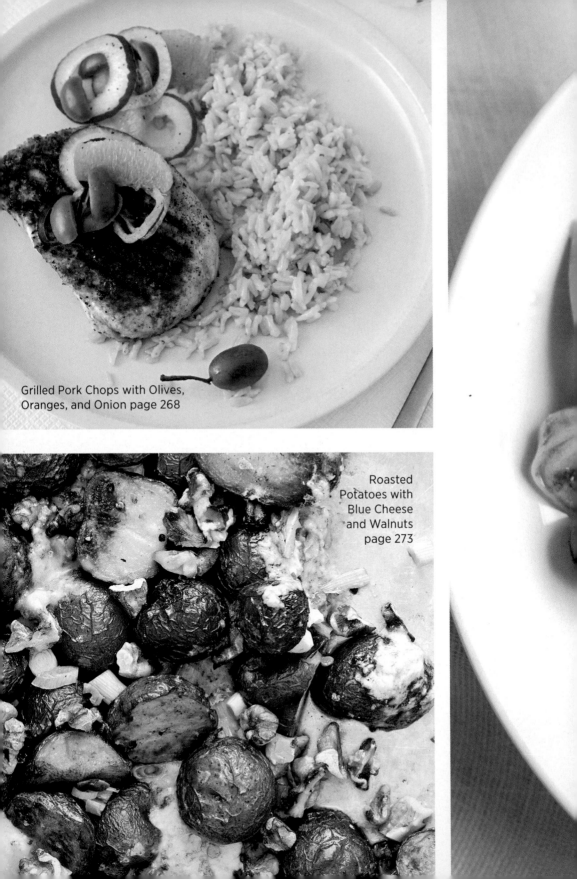

Grilled Pork Chops with Olives,
Oranges, and Onion page 268

Roasted
Potatoes with
Blue Cheese
and Walnuts
page 273

Tortellini Pasta Salad page 222

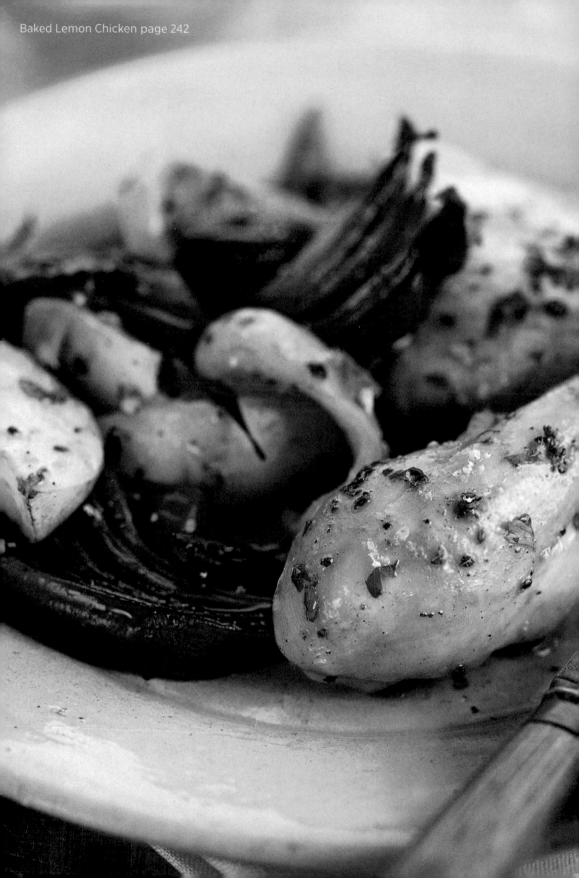

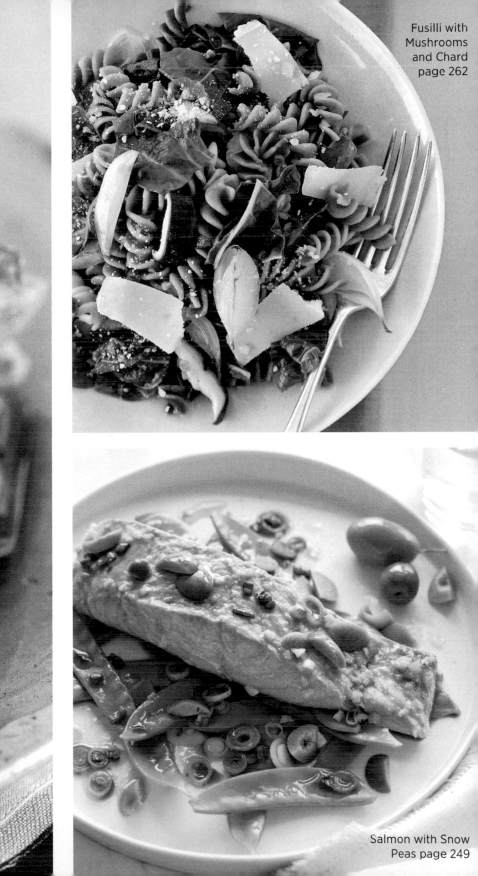

Fusilli with Mushrooms and Chard page 262

Salmon with Snow Peas page 249

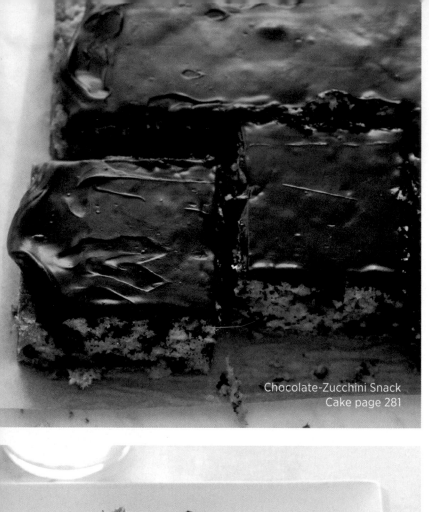

Chocolate-Zucchini Snack
Cake page 281

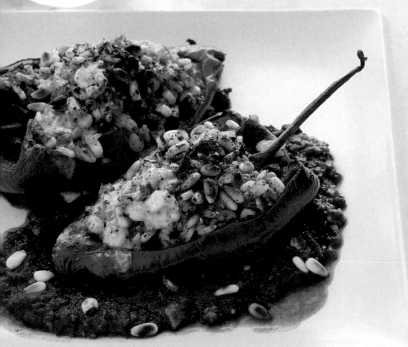

Mexican-Style Stuffed Peppers
page 263

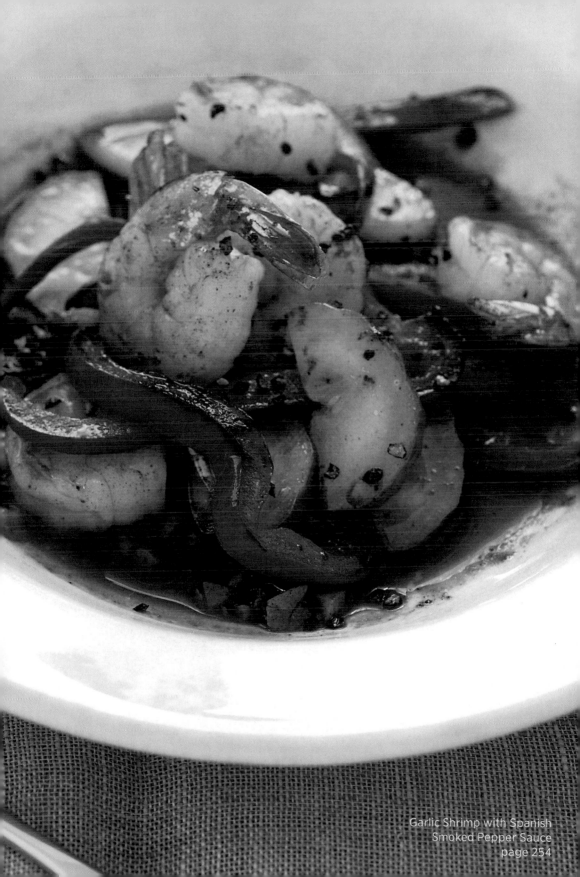

Garlic Shrimp with Spanish
Smoked Pepper Sauce
page 254

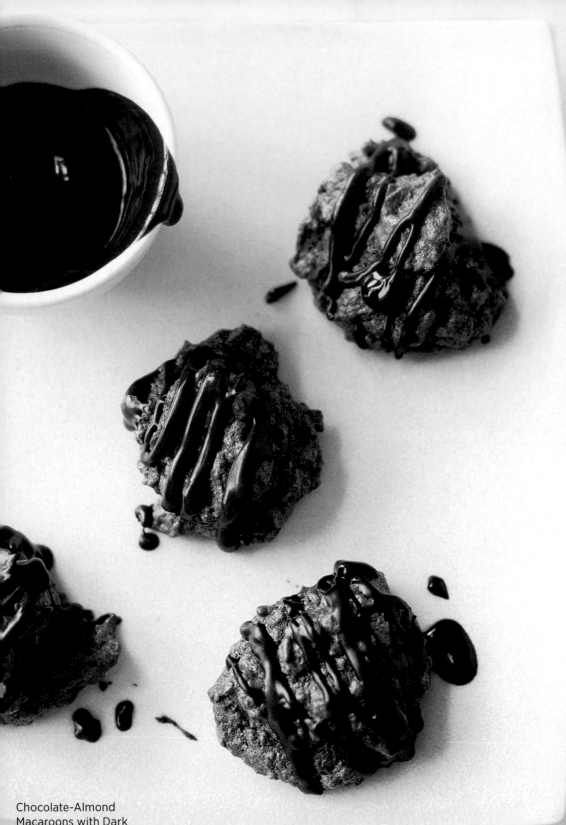

Chocolate-Almond
Macaroons with Dark
Chocolate Dunking Sauce
page 283

Salmon with Snow Peas

Cooking time: 30 minutes / Makes 4 servings

4 skinless salmon fillets, about 1½" thick (1 pound)
1 teaspoon grated fresh ginger
1 clove garlic, minced
1 tablespoon freshly squeezed lime juice (about 2 limes)
2 teaspoons reduced-sodium soy sauce
1 teaspoon toasted sesame oil
2 scallions, thinly sliced
1 pound snow peas, trimmed

MUFA: 40 black olives, sliced

1. Rub the fillets with the ginger and garlic. Coat a steamer basket with cooking spray and arrange the fillets in the basket.

2. Bring 2" of water to a boil in a saucepan. Place the steamer basket in the saucepan and cover. Cook for 8 minutes.

3. Meanwhile, whisk together the lime juice, soy sauce, sesame oil, and scallions in a small bowl. Set aside.

4. After the salmon has cooked for 8 minutes, top with the snow peas and cover. Cook for about 4 more minutes, or until the salmon is opaque and the snow peas are crisp-tender.

5. Make a bed of the snow peas on 4 plates, top with the salmon, scatter one-quarter of the olives over each portion, and drizzle with the reserved sauce.

■ Eat One Serving:

333

calories, 26 g protein, 13 g carbohydrates, 20 g fat, 3.5 g saturated fat*, 65 mg cholesterol, 650 mg sodium*, 5 g fiber

MAKE IT A FLAT BELLY DIET MEAL:

Serve with 1 medium orange (69).

■ Total Meal:

402

calories, 26 g protein, 30 g carbohydrates, 20 g fat, 3.5 g saturated fat*, 65 mg cholesterol, 650 mg sodium*, 8 g fiber

* Limit saturated fat to no more than 10 percent of total calories—about 17 grams per day for most women or 21 grams for most men—and sodium intake to no more than 2,300 milligrams.

Zucchini-Stuffed Sole with Lemon-Butter Sauce

Cooking time: 20 minutes / Makes 4 servings

2 teaspoons extra-virgin olive oil

1 cup thinly sliced zucchini

1 clove garlic, chopped

½ teaspoon salt

¼ teaspoon freshly ground black pepper

1 pound sole fillets

¼ cup dry white wine, or 2 tablespoons freshly squeezed lemon juice mixed with 2 tablespoons vegetable broth

1 tablespoon butter

Juice of a freshly squeezed lemon (about 2 teaspoons)

½ teaspoon freshly grated lemon zest

1 teaspoon finely chopped fresh parsley

MUFA: ½ cup pine nuts, toasted

1. Heat 1 teaspoon of the oil in a large nonstick skillet over medium-high heat. Add the zucchini and garlic. Stir constantly for 2 to 3 minutes, or until softened. Remove from heat and season with ¼ teaspoon salt and ⅛ teaspoon pepper.

2. Season both sides of the fish with remaining ¼ teaspoon salt and ⅛ teaspoon pepper. Place each fillet on a flat surface and spread ¼ of the squash mixture evenly over the top, leaving a ½" margin on both ends. Roll the fillet into a cylinder and secure with a wooden pick.

3. Add the remaining teaspoon of oil to the skillet and place over medium heat. Add the fish rolls, seam side up. Cook for 2 minutes. Add the wine or lemon juice–broth mixture. Reduce the heat to medium-low, cover, and cook 5 minutes longer, or until the fish flakes easily with a fork.

4. Transfer the fish to a plate and tent loosely with foil. Add the butter, lemon juice, and lemon zest to the skillet. Remove from the heat, swirl until the butter melts, and spoon over the fish. Remove the picks from the fish. Sprinkle with the parsley and pine nuts.

■ Eat One Serving:

282

calories, 24 g protein, 4 g carbohydrates, 18 g fat*, 3.5 g saturated fat, 60 mg cholesterol, 410 mg sodium, 1 g fiber

MAKE IT A FLAT BELLY DIET MEAL:

Serve with 4 ounces roasted baby red potatoes (93) dressed with 1 tablespoon reduced-fat sour cream (20).

■ Total Meal:

395

calories, 27 g protein, 25 g carbohydrates, 20 g fat, 4.5 g saturated fat*, 70 mg cholesterol, 420 mg sodium, 2 g fiber

* Limit saturated fat to no more than 10 percent of total calories—about 17 grams per day for most women or 21 grams for most men—and sodium intake to no more than 2,300 milligrams.

Roasted Flounder with Artichokes

Cooking time: 50 minutes / Makes 4 servings

2 large red onions, cut into ¼" wedges

MUFA: ¼ cup sunflower oil

1 package (10 ounces) frozen artichoke hearts, thawed (about 2 cups)

1 cup small cherry or grape tomatoes

2 tablespoons chopped parsley

1 teaspoon freshly grated orange zest

1 clove garlic, minced

4 skinless flounder fillets (1–1½ pounds total)

1. Preheat the oven to 400°F.

2. Combine the onions and oil in a 13" x 9" baking dish. Toss and then spread in an even layer.

3. Roast the onions for about 35 minutes, or until very soft. Remove from the oven and stir in the artichokes and tomatoes.

4. Mix the parsley, orange zest, and garlic in a small bowl. Set aside.

5. Increase the oven temperature to 450°F. Push the vegetables to one side of the dish and add the flounder, arranging it evenly in the pan. Spoon the vegetables over the fish and sprinkle with the parsley mixture.

6. Return the baking dish to the oven and roast until the fish flakes easily with a fork (about 5 minutes for thin fillets; 10 to 12 minutes for thicker fillets).

■ **Eat One Serving:**

296

calories, 24 g protein, 15 g carbohydrates, 16 g fat, 2 g saturated fat, 55 mg cholesterol, 180 mg sodium, 6 g fiber

MAKE IT A FLAT BELLY DIET MEAL: Serve with ½ cup steamed brown rice (109).

■ **Total Meal:**

405

calories, 27 g protein, 38 g carbohydrates, 17 g fat, 2 g saturated fat, 55 mg cholesterol, 180 mg sodium, 8 g fiber

Roasted Cod with Fennel and Olive Salad

Cooking time: 30 minutes / Makes 4 servings

MUFA: ¼ cup sun-dried tomato pesto

1½ pounds cod fillets, cut into 4 portions
2 bunches fennel (¾ pound), trimmed, halved, and very thinly sliced crosswise
2 tablespoons chopped fennel fronds
⅓ cup pitted kalamata olives, halved
1 cup whole fresh parsley leaves, stems removed
1½ teaspoons lemon juice
1½ teaspoons olive oil
⅛ teaspoon salt

1. Preheat the oven to 400°F. Coat an ovenproof skillet with cooking spray.

2. Spoon 1 tablespoon of the pesto on each fillet. Arrange in the prepared skillet with space in between. Roast for 9 minutes, or until the fish flakes easily. Remove from the oven.

3. Meanwhile, combine the sliced fennel and fronds, olives, parsley, lemon juice, oil, and salt in a large bowl. Toss to mix.

4. Divide the salad among 4 plates and top each with fish.

■ **Eat One Serving:**

219

calories, 32 g protein, 9 g carbohydrates, 6 g fat, 1 g saturated fat, 50 mg cholesterol, 520 mg sodium, 3 g fiber

MAKE IT A FLAT BELLY DIET MEAL:
Serve with 1 cup whole wheat couscous (140) and half of an orange (34).

■ **Total Meal:**

393

calories, 38 g protein, 48 g carbohydrates, 6 g fat, 1 g saturated fat, 75 mg cholesterol, 520 mg sodium, 9 g fiber

Steamed Tilapia with Pesto

Cooking time: 25 minutes / Makes 4 servings

6 cups baby spinach

1 red bell pepper, thinly sliced

4 tilapia fillets (6 ounces each)

½ teaspoon salt

¼ teaspoon freshly ground black pepper

MUFA: 4 tablespoons pesto

1. Preheat the oven to 450°F. Coat one side of four 12" x 20" sheets of foil with cooking spray.

2. Top half of each foil sheet with 1½ cups of the spinach, one-quarter of the bell pepper, and 1 tilapia fillet. Sprinkle with the salt and black pepper. Fold the other half of each foil sheet over the filling and crimp the edges to make a tight seal.

3. Arrange the packets on a large baking sheet. Bake for 10 to 12 minutes, or until the packets are puffed. Transfer each packet to a serving plate. Carefully slit the top of each to allow the steam to escape. After a minute, peel back the foil to reveal the fish. Check to make sure the fish flakes easily when tested with a fork.

4. Top each portion with 1 tablespoon of pesto before serving.

■ Eat One Serving:

256

calories, 37 g protein, 6 g carbohydrates, 10 g fat, 2.5 g saturated fat, 85 mg cholesterol, 560 mg sodium, 2 g fiber

MAKE IT A FLAT BELLY DIET MEAL:

Serve with 4 ounces roasted baby red potatoes (93) and 1 cup steamed broccoli (44) tossed with 1 fresh plum tomato, chopped (12).

■ Total Meal:

405

calories, 45 g protein, 37 g carbohydrates, 11 g fat, 2.5 g saturated fat, 85 mg cholesterol, 610 mg sodium*, 9 g fiber

* Limit saturated fat to no more than 10 percent of total calories—about 17 grams per day for most women or 21 grams for most men—and sodium intake to no more than 2,300 milligrams.

Garlic Shrimp with Spanish Smoked Pepper Sauce

Cooking time: 25 minutes / Makes 4 servings

MUFA: 4 tablespoons safflower oil

2 red bell peppers, cut into thin strips
½ seedless cucumber, thinly sliced (1½ cups)
¼ teaspoon salt
4 large cloves garlic, minced
1 pound peeled and deveined shrimp, thawed if frozen
1 tablespoon smoked paprika
½ teaspoon freshly ground black pepper
2 tablespoons medium-dry sherry (optional)
2 tablespoons freshly squeezed lemon juice

1. Warm 1 tablespoon of the oil in a large, deep, heavy skillet over medium heat. Add the bell peppers, cover, and cook, stirring often, for about 5 minutes, or until tender. Add the cucumber and ⅛ teaspoon of the salt, cover, and cook, stirring often, for 3 minutes, or until tender and becoming translucent. Transfer the vegetables to a serving dish. Cover to keep warm.

2. Combine the garlic and remaining 3 tablespoons oil in the same skillet over medium heat. Cook, stirring, for about 1 minute, or until fragrant.

3. Stir in the shrimp and sprinkle with the paprika, black pepper, and remaining ⅛ teaspoon salt. Cook, stirring often, for 5 to 7 minutes, or until the shrimp are opaque. (If the pan becomes very dry, add 1 to 2 tablespoons water.)

4. Add the sherry, if using, and lemon juice. Cook, stirring, for 1 minute, or until the pan juices are bubbly and thickened. Serve the shrimp over the vegetables.

■ Eat One Serving:

277

calories, 24 g protein, 8 g carbohydrates, 16 g fat, 1.5 g saturated fat, 170 mg cholesterol, 320 mg sodium, 2 g fiber

MAKE IT A FLAT BELLY DIET MEAL:

Serve with the Saffron Rice on page 271, but omit the pistachios (138).

■ Total Meal:

415

calories, 27 g protein, 33 g carbohydrates, 18 g fat, 1.5 g saturated fat, 170 mg cholesterol, 620 mg sodium*, 4 g fiber

* Limit saturated fat to no more than 10 percent of total calories—about 17 grams per day for most women or 21 grams for most men—and sodium intake to no more than 2,300 milligrams.

Jamaican-Style Scallops with Black Bean Salsa

Cooking time: 45 minutes / Makes 4 servings

16 sea scallops
(1 ounce each),
preferably dry-
packed
1 teaspoon
Caribbean jerk
seasoning
1 can (14½
ounces) no-salt-
added black
beans, rinsed
and drained
1 tomato, chopped
1 red bell pepper,
chopped
1 mango, peeled
and cubed
½ red onion, finely
chopped
1 small jalapeño
chile pepper,
finely chopped
2 tablespoons
lime juice
2 tablespoons
canola oil
1 tablespoon
chopped cilantro
¼ teaspoon
ground cumin
⅛ teaspoon salt
Freshly ground
black pepper

**MUFA: ½ cup
macadamia nuts,
chopped**

4 lime wedges

1. Place the scallops on a work surface. Pat dry. Dust with the jerk seasoning and toss to coat evenly. Set aside.

2. Combine the beans, tomato, bell pepper, mango, onion, jalapeño pepper, lime juice, 1 tablespoon canola oil, cilantro, cumin, salt, and pepper to taste in a medium bowl, mixing well. Let stand to blend flavors.

3. Meanwhile, heat a skillet over medium-high heat. Add the remaining tablespoon of oil and heat for 1 minute. Add the scallops to the skillet. Cook for 1 to 2 minutes on each side, until well browned all over and opaque in the center. Remove to a plate.

4. Spoon the salsa onto 4 dinner plates. Top with the scallops and scatter 2 tablespoons macadamia nuts over each serving. Garnish with a lime wedge.

■ Eat One Serving:

386

calories, 24 g protein, 30 g carbohydrates, 21 g fat, 2.5 g saturated fat, 35 mg cholesterol, 560 mg sodium, 7 g fiber

A SINGLE SERVING OF THIS RECIPE COUNTS as a Flat Belly Diet Meal without any add-ons!

Lemon Linguine with Scallops and Asparagus

Cooking time: 35 minutes / Makes 4 servings

1 bunch asparagus, cut diagonally into 2" pieces

8 ounces multigrain linguine

16 sea scallops (1 ounce each), preferably dry-packed Ground black pepper

¼ teaspoon salt

2 teaspoons olive oil

2 tablespoons lemon juice Strip lemon peel, ½" × 3", thinly sliced

¼ cup water

¼ cup chopped fresh basil + additional leaves for garnish

MUFA: ½ cup walnuts, toasted and chopped

1. Bring 3 quarts of water to a boil in a large pot. Add the asparagus and cook for 1 minute, or until bright green and crisp-tender. Remove with tongs, rinse in cool water, and set aside.

2. In the same pot, cook the linguine for about 10 minutes, or until al dente.

3. Meanwhile, season the scallops with pepper to taste and ⅛ teaspoon salt. Heat a large skillet over medium-high heat. Add the oil to the pan. Cook scallops for 1 to 2 minutes on each side, until well browned all over and opaque in the center. Remove and set aside.

4. In the same skillet, combine the lemon juice, lemon peel, ¼ cup of water, and the remaining ⅛ teaspoon of salt. Cook, stirring, for about 1 minute, or until slightly reduced.

5. Drain the pasta and toss with the asparagus, chopped basil, walnuts, and lemon juice mixture. Serve in pasta bowls topped with the scallops and garnished with basil leaves.

■ **Eat One Serving:**

430

calories, 32 g protein, 45 g carbohydrates, 14 g fat, 1.5 g saturated fat, 36 mg cholesterol, 360 mg sodium, 6 g fiber

A SINGLE SERVING OF THIS RECIPE COUNTS as a Flat Belly Diet Meal without any add-ons!

Tofu Stir-Fry with Broccoli and Toasted Almonds

Cooking time: 40 minutes (including draining time) / Makes 4 servings

1 package
  (16 ounces)
  firm tofu
4 cups broccoli
  florets
2 teaspoons
  sesame oil
2 teaspoons
  canola oil
1 bunch scallions,
  thinly sliced
1 tablespoon
  minced garlic
1 small jalapeño
  chile pepper,
  halved, seeded,
  and finely
  chopped (wear
  plastic gloves
  when handling)
3½ teaspoons soy
  sauce

MUFA: ½ cup sliced almonds, lightly toasted

1. Place the tofu on a plate, and top with a cutting board. Place several cans of food on the board to weight it down. Let the tofu rest for 30 minutes while water is squeezed out. Cut the tofu into small cubes.

2. While the tofu drains, lightly steam the broccoli for about 5 minutes, or until crisp-tender. Set aside.

3. Coat a wok or large skillet with cooking spray. Set over high heat for 1 minute. Add 1 teaspoon of each oil. When hot, add the tofu and cook for about 5 minutes, stirring constantly, until browned. Transfer to a shallow bowl.

4. Add the remaining 2 teaspoons of oil to the wok, followed by the scallions, garlic, pepper, and broccoli. Stir-fry over medium-high heat for 2 minutes. Stir in the soy sauce, almonds, and tofu. Gently toss to combine.

■ Eat One Serving:

309

calories, 16 g protein, 33 g carbohydrates, 14 g fat, 1.5 g saturated fat, 0 mg cholesterol, 250 mg sodium, 6 g fiber

MAKE IT A FLAT BELLY DIET MEAL:

Serve with ½ cup steamed brown rice (109).

■ Total Meal:

418

calories, 18 g protein, 56 g carbohydrates, 14 g fat, 1.5 g saturated fat, 0 mg cholesterol, 250 mg sodium, 8 g fiber

Coconut Curried Tofu with Macadamia Nuts

Cooking time: 1 hour (including standing time) / Makes 6 servings

- 1 cup brown basmati rice
- 1 package (14 ounces) firm tofu, drained and cut into $3/4$" cubes
- 1 tablespoon canola oil
- $1/2$ teaspoon salt
- 1 large onion, halved and thinly sliced
- 1 –2 tablespoons red curry paste
- $1/2$ teaspoon curry powder
- 4 cups broccoli florets
- 1 cup light coconut milk
- $3/4$ cup reduced-sodium vegetable broth
- 1 cup frozen green peas
- 1 large tomato, cut into $3/4$" pieces
- 2 tablespoons lime juice

MUFA: $3/4$ cup chopped macadamia nuts

1. Cook the rice according to package directions. Place the tofu between layers of paper towels and let stand for 10 minutes.

2. Heat the oil in a large nonstick skillet over medium-high heat. Add the tofu and cook, turning once, for 6 to 8 minutes, or until golden brown. Sprinkle with $1/4$ teaspoon of the salt. With a slotted spoon, remove to a plate.

3. Add the onion to the skillet and cook, stirring frequently, for 3 to 4 minutes, or until browned. Stir in 1 tablespoon of the curry paste, curry powder, and the remaining $1/4$ teaspoon salt. Taste and add more curry paste if desired. Add the broccoli, coconut milk, broth, and peas. Bring to a boil.

4. Reduce the heat to low. Cover and simmer for 3 to 4 minutes, or until the broccoli is crisp-tender. Stir in the tomato, lime juice, and the reserved tofu. Simmer, stirring occasionally, for 2 to 3 minutes, or until the tofu is hot. Serve over the rice. Sprinkle with the macadamia nuts.

■ **Eat One Serving:**

417

calories, 18 g protein, 38 g carbohydrates, 25 g fat, 5 g saturated fat*, 0 mg cholesterol, 370 mg sodium, 7 g fiber

A SINGLE SERVING OF THIS RECIPE COUNTS as a Flat Belly Diet Meal without any add-ons!

* Limit saturated fat to no more than 10 percent of total calories—about 17 grams per day for most women or 21 grams for most men—and sodium intake to no more than 2,300 milligrams.

Lentil and Cauliflower Curry

Cooking time: 1 hour 15 minutes / Makes 4 servings

3 teaspoons
canola oil

4 cups cauliflower
florets, cut into
small pieces
(12–16 ounces)

½ cup chopped
onion (1 small)

½ cup chopped
carrot
(1 medium)

1 cup dried
brown lentils

2 teaspoons
minced garlic

1 teaspoon curry
powder

1½ cups reduced-
sodium
vegetable broth

¼ teaspoon salt

½ cup fat-free
plain yogurt

**MUFA: ½ cup pine
nuts, toasted if
desired**

Fresh cilantro
leaves

1. Heat a large, deep skillet
over medium-high heat. Add
2 teaspoons of the oil. Heat for
1 minute. Add the cauliflower.
Cover and cook, tossing
occasionally, for 5 minutes, or
until the cauliflower is lightly
charred. Reduce the heat if the
cauliflower is browning too
quickly. Remove the cauliflower to
a plate. Set aside.

2. Return the skillet to medium
heat. Add the remaining 1 teaspoon
oil and the onion and carrot. Cook,
stirring, for 3 minutes, or until the
vegetables start to soften. Stir in
the lentils, garlic, and curry powder.
Cook, stirring, for 3 minutes to coat
the lentils with the seasonings.
Add the broth. Bring almost to a
boil. Partially cover the pan and
reduce the heat. Simmer for about
20 minutes, or until the lentils are
almost tender.

3. Add the cauliflower to the skillet.
Partially cover and simmer for
about 5 minutes, or until the
cauliflower is tender and the lentils
are cooked. Stir in the salt. Spoon
onto 4 pasta plates. Divide and
dollop on the yogurt and sprinkle
with pine nuts. Garnish with
cilantro.

■ **Eat One Serving:**

356

calories, 16 g protein,
42 g carbohydrates, 16
g fat, 1 g saturated fat,
0 mg cholesterol, 260
mg sodium, 11 g fiber

**MAKE IT A FLAT
BELLY DIET MEAL:**
Serve with ½ sliced
apple (39).

■ **Total Meal:**

395

calories, 16 g protein,
52 g carbohydrates, 17
g fat, 1 g saturated fat,
0 mg cholesterol, 260
mg sodium, 15 g fiber

Vegetarian Picadillo with Cashews

Cooking time: 30 minutes / Makes 4 servings

MUFA: ½ cup cashews, chopped

1 tablespoon olive oil
1 large onion, chopped
3 cloves garlic, minced
8 ounces meatless burger crumbles
1½ teaspoons ground cumin
¼–½ teaspoon red-pepper flakes
½ teaspoon salt
1½ pounds plum tomatoes, coarsely chopped
¾ cup no-salt-added canned black beans, rinsed and drained
2 tablespoons raisins
2 tablespoons chopped black olives

1. Toast the cashews in a large, deep skillet over medium heat, stirring often, for about 3 minutes, or until lightly golden. Tip into a bowl. Wipe out the skillet.

2. Warm the oil in the same skillet over medium-high heat. Add the onion and garlic and cook, stirring often, for about 4 minutes, or until tender. Stir in the crumbles, cumin, red-pepper flakes, and salt. Cook and stir for 30 seconds.

3. Add the tomatoes and stir well, scraping the bottom of the skillet. Cook for about 2 minutes, or until the tomatoes start to release juice.

4. Reduce the heat to low. Stir in the beans and raisins. Cover and cook for 5 minutes, or until heated through and the tomatoes are cooked down. Add the olives and toasted cashews. Simmer, uncovered, for about 2 minutes, or until heated through.

■ Eat One Serving:

315

calories, 21 g protein, 33 g carbohydrates, 15 g fat, 2.5 g saturated fat, 0 mg cholesterol, 620 mg sodium*, 9 g fiber

MAKE IT A FLAT BELLY DIET MEAL:
Serve with 2 (6") corn tortillas, warmed (105).

■ Total Meal:

420

calories, 23 g protein, 55 g carbohydrates, 16 g fat, 2.5 g saturated fat, 0 mg cholesterol, 640 mg sodium*, 12 g fiber

* Limit saturated fat to no more than 10 percent of total calories—about 17 grams per day for most women or 21 grams for most men—and sodium intake to no more than 2,300 milligrams.

Soba Noodles with Peanut Sauce

Cooking time: 25 minutes / Makes 4 servings

MUFA: ½ cup peanut butter

¼ cup water
1 tablespoon honey
3 tablespoons rice vinegar
2 tablespoons reduced-sodium soy sauce
1 teaspoon grated fresh ginger
1 tablespoon sesame oil
⅛ teaspoon crushed red-pepper flakes
8 ounces soba or whole wheat noodles
3 carrots, cut into small matchsticks (about 2 cups)
2 scallions, chopped

1. Combine the peanut butter, water, honey, vinegar, soy sauce, ginger, oil, and pepper flakes in a small saucepan over medium-high heat. Bring to a boil and cook, stirring constantly, for 1 minute. Set aside.

2. Bring a pot of water to a boil. Add the noodles and return to a boil. Cook the noodles for 4 minutes, then stir in the carrots. Cook for 2 minutes longer, or until the carrots are crisp-tender. Drain the noodles and carrots and transfer to a large bowl.

3. Toss the noodles and carrots with the scallions and peanut sauce. Serve immediately.

■ **Eat One Serving:**

447

calories, 17 g protein, 58 g carbohydrates, 19 g fat*, 4 g saturated fat, 0 mg cholesterol, 439 mg sodium, 10 g fiber

A SINGLE SERVING OF THIS RECIPE COUNTS as a Flat Belly Diet Meal without any add-ons!

* Limit saturated fat to no more than 10 percent of total calories—about 17 grams per day for most women or 21 grams for most men—and sodium intake to no more than 2,300 milligrams.

VEGETARIAN

Fusilli with Mushrooms and Chard

Cooking time: 25 minutes / Makes 6 servings

8 ounces tricolor or whole wheat fusilli pasta

MUFA: 6 tablespoons olive oil

12 ounces frozen meatless burger crumbles

4 large shallots, peeled and quartered lengthwise

1 large bunch green chard, trimmed; stems cut into $\frac{1}{2}$"-thick slices; leaves (inner stems removed) sliced into long strips

10 ounces shiitake or brown mushrooms, stems removed and caps sliced

$\frac{1}{4}$ teaspoon salt

$\frac{1}{4}$ teaspoon ground black pepper

2 tablespoons chopped fresh parsley

$\frac{1}{3}$ cup (about $2\frac{3}{4}$ ounces) grated or shaved Parmesan cheese

1. Cook the pasta according to the package directions.

2. Meanwhile, in a large skillet, heat 3 tablespoons of the oil over medium heat and cook the burger crumbles until thawed and heated through. Transfer to a plate and keep warm. Add the remaining 3 tablespoons of oil to the pan. Add the shallots. Cook, tossing or stirring, for about 5 minutes, or until tender and golden brown. Add the chard stems. Cook for about 4 minutes, stirring often, until softened. Add the mushrooms, salt, and pepper. Cook for 2 to 3 minutes. Stir in the parsley and chard leaves and cook 1 minute longer, or until most of the liquid has evaporated and the leaves are wilted.

3. Drain the pasta, reserving $\frac{1}{3}$ cup of the cooking water. Return the pasta and the reserved water to the pot. Add the chard mixture, burger crumbles, and cheese. Toss well and serve immediately.

■ **Eat One Serving:**

385

calories, 20 g protein, 39 g carbohydrates, 18 g fat, 3 g saturated fat, 5 mg cholesterol, 520 mg sodium, 5 g fiber

A SINGLE SERVING OF THIS RECIPE COUNTS as a Flat Belly Diet Meal without any add-ons!

Mexican-Style Stuffed Peppers

Cooking time: 1 hour 15 minutes / Makes 4 servings

MUFA: ½ cup pine nuts

- 1 jalapeño chile pepper, stemmed, halved, and seeded (wear plastic gloves when handling)
- 2 large cloves garlic
- 1 can (14½ ounces) no-salt-added stewed tomatoes
- ¼ cup vegetable broth or water
- 2 tablespoons chili powder
- 2 cups cooked brown rice
- ¾ cup frozen corn kernels
- 2 plum tomatoes, chopped
- ½ onion, chopped
- 2 egg whites
- ¼ teaspoon salt
- 4 large poblano or Cubanelle peppers
- ¾ cup shredded reduced-fat Monterey Jack cheese

1. Preheat the oven to 400°F. Put the pine nuts in a small baking dish or skillet for about 8 minutes to lightly toast while the oven heats. Tip onto a plate.

2. Combine the jalapeño pepper, garlic, stewed tomatoes with juice, broth or water, and 1 tablespoon plus 2 teaspoons of the chili powder in the bowl of a food processor fitted with a metal blade. Process to a medium-coarse texture. Pour into a 9" × 13" glass baking dish and set aside.

3. Mix the rice, corn, plum tomatoes, onion, egg whites, salt, toasted nuts, and remaining 1 teaspoon chili powder in a medium bowl. Halve the poblano or Cubanelle peppers lengthwise and remove the stems and seeds. Spoon about ½ cup of the stuffing into each pepper half and place stuffed side up in the reserved sauce in the baking dish.

4. Cover the dish with foil and bake for 40 to 45 minutes, or until the peppers are tender.

5. Remove the foil and sprinkle the peppers evenly with the cheese. Bake for 5 to 8 minutes longer, or until the cheese has melted. Serve the peppers with the sauce.

■ **Eat One Serving:**

395

calories, 16 g protein, 45 g carbohydrates, 20 g fat, 4 g saturated fat*, 15 mg cholesterol, 435 mg sodium, 8 g fiber

A SINGLE SERVING OF THIS RECIPE COUNTS as a Flat Belly Diet Meal without any add-ons!

* Limit saturated fat to no more than 10 percent of total calories—about 17 grams per day for most women or 21 grams for most men—and sodium intake to no more than 2,300 milligrams.

Gnocchi Casserole

Cooking time: 1 hour + standing time / Makes 6 servings

¾ cup part-skim ricotta cheese

¼ cup fresh basil, thinly sliced

MUFA: ¾ cup almonds, finely chopped

½ cup grated reduced-fat mozzarella

2 tablespoons grated Parmesan cheese

1 egg, lightly beaten

3 cups prepared marinara sauce

1 package (16 ounces) potato gnocchi

2 cups spinach leaves, thinly sliced

1. Preheat the oven to 400°F. Lightly coat a 1½-quart casserole or gratin dish with vegetable oil spray and set aside.

2. Combine the ricotta, basil, almonds, ¼ cup of the mozzarella, Parmesan, and egg in a small bowl. Stir until blended. Set aside.

3. Spread a thin layer of the marinara sauce in the baking dish. On top of the sauce, layer half of the gnocchi and spinach. Using half of the ricotta mixture, place small dollops on top of the spinach. Cover with another thin layer of sauce. Repeat the process, ending with sauce. Sprinkle on the remaining ¼ cup mozzarella.

4. Bake for 40 minutes, or until the top is bubbly and the cheese is lightly browned. Let stand for 15 minutes before serving.

■ **Eat One Serving:**

334

calories, 14 g protein, 28 g carbohydrates, 19 g fat, 7 g saturated fat*, 65 mg cholesterol, 710 mg sodium*, 4 g fiber

MAKE IT A FLAT BELLY DIET MEAL:

Serve with ¼ pound steamed asparagus (23) tossed with 1 teaspoon olive oil (40) and a squeeze of fresh lemon juice (0).

■ **Total Meal:**

397

calories, 16 g protein, 33 g carbohydrates, 23 g fat, 8 g saturated fat*, 65 mg cholesterol, 720 mg sodium*, 7 g fiber

* Limit saturated fat to no more than 10 percent of total calories—about 17 grams per day for most women or 21 grams for most men—and sodium intake to no more than 2,300 milligrams.

Filet Mignon with Mustard-Horseradish Sauce and Roasted Potatoes

Cooking time: 1 hour + standing time / Makes 4 servings

1½ pounds small red potatoes, halved or quartered

MUFA: ¼ cup olive oil

½ teaspoon salt
4 boneless beef tenderloin steaks (4 ounces each), well-trimmed
¾ teaspoon coarsely ground black pepper
1 tablespoon + 1 teaspoon grainy mustard
3 tablespoons reduced-fat sour cream
1 small plum tomato, finely chopped
2 tablespoons snipped fresh chives or scallion greens
1 tablespoon prepared horseradish
1 small shallot, minced

1. Preheat the oven to 425°F. Coat a broiler-pan rack with olive oil cooking spray and set aside.

2. Place potatoes, oil, and ¼ teaspoon salt in a 9" x 9" baking dish and toss to coat. Bake for 30 minutes, removing from the oven a few times to toss, until they are golden and tender. Loosely tent with foil and set aside.

3. Sprinkle the steaks on both sides with the pepper and remaining ¼ teaspoon salt. Place on the prepared broiler pan. Broil 2" to 4" from the heat for 4 to 5 minutes, until browned. Turn and spread the tops with 1 tablespoon of the mustard. Cook 3 to 4 minutes longer for medium-rare, or until desired doneness. Remove from the heat, transfer to a plate, and let rest for 10 minutes.

4. While the steaks rest, make the sauce by mixing the sour cream, tomato, chives or scallion greens, horseradish, shallot, and remaining teaspoon of mustard in a small bowl until well blended. Divide sauce evenly among 4 dinner plates and arrange steak and potatoes on top.

■ Eat One Serving:

448

calories, 29 g protein, 30 g carbohydrates, 23 g fat, 6 g saturated fat*, 80 mg cholesterol, 300 mg sodium, 3 g fiber

A SINGLE SERVING OF THIS RECIPE COUNTS as a Flat Belly Diet Meal without any add-ons!

* Limit saturated fat to no more than 10 percent of total calories—about 17 grams per day for most women or 21 grams for most men—and sodium intake to no more than 2,300 milligrams.

Greek Eggplant Casserole

Cooking time: 45 minutes / Makes 6 servings

1 onion, chopped
2 cloves garlic, minced
¾ pound 97% lean ground beef
1 can (14½ ounces) no-salt-added diced tomatoes
¼ cup tomato paste
½ teaspoon ground cinnamon
¼ teaspoon ground allspice
2 eggplants, peeled and cut lengthwise into ¼"-thick slices

MUFA: 6 tablespoons safflower oil

2 cups 1% milk
3 tablespoons cornstarch
½ cup grated Romano cheese

1. Heat the broiler. Coat a 9" x 9" baking dish and a large baking sheet with olive oil cooking spray.

2. Heat a large skillet coated with cooking spray over medium-high heat. Cook the onion and garlic for 3 minutes, or until the onion begins to soften. Add the beef and cook for 5 to 7 minutes, stirring often, or until the beef is browned and cooked through. Stir in the tomatoes (with juice), tomato paste, cinnamon, and allspice. Bring to a boil. Reduce the heat to low and simmer for 10 minutes.

3. Place half of the eggplant on the prepared baking sheet and brush with 3 tablespoons of the oil. Broil 6" from the heat for 10 minutes or until browned, turning once. Repeat.

4. Whisk together the milk and cornstarch in a small saucepan. Bring to a simmer over medium heat and cook, whisking, for 8 minutes, or until thickened. Remove from the heat and stir in the cheese.

5. Layer half of the eggplant in the baking dish, then half of the meat sauce. Repeat. Spread the cheese sauce on top. Broil for 3 minutes, or until just starting to brown.

■ **Eat One Serving:**

350

calories, 19 g protein, 21 g carbohydrates, 21 g fat, 4.5 g saturated fat*, 45 mg cholesterol, 340 mg sodium, 5 g fiber

MAKE IT A FLAT BELLY DIET MEAL:
Serve with ½ cup fat-free Greek-style yogurt (60).

■ **Total Meal:**

410

calories, 29 g protein, 25 g carbohydrates, 21 g fat, 4.5 g saturated fat*, 45 mg cholesterol, 380 mg sodium, 5 g fiber

* Limit saturated fat to no more than 10 percent of total calories—about 17 grams per day for most women or 21 grams for most men—and sodium intake to no more than 2,300 milligrams.

Five-Spice Pecan Pork

Cooking time: 20 minutes + standing time: 5 minutes / Makes 4 servings

1 pound pork tenderloin, trimmed of all visible fat

2 teaspoons five-spice powder (see note)

¼ teaspoon salt + pinch of salt

2 teaspoons trans-free margarine

3 large Granny Smith apples, cored and sliced in ½" wedges

½ cup dried cranberries

MUFA: ½ cup chopped pecans

½ cup water

1. Cut the tenderloin in half to create two equal pieces. Rub the spice powder and ¼ teaspoon salt over all sides of each piece.

2. Melt 1 teaspoon of the margarine in a small nonstick skillet over medium-high heat. Add the meat and cook, turning as needed, for about 4 minutes, or until browned on all sides. Cover and continue to cook, turning occasionally, for about 12 minutes, or until a thermometer inserted in the center reaches 155°F and the juices run clear. Remove and let stand for 5 minutes. Cut each piece into 6 medallions.

3. Meanwhile, combine the apples, cranberries, remaining teaspoon of margarine, the pecans, water, and the remaining pinch of salt in a heavy skillet set over medium-high heat. Cook, shaking the pan occasionally, until the liquid has almost evaporated and the apples soften. Serve with the pork medallions.

■ **Eat One Serving:**

328

calories, 25 g protein, 26 g carbohydrates, 15 g fat, 2 g saturated fat, 75 mg cholesterol, 220 mg sodium, 4 g fiber

MAKE IT A FLAT BELLY DIET MEAL:
Serve with ½ cup steamed brown rice (109).

■ **Total Meal:**

437

calories, 28 g protein, 48 g carbohydrates, 15 g fat, 2 g saturated fat, 75 mg cholesterol, 220 mg sodium, 4 g fiber

NOTE: Five-spice powder is a Chinese seasoning mixture comprised of cinnamon, cloves, fennel seed, star anise, and Szechuan peppercorns. Look for it in the spice section of the supermarket.

Grilled Pork Chops with Olives, Oranges, and Onion

Cooking time: 25 minutes / Makes 4 servings

2 oranges

MUFA: 40 green olives (about 1⅓ cups), quartered lengthwise

½ small red onion, thinly sliced
½ teaspoon cracked black pepper
½ teaspoon smoked paprika
½ teaspoon salt
4 boneless pork chops (about 4 ounces each)

1. Coat a grill rack or rack in a broiler pan with cooking spray. Preheat the grill or broiler.

2. Cut the peel and white pith from the oranges. Holding the oranges over a medium bowl to catch the juice, cut between the membranes to release the segments, allowing them to drop into the bowl. Squeeze the membranes to release any juices into the bowl. Add the olives, onion, and pepper to the bowl. Toss to combine.

3. Combine the paprika and salt in a small bowl. Rub onto both sides of the chops. Grill or broil, turning once, for 6 to 10 minutes, or until a thermometer inserted in the center of a chop registers 155°F. Serve the chops topped with the orange mixture.

■ **Eat One Serving:**

246

calories, 26 g protein, 10 g carbohydrates, 12 g fat, 1.5 g saturated fat, 80 mg cholesterol, 490 mg sodium, 2 g fiber

MAKE IT A FLAT BELLY DIET MEAL: Serve with the Saffron Rice on page 271, but omit the pistachios (138).

■ **Total Meal:**

384

calories, 29 g protein, 35 g carbohydrates, 14 g fat, 1.5 g saturated fat, 80 mg cholesterol, 790 mg sodium*, 3 g fiber

* Limit saturated fat to no more than 10 percent of total calories—about 17 grams per day for most women or 21 grams for most men—and sodium intake to no more than 2,300 milligrams.

Slow-Cooked Barbecue Pulled Pork

Cooking time: 2 hours / Makes 6 servings

MUFA: 6 tablespoons olive oil

- 1½ pounds boneless pork loin, trimmed of all visible fat
- 1 medium onion, chopped (about ½ cup)
- ⅔ cup ketchup
- 1 tablespoon cider vinegar
- 1 tablespoon molasses
- 2 teaspoons packed brown sugar
- 2 teaspoons mustard powder
- 1½ teaspoons garlic powder
- 1 teaspoon Worcestershire sauce
- ¼ teaspoon freshly ground black pepper
- 1½ cups chicken or vegetable broth
- 6 whole wheat hamburger buns

1. Heat the oil in a 4- to 6-quart pot over medium-high heat. Add the pork loin and brown, turning occasionally, for 5 minutes.

2. Add the onion and cook for 5 minutes more, or until the onion starts to turn golden. Add the ketchup, vinegar, molasses, sugar, mustard powder, garlic powder, Worcestershire sauce, black pepper, and broth.

3. Stir well to combine and bring to a boil over medium-high heat. Reduce the heat to low, cover, and simmer, stirring occasionally, for 1½ hours.

4. Uncover the pot and simmer 10 minutes longer, or until the sauce has thickened slightly and the pork is very tender. Remove from the heat.

5. Pull the pork into shreds with two forks and serve on whole wheat hamburger buns.

■ **Eat One Serving:**

419

calories, 29 g protein, 35 g carbohydrates, 19 g fat, 3 g saturated fat, 75 mg cholesterol, 810 mg sodium*, 4 g fiber

A SINGLE SERVING OF THIS RECIPE COUNTS as a Flat Belly Diet Meal without any add-ons!

* Limit saturated fat to no more than 10 percent of total calories—about 17 grams per day for most women or 21 grams for most men—and sodium intake to no more than 2,300 milligrams.

Pork and Almond Meatballs

Cooking time: 40 minutes / Makes 4 servings

MUFA: ½ cup almonds

1 pound pork tenderloin, trimmed and cut into small chunks
1½ teaspoons crumbled dried sage
2 cloves garlic, minced
2 teaspoons red wine vinegar
¼ teaspoon salt
¼ teaspoon freshly ground black pepper
Olive oil in a spritzer

1. Preheat the oven to 375°F. Coat a large baking pan with cooking spray. Set aside.

2. Pulse the almonds in the bowl of a food processor fitted with a metal blade until coarsely chopped. Add the pork, sage, garlic, vinegar, salt, and pepper. Pulse until evenly ground.

3. Divide the mixture into 12 equal portions and roll into meatballs. Arrange on the prepared pan. Spritz lightly with the oil.

4. Bake for about 25 minutes, or until cooked through.

■ Eat One Serving:

205

calories, 27 g protein, 4 g carbohydrates, 9 g fat, 1.5 g saturated fat, 75 mg cholesterol, 210 mg sodium, 2 g fiber

MAKE IT A FLAT BELLY DIET MEAL: Serve with 1 cup steamed zucchini (29) drizzled with 1 teaspoon olive oil (40) and tossed with ½ cup multigrain penne, cooked (101).

■ Total Meal:

375

calories, 31 g protein, 32 g carbohydrates, 14 g fat, 2 g saturated fat, 75 mg cholesterol, 210 mg sodium, 5 g fiber

Saffron Rice with Pistachios

Cooking time: 30 minutes / Makes 4 servings

½ teaspoon
saffron threads
1 tablespoon +
2¼ cups water

**MUFA: ½ cup
pistachios**

1 teaspoon olive
oil
½ teaspoon salt
1½ cups instant
brown rice

1. Soak the saffron in 1 tablespoon of the water in a small bowl for 20 minutes. Use the back of a spoon to mash the threads.

2. Toast the pistachios in a large nonstick skillet over medium heat, stirring often, for 3 to 4 minutes, or until lightly browned and fragrant. Tip onto a plate and let cool.

3. Bring the oil, salt, and remaining 2¼ cups water to a boil over medium-high heat. Reduce the heat to low, add the rice and the saffron mixture, and cook, covered, for 5 minutes. Turn off the heat and let the rice sit for 5 minutes.

4. Fluff the rice with a fork and stir in the pistachios.

■ Eat One Serving:

229

calories, 6 g protein, 30 g carbohydrates, 10 g fat, 1 g saturated fat, 0 mg cholesterol, 300 mg sodium, 3 g fiber

MAKE IT A FLAT BELLY DIET MEAL:

Serve with 4 ounces broiled shrimp (112) and ½ cup fat-free Greek-style yogurt (60). To serve as part of another FBD meal, omit the pistachios (138).

■ Total Meal:

401

calories, 40 g protein, 34 g carbohydrates, 11 g fat, 1.5 g saturated fat, 220 mg cholesterol, 600 mg sodium*, 3 g fiber

* Limit saturated fat to no more than 10 percent of total calories—about 17 grams per day for most women or 21 grams for most men—and sodium intake to no more than 2,300 milligrams.

Balsamic Roasted Carrots

Cooking time: 30 minutes / Makes 2 servings

8 medium carrots, quartered lengthwise

MUFA: 2 tablespoons extra-virgin olive oil

1 tablespoon balsamic vinegar
½ teaspoon salt
¼ teaspoon freshly ground black pepper

1. Preheat the oven to 450°F.

2. Combine the carrots, 1 tablespoon oil, vinegar, salt, and pepper in a roasting pan. Toss to coat. Roast for 20 to 25 minutes, tossing occasionally, until lightly caramelized and tender but still firm. Drizzle with the remaining tablespoon of oil.

■ **Eat One Serving:**

232

calories, 2 g protein, 25 g carbohydrates, 15 g fat, 2 g saturated fat, 0 mg cholesterol, 650 mg sodium*, 7 g fiber

MAKE IT A FLAT BELLY DIET MEAL:
Serve with 2 cups organic mixed baby greens (20), 1 cup cherry tomatoes (27), and 4 ounces roasted cod (93).

■ **Total Meal:**

396

calories, 31 g protein, 34 g carbohydrates, 16.5 g fat, 2.5 g saturated fat, 62 mg cholesterol, 775 mg sodium*, 11 g fiber

* Limit saturated fat to no more than 10 percent of total calories—about 17 grams per day for most women or 21 grams for most men—and sodium intake to no more than 2,300 milligrams.

Roasted Potatoes with Blue Cheese and Walnuts

Cooking time: 45 minutes / Makes 4 servings

1 pound thin-skinned baby potatoes, halved
1½ teaspoons olive oil
¼ teaspoon freshly ground black pepper
⅛ teaspoon salt

MUFA: 1/2 cup coarsely chopped walnuts

2 ounces crumbled blue cheese
2 scallions, thinly sliced

1. Preheat the oven to 425°F. Coat a 9″ x 9″ baking dish with cooking spray or line with parchment paper. Place the potatoes in the prepared dish and toss with the oil, pepper, and salt. Turn cut side down in the pan. Roast for 30 to 35 minutes, or until very tender and lightly golden on the underside.

2. Meanwhile, put the walnuts in a small baking pan or ovenproof skillet and place in the oven to toast for 6 to 8 minutes. Tip into a bowl and let cool. Add the blue cheese and scallions and crumble with your fingers.

3. When the potatoes are done, turn them over and sprinkle evenly with the walnut mixture. Bake for 5 minutes longer, or until the cheese is melted.

■ **Eat One Serving:**

243

calories, 8 g protein, 21 g carbohydrates, 15 g fat, 4 g saturated fat*, 10 mg cholesterol, 280 mg sodium, 3 g fiber

MAKE IT A FLAT BELLY DIET MEAL:

Add 3 ounces lean broiled flank steak (165). Serve with ½ sliced apple (39).

■ **Total Meal:**

447

calories, 31 g protein, 30 g carbohydrates, 23 g fat, 7 g saturated fat*, 55 mg cholesterol, 330 mg sodium, 3 g fiber

* Limit saturated fat to no more than 10 percent of total calories—about 17 grams per day for most women or 21 grams for most men—and sodium intake to no more than 2,300 milligrams.

Cheesy Squash Casserole

Cooking time: 1 hour 25 minutes / Makes 6 servings

1 spaghetti squash, halved and seeded
2 tablespoons olive oil
1 small onion, chopped
2 cloves garlic, chopped
1 tablespoon chopped fresh basil, or 1 teaspoon dried
2 plum tomatoes, chopped
1 cup 1% cottage cheese
½ cup shredded low-fat mozzarella cheese
¼ cup chopped fresh parsley
¼ teaspoon salt

MUFA: ¾ cup pine nuts

¼ cup grated Parmesan cheese
3 tablespoons whole wheat bread crumbs

1. Preheat the oven to 400°F. Coat a 13" x 9" baking dish and a baking sheet with cooking spray. Place the squash, cut side down, on the prepared baking sheet. Bake for 30 minutes, or until tender. With a fork, scrape the squash strands into a large bowl.

2. Meanwhile, heat the oil in a medium skillet over medium heat. Add the onion, garlic, and basil, and cook for 4 minutes. Add the tomatoes and cook for 3 minutes.

3. Add the cottage cheese, mozzarella, parsley, salt, and the tomato mixture to the bowl with the squash. Toss to coat. Place in the prepared baking dish. Scatter the pine nuts, Parmesan, and bread crumbs over the top.

4. Bake for 30 minutes, or until hot and bubbly.

■ **Eat One Serving:**

286

calories, 14 g protein, 13 g carbohydrates, 21 g fat, 4.5 g saturated fat*, 15 mg cholesterol, 480 mg sodium, 2 g fiber

MAKE IT A FLAT BELLY DIET MEAL:
Serve with 1 medium pear (103).

■ **Total Meal:**

389

calories, 15 g protein, 41 g carbohydrates, 21 g fat, 4.5 g saturated fat*, 15 mg cholesterol, 480 mg sodium, 8 g fiber

* Limit saturated fat to no more than 10 percent of total calories—about 17 grams per day for most women or 21 grams for most men—and sodium intake to no more than 2,300 milligrams.

Chips and Guacamole

Cooking time: 15 minutes / Makes 8 servings

MUFA: 2 cups mashed Hass avocado

- 1 large tomato, chopped
- ¼ white onion, diced
- ¼ cup chopped fresh cilantro
- ¼ cup freshly squeezed lime juice
- 1 fresh jalapeño chile pepper, minced (wear gloves when handling)
- ¼ teaspoon salt
- ½ teaspoon green or red hot sauce, such as Tabasco (optional)
- 8 whole wheat tortillas (8" diameter) Vegetable oil spray Chili powder

1. Place the avocado, tomato, onion, cilantro, lime juice, pepper, salt, and hot sauce (if using) in a medium bowl. Stir until combined.

2. Preheat the oven to 350°F. Spread the tortillas on a work surface. Coat lightly with vegetable oil spray. Sprinkle lightly with chili powder. Flip the tortillas and repeat with the spray and chili powder.

3. Place the tortillas in a stack. With a serrated knife, cut the stack into 8 equal wedges. Spread the triangles out on a baking sheet or sheets so they are not touching. Bake for about 10 minutes, or until crisp and starting to puff. Let stand to cool. Serve right away with the guacamole or store in an airtight container.

■ Eat One Serving (8 chips per serving):

206

calories, 3 g protein, 25 g carbohydrates, 11 g fat, 1 g saturated fat, 0 mg cholesterol, 450 mg sodium, 7 g fiber

MAKE IT A FLAT BELLY DIET MEAL:

Serve with ½ cup mashed black beans (110) and ½ fresh mango (67).

■ Total Meal:

383

calories, 11 g protein, 51 g carbohydrates, 13 g fat, 1 g saturated fat, 0 mg cholesterol, 969 mg sodium*, 17 g fiber

* Limit saturated fat to no more than 10 percent of total calories—about 17 grams per day for most women or 21 grams for most men—and sodium intake to no more than 2,300 milligrams.

Spicy Snack Mix

Cooking time: 2–3 hours / Makes 18 servings

½ cup canola oil
1 tablespoon chili powder
1 teaspoon ground cumin
1 teaspoon dried oregano
½ teaspoon salt
¼ teaspoon ground red pepper
3 cups multigrain square cereal

MUFA: 2¼ cups unsalted sunflower seeds

2 cups oat or multigrain cereal
2 cups multigrain pretzel sticks

1. Combine the oil, chili powder, cumin, oregano, salt, and pepper in a small measuring cup.

2. Combine the cereal squares, sunflower seeds, oat cereal, and pretzels in a 3½- to 5-quart slow cooker. Drizzle with the oil mixture, tossing to coat well. Cover and cook on low for 2 to 3 hours, stirring twice during the cooking time. Be sure to check the mixture after 2 hours, as slow cooker times can vary.

3. Remove the lid during the last half hour of cooking to allow the mix to dry.

■ **Eat One Serving** (½ cup per serving):

230

calories, 5 g protein, 22 g carbohydrates, 15 g fat, 1.5 g saturated fat, 0 mg cholesterol, 320 mg sodium, 3 g fiber

MAKE IT A FLAT BELLY DIET MEAL: Serve with 4 ounces broiled shrimp (112) and ½ cup seedless red grapes (52).

■ **Total Meal:**

394

calories, 29 g protein, 36 g carbohydrates, 16 g fat, 1.5 g saturated fat, 220 mg cholesterol, 580 mg sodium, 4 g fiber

Granola Bars with Cashews and Dried Cherries

Cooking time: 50 minutes / Makes 12 servings

MUFA: 1½ cups cashews, chopped

1½ cups dry plain oats
1 tablespoon all-purpose flour
⅔ cup chopped dried unsweetened cherries
2 eggs
1 cup packed light brown sugar
1 tablespoon canola oil
1 teaspoon ground cinnamon
¼ teaspoon salt
1 teaspoon vanilla extract

1. Preheat the oven to 325°F. Line a 9" x 9" pan with foil, allowing about a 1" overhang from the sides. Coat with cooking spray.

2. Place 1 cup of the cashews and ½ cup of the oats on a large baking sheet with sides. Bake for 10 minutes, or until toasted, stirring once. Set aside.

3. Place the flour and remaining 1 cup oats and ½ cup cashews in a food processor fitted with a metal blade. Process until smooth. Transfer to a medium bowl and combine with the cherries and reserved cashews and oats.

4. Whisk together the eggs, brown sugar, oil, cinnamon, salt, and vanilla in a large bowl. Stir in the oats-cashew mixture until well blended. Spread in the prepared pan.

5. Bake for 30 minutes, or until golden brown. Remove from the pan, using the foil as a guide, and cool completely on a rack. Cut into 12 rectangles with a serrated knife.

■ Eat One Serving:

261

calories, 6 g protein, 37 g carbohydrates, 11 g fat, 2 g saturated fat, 35 mg cholesterol, 70 mg sodium, 2 g fiber

MAKE IT A FLAT BELLY DIET MEAL:

Serve with 1 cup fat-free milk (83).

■ Total Meal:

344

calories, 15 g protein, 51 g carbohydrates, 11 g fat, 2 g saturated fat, 38 mg cholesterol, 199 mg sodium, 3 g fiber

Fruit and Nut Muffins

Cooking time: 30 minutes / Makes 12 servings

1¾ cups whole grain pastry flour
1½ teaspoons baking powder
1½ teaspoons ground cinnamon
½ teaspoon baking soda
¼ teaspoon salt
1 cup fat-free vanilla yogurt
½ cup brown sugar
1 egg
2 tablespoons canola oil
1 teaspoon vanilla extract

MUFA: 1½ cups pecans, chopped

½ cup crushed pineapple in juice, drained
⅓ cup currants or raisins
¼ cup grated carrots

1. Preheat the oven to 400°F.

2. Combine the flour, baking powder, cinnamon, baking soda, and salt in a large bowl. Combine the yogurt, brown sugar, egg, oil, and vanilla in a medium bowl. Stir the yogurt mixture into the flour mixture just until blended. (Lumps are okay.) Fold in the pecans, pineapple, currants or raisins, and carrots.

3. Divide the batter evenly among 12 muffin cups coated with cooking spray.

4. Bake for 20 minutes, or until a toothpick inserted in the center of a muffin comes out clean.

5. Cool in the pan on a wire rack for 5 minutes. Remove muffins from the pan to cool completely on the wire rack.

■ Eat One Serving:

250

calories, 5 g protein, 30 g carbohydrates, 14 g fat, 1 g saturated fat, 20 mg cholesterol, 180 mg sodium, 3 g fiber

MAKE IT A FLAT BELLY DIET MEAL: Serve with ¾ cup fat-free Greek-style yogurt (92) and ½ cup blueberries (42).

■ Total Meal:

384

calories, 20 g protein, 47 g carbohydrates, 14 g fat, 1.5 g saturated fat, 20 mg cholesterol, 240 mg sodium, 5 g fiber

Double Pumpkin Snack Bars

Cooking time: 40 minutes / Makes 12 servings

MUFA: 1½ cups shelled pumpkin seeds

- 1 cup canned solid-pack pumpkin
- 1 cup shredded carrot
- ½ cup sugar
- ⅓ cup dried cranberries or raisins, chopped
- ¼ cup canola oil
- 2 large eggs
- 1 cup whole grain pastry flour
- 1 teaspoon baking powder
- 1 teaspoon ground cinnamon
- ½ teaspoon baking soda
- ¼ teaspoon salt

1. Preheat the oven to 350°F. Coat a 13" x 9" x 2" baking pan with cooking spray.

2. Measure 1 cup of the pumpkin seeds into a blender or food processor and process until finely ground. Set aside. Coarsely chop the remaining seeds and set aside.

3. Combine the pumpkin, carrot, sugar, cranberries or raisins, oil, and eggs in a large bowl and stir until well blended. Add the flour, ground pumpkin seeds, baking powder, cinnamon, baking soda, and salt. Mix until blended.

4. Pour the batter into the prepared pan and spread evenly. Sprinkle with the reserved chopped pumpkin seeds. Bake for 22 to 25 minutes, or until the top springs back when pressed lightly. Cool completely in the pan on a rack before cutting into 12 bars.

■ **Eat One Serving:**

285

calories, 12 g protein, 24 g carbohydrates, 18 g fat, 3 g saturated fat, 35 mg cholesterol, 105 mg sodium, 3 g fiber

MAKE IT A FLAT BELLY DIET MEAL:
Serve with ½ cup 1% cottage cheese (81) and ¼ cup pineapple chunks canned in own juice (27).

■ **Total Meal:**

393

calories, 26 g protein, 34 g carbohydrates, 19 g fat, 3.5 g saturated fat, 40 mg cholesterol, 570 mg sodium, 4 g fiber

Harvest Apple Cake

Cooking time: 1 hour 15 minutes (including standing time) / Makes 8 servings

2 Granny Smith apples, peeled, cored, and cut into ½" cubes

¾ cup packed brown sugar

1½ cups whole grain pastry flour

1 teaspoon baking soda

1 teaspoon ground cinnamon

1 teaspoon ground ginger

½ teaspoon ground nutmeg

½ teaspoon salt

⅓ cup low-fat buttermilk

⅓ cup canola oil

1 large egg

1 teaspoon vanilla extract

MUFA: 1 cup pecans, chopped

½ cup raisins

1. Preheat the oven to 350°F. Coat a 9" x 9" baking pan with cooking spray.

2. Combine the apples and brown sugar in a large bowl and stir to coat the apples well. Let stand for 30 minutes, stirring occasionally.

3. Combine the flour, baking soda, cinnamon, ginger, nutmeg, and salt in a separate bowl.

4. Mix the buttermilk, oil, egg, and vanilla in a small bowl until blended. Pour the buttermilk mixture over the apple mixture and add the pecans and raisins. Stir until combined. Add the flour mixture and stir until batter is blended. Pour into the prepared pan and spread evenly. Bake for 35 to 40 minutes, or until a wooden pick inserted into the center comes out clean.

5. Cool in the pan on a rack. Serve warm or at room temperature.

■ **Eat One Serving:**

422

calories, 6 g protein, 45 g carbohydrates, 26 g fat, 2.5 g saturated fat, 25 mg cholesterol, 330 mg sodium, 4 g fiber

A SINGLE SERVING OF THIS RECIPE COUNTS as a Flat Belly Diet Meal without any add-ons!

Chocolate-Zucchini Snack Cake

Cooking time: 45 minutes / Makes 12 servings

1¾ cups whole wheat pastry flour
1½ teaspoons baking powder
½ teaspoon baking soda
¼ teaspoon salt
2 eggs
½ cup sugar
½ cup low-fat vanilla yogurt
⅓ cup canola oil
1 teaspoon vanilla extract
1½ cups shredded zucchini

MUFA: 3 cups semisweet chocolate chips

1. Preheat the oven to 350°F. Coat an 11" x 7" baking pan with cooking spray.

2. Combine the flour, baking powder, baking soda, and salt in a large bowl.

3. Whisk the eggs, sugar, yogurt, oil, and vanilla in a medium bowl. Whisk in the zucchini and 1½ cups of the chips. Stir into the flour mixture just until blended. Spread into the prepared pan and bake for 30 minutes, or until lightly browned and a wooden pick inserted into the center comes out clean.

4. Remove from the oven and sprinkle the remaining 1½ cups of chips over the cake. Spread with a small spatula as they melt to form an icing, placing back into the warm oven, if needed, for about 1 minute.

■ **Eat One Serving:**

361

calories, 5 g protein, 47 g carbohydrates, 20 g fat, 8 g saturated fat*, 36 mg cholesterol, 175 mg sodium, 4 g fiber

A SINGLE SERVING OF THIS RECIPE COUNTS as a Flat Belly Diet Meal without any add-ons!

* Limit saturated fat to no more than 10 percent of total calories—about 17 grams per day for most women or 21 grams for most men—and sodium intake to no more than 2,300 milligrams.

Dunking Cookies with Sweet Peanut Sauce

Cooking time: 35 minutes / Makes 10 servings

2 cups whole wheat pastry flour
½ teaspoon baking soda
¼ teaspoon salt
1 teaspoon ground cinnamon
½ teaspoon ground ginger
4 tablespoons trans-free margarine, softened
2 tablespoons canola oil
⅓ cup packed dark brown sugar
⅓ cup + 2 tablespoons honey
1 large egg

MUFA: ½ cup creamy natural unsalted peanut butter

½ cup fat-free evaporated milk

1. Preheat the oven to 350°F. Coat 2 baking sheets with cooking spray.

2. Combine the flour, baking soda, salt, cinnamon, and ginger in a medium bowl. Set aside.

3. Cream the margarine, oil, brown sugar, ⅓ cup honey, and egg with a hand mixer. Add the reserved dry ingredients and stir until combined.

4. Drop by rounded tablespoons onto the prepared baking sheets and bake for 10 to 12 minutes, or until golden. Let cool on the trays for 5 minutes. Transfer to a rack to cool completely.

5. Make the sauce by heating the peanut butter, milk, and remaining 2 tablespoons honey in a small saucepan over low heat. Stir constantly until melted and smooth. Serve warm.

■ **Eat One Serving (3 cookies + 4 Tbsp sauce per serving):**

453

calories, 13 g protein, 49 g carbohydrates, 23 g fat, 3.5 g saturated fat*, 21 mg cholesterol, 141 mg sodium, 4 g fiber

A SINGLE SERVING OF THIS RECIPE COUNTS as a Flat Belly Diet Meal without any add-ons!

* Limit saturated fat to no more than 10 percent of total calories—about 17 grams per day for most women or 21 grams for most men—and sodium intake to no more than 2,300 milligrams.

Chocolate-Almond Macaroons with Dark Chocolate Dunking Sauce

Cooking time: 50 minutes + cooling time / Makes 6 servings

¾ cup blanched almonds

½ cup sugar

4 egg whites

¼ cup unsweetened cocoa powder

1 teaspoon vanilla extract

½ teaspoon almond extract

¼ teaspoon salt

MUFA: 4 ounces bittersweet or semisweet chocolate

½ cup whole milk

2 tablespoons packed brown sugar

1. Preheat the oven to 325°F. Line 2 large baking sheets with parchment paper.

2. Toast the almonds in a large, deep skillet over medium heat, stirring often, for about 3 minutes, or until golden. Tip into the bowl of a food processor fitted with a metal blade.

3. Add 1 tablespoon of the sugar. Process until the almonds are finely ground.

4. Beat the egg whites with an electric mixer on high speed until the whites hold soft peaks. Gradually beat in the remaining sugar until the whites hold stiff peaks. Beat in the cocoa, vanilla, almond extract, and salt. Gently fold in the almonds.

5. Drop the mixture by rounded tablespoons onto the prepared baking sheets, leaving 1″ between each macaroon. Bake for 27 to 30 minutes, or until very lightly browned. Place baking sheets on a rack and let macaroons cool until firm.

6. Make the sauce by heating the chocolate, milk, and brown sugar in a small saucepan over low heat. Stir constantly until melted and smooth. Serve warm.

■ **Eat One Serving (5 cookies + 3 tbsp sauce per serving):**

373

calories, 9 g protein, 49 g carbohydrates, 19 g fat, 7 g saturated fat*, 5 mg cholesterol, 160 mg sodium, 5 g fiber

A SINGLE SERVING OF THIS RECIPE COUNTS as a Flat Belly Diet Meal without any add-ons!

* Limit saturated fat to no more than 10 percent of total calories—about 17 grams per day for most women or 21 grams for most men—and sodium intake to no more than 2,300 milligrams.

Chocolate-Cranberry Oatmeal Cookies

Cooking time: 20 minutes / Makes 24 servings

2 cups rolled oats
½ cup whole grain pastry flour
¾ teaspoon baking soda
½ teaspoon ground cinnamon
¼ teaspoon salt
½ cup brown sugar
⅓ cup canola oil
3 large egg whites
2 teaspoons vanilla extract
¾ cup cranberries, coarsely chopped

MUFA: 2¼ cups chopped walnuts

1 cup semisweet chocolate chips

1. Preheat the oven to 350°F. Coat 2 large baking sheets with cooking spray.

2. Combine the oats, flour, baking soda, cinnamon, and salt in a large bowl. Whisk together the brown sugar, oil, egg whites, and vanilla in a separate bowl. Pour sugar mixture into flour mixture and stir until well blended. Fold in the cranberries, walnuts, and chocolate chips.

3. Drop the batter by tablespoons onto the prepared baking sheets. Bake cookies for 10 minutes, or until golden brown. Transfer to a wire rack to cool completely.

■ **Eat One Serving (2 cookies per serving):**

376

calories, 8 g protein, 30 g carbohydrates, 24 g fat, 3 g saturated fat, 0 mg cholesterol, 140 mg sodium, 4 g fiber

A SINGLE SERVING OF THIS RECIPE COUNTS as a Flat Belly Diet Meal without any add-ons!

Orange Frappé with Strawberries

Cooking time: 5 minutes / Makes 1 serving

¼ cup reduced-fat ricotta cheese
1 tablespoon nonfat dry milk
1½ teaspoons honey

MUFA: 1 tablespoon flaxseed oil

1 teaspoon orange zest
¼ cup sliced fresh or partially thawed loose-pack frozen strawberries

Combine the cheese, dry milk, honey, flaxseed oil, and orange zest in a blender. Process until very smooth. Top with the strawberries.

■ Drink One Serving:

268

calories, 9 g protein, 18 g carbohydrates, 19 g fat, 4 g saturated fat*, 20 mg cholesterol, 102 mg sodium, 1 g fiber

MAKE IT A FLAT BELLY DIET MEAL: Serve with 1 slice whole wheat toast (70) topped with ¼ cup reduced-fat ricotta cheese (60) and ½ teaspoon cinnamon (0).

■ Total Meal:

398

calories, 18 g protein, 36 g carbohydrates, 22 g fat, 6 g saturated fat, 35 mg cholesterol, 217 mg sodium, 3 g fiber

* Limit saturated fat to no more than 10 percent of total calories—about 17 grams per day for most women or 21 grams for most men—and sodium intake to no more than 2,300 milligrams.

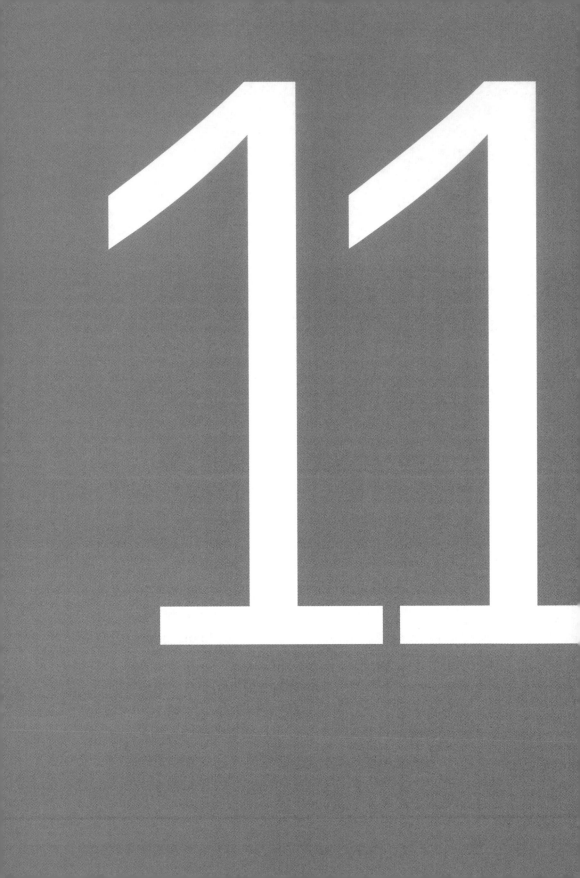

THE FLAT BELLY DIET
DIABETES
WORKOUT

A FLAT BELLY, no crunches required. With the Flat Belly Diet Diabetes, that's not just a promise, it's a scientific fact.

When researchers in the Biomechanics Lab at San Diego State University measured the effectiveness of exercises touted to trim the human torso, traditional crunches came in 11th out of 13 moves they tested. That means 10 exercises were better, in some cases *three times better,* at working the rectus abdominus and oblique muscles of the midsection.[1] I found these results intriguing and, on a personal level, very validating—I used to skip out on the crunches at the end of my step classes because they didn't feel good (all that huffing and puffing) and didn't seem to be doing much, either!

Prevention magazine's fitness director Michele Stanten, who brought this research to my attention, incorporated some of those better moves into the Flat Belly Diet Diabetes Workout.

Think of this chapter as your workout instruction manual. (For day-to-day exercise "assignments" during Phase 1 and Phase 2 of the Flat Belly Diet Diabetes, turn to Chapters 7 and 8.) But it's more than "do this, do that." This plan works because we made it "life proof." It doesn't take much time, it doesn't require scads of special equipment or special clothing, and most moves can be done anywhere. We also built in plenty of features that allow you to tailor routines and moves to your fitness level, thereby abolishing frustration and achy overworked muscles—the lingering OUCH! that leads to skipped workouts the next day.

The Flat Belly Workout: Fast, Effective, Custom-Fit

THIS "DONE-IN-NO-TIME-FLAT" WORKOUT IS customized to fit your schedule and your fitness level. The result: more flexibility for greater success and less frustration. As you learned in Chapter 8, there are three key components to your Flat Belly Workout:

If You Have Diabetes

Exercise safely. Wearing a medical-alert bracelet is a smart move if you have diabetes—it could help get you the right care in the event of an emergency while you're out walking or are exercising away from home. If you use insulin or take diabetes medications that raise risk for low blood sugar, be sure to carry quickly absorbed carbs such as hard candy or glucose tablets, and tell your exercise companions how to help you spot and treat signs of low blood sugar, pronto. (Turn to Chapter 4 for all the details on avoiding and treating low blood sugar episodes during exercise.)

- Cardio exercise—walking or an activity of your choice—to burn calories, shed fat, and improve blood sugar. If you're new to cardio exercise, you'll do just 15 minutes a day at first, while experienced exercisers will aim for 30—which you can split into two 15-minute sessions if you'd like. You'll alternate between Fat Blast Walks (at a steady pace) and Calorie Torch Walks (during which you do intervals at different intensities) to maximize your results.

- Strength training with weights to build muscle, boost metabolism, and, again, improve blood sugar. You'll pick the weights that are just heavy enough to get the job done—for you. You'll also choose one of three versions of each move—basic, easier, and harder—for maximum effectiveness. The four exercises of your Metabolism Boost Routine multitask beautifully, working several muscle groups at once so you can whittle your middle in 10 minutes or less.

- Core-focused moves to tone and tighten your torso. Again, you'll have three options from which to choose for each of the five exercises, so you can customize a Belly Routine that's challenging enough to see results—and doable enough that moves feel easy and can be mastered. And it's speedy. You'll be done in 10 minutes or less.

6 Days a Week: Take a Calorie-Burning Walk

THE ONLY WAY TO shrink the layer of subcutaneous fat covering your tummy muscles *and* the visceral fat lurking inside your abdomen is by burning calories. Ab exercises alone won't burn off this stuff. No spot-reducing exercise can—you have to burn calories and fat to get the job done!

We recommend walking as your cardio exercise of choice because it's easy and can be done virtually anywhere. But—and here's where the customizing begins—you can do anything you like: cycling, swimming, jogging, or using machines like treadmills, stairclimbers, and elliptical trainers. If you have foot or leg problems due to diabetes, you can substitute a "pedaler"—an inexpensive and small piece of equipment that lets you get a workout while seated in a chair at home. These can be purchased online or in some exercise-equipment stores for as little as $30.

The Flat Belly Diet Diabetes includes two types of cardio walks: Fat Blast and Calorie Torch Walks. Fat Blast Walks, which you start in Week 1, are steadily paced walks guaranteed to burn off belly fat. As you become fitter, you should be able to walk faster (and burn fat faster!) without feeling any extra effort. Calorie Torch Walks, which you begin in Week 3, include intervals, meaning bursts of faster-paced walking interspersed with a moderate pace. Studies show that interval training keeps metabolism revved up long after the workout is done. The upshot? You burn more calories throughout the day.

You'll walk 6 days a week. Our Flat Belly Diet Diabetes plan gives you Sundays off, but feel free to use your "free" day whenever you'd like, or when a need arises. If you're new to walking and to exercise, opt for our beginner walks—15 minutes a day in Weeks 1 through 4, 20 minutes a day in Week 5. If you've already been walking or exercising, go for our "advanced" walks—30 minutes a

Ensure Your Safety Outside

- Walk with a buddy.
- Choose routes with which you're familiar.
- Wear reflective clothing and carry a flashlight in the dark and at dawn and dusk. Wear bright colors during the day.
- Try to avoid rush hour to reduce your exposure to carbon monoxide.
- Walk facing traffic so you can see cars coming.
- Carry a cell phone and an ID.
- If you listen to music, keep the volume low enough so you can hear if a car or person is approaching you.

day in Weeks 1 through 4, 35 minutes in Week 5. Of course, if you have an established fitness routine that keeps you moving for at least that many minutes, you can stick with that instead.

THE IMPORTANCE OF SPEED AND INTENSITY

As you become fitter and your muscles grow stronger, you'll naturally walk faster and burn more calories, without it feeling any harder. For instance, a 2-mile walk at 2 mph burns 170 calories (based on a 150-pound person). But when you ratchet it up to 3 mph in that same hour, you'll burn 224 calories—a third more calories, and not an extra minute of exercise time. A win-win situation, don't you agree?

You'll get a feel for faster-paced walking when you do the interval walks—aka Calorie Torch Walks, which alternate brisk-paced bouts with faster, higher-intensity bursts. How fast? Here's another example of how customized this plan is. You can and should start with the level that is the most comfortable for you and work your way up as you gain more endurance. *No matter what your fitness level, you can get a high-intensity workout simply by pushing yourself just a little out of your comfort zone.* Working at higher intensity can burn from 25 to 75 percent more calories than exercising at low intensity.

We do have some guidelines for speed and intensity. As a general rule, move at a "brisk" pace for Fat Blast Walks—a pace that allows you to talk freely with a companion, but makes it difficult to sing. On an exercise intensity scale of 1 to 10 (with 1 being barely moving and 10 being "I'm climbing Mount Everest without oxygen!"), that's a 5 to 6. Your Calorie Torch Walks will alternate brisk walking (5–6 intensity level) with short bursts of faster walking (7–8 intensity level) at a pace that allows you to speak in short phrases, but with an effort.

Here's a breakdown of speeds and intensities for all phases of our Flat Belly Workout walks. Use these pace and intensity levels (based on a 1 to 10 scale) to ensure that you're working out at the right intensity level for your Fat Blast and Calorie Torch Walks.

	HOW IT FEELS	INTENSITY LEVEL	SPEED (MPH) *
WARMUP, COOLDOWN	Easy enough that you can sing	3–4	2.8–3.2
BRISK	You can talk freely, but no more singing	5–6	3.5–3.8
FAST	You can talk in brief phrases, but you'd rather not	7–8	3.8+

* Note that these walking speeds are merely guidelines. The fitter you get, the faster you'll walk at each of these levels.

TUNE UP YOUR WALKING FORM

The secret to turning your everyday stroll into a fat-blasting stride is proper walking form and technique. The most common mistake people make when they try to pick up the pace is that they take longer strides. This can actually slow you down because your outstretched leg acts like a brake, and it can cause injuries due to increased stress on your joints. Instead, take shorter, quicker steps, rolling from heel to toes and pushing off with your toes. Next, bend your

Gear Up for Your Walks

Everyone needs good shoes and socks for exercising, but it's even more important if you have diabetes. Worn-out shoes can contribute to foot, knee, and back pain. If you have diabetes, the added risk for circulation and nerve problems means it's also important to protect against blisters, sores, and chafing. Follow these steps for the perfect footwear:

1: Find a knowledgeable salesperson. Unlike mass-market retailers, specialty stores often employ trained shoe fitters who will ask you about your walking habits and watch you walk. This information will improve your chances of getting the right shoe for your feet.

2: Get your feet measured. Your size can change over time, and footwear that's too small or too narrow can set you up for an array of problems. Make arms at about 90-degree angles and swing them forward (no higher than chest height) and back so your hand is almost skimming your hip. Letting your arms flail across your body will slow your forward momentum. Practice these techniques and you'll be cruising past other walkers in no time.

3 Days a Week: Build Muscle with the Metabolism Boost

IN ADDITION TO THE daily walk, you'll perform four strength-training moves—our Metabolism Boost Routine—3 days a week starting in Week 2.

Strength training isn't just for Olympic power-lifters and sweaty, bulked-up bodybuilders. It's for any woman or man, at any age, who wants to stay strong, flexible, healthy, and slim. How? Strength training preserves and even rebuilds precious muscle—the body's calorie-burning engine that fuels metabolism. Beginning as early as in your thirties, you start to lose about half a pound of muscle a year. (For women, those losses can double by the time you hit menopause.) With every pound of muscle lost, your body burns fewer calories, which explains why gaining weight gets easier and losing it gets tougher

sure you have a thumb's width of room in front of the end of your big toe while you're standing rather than sitting. And make sure the width of the shoes is comfortable, too.

3: Replace your shoes every 300 to 500 miles. That's about every 5 to 8 months if you're walking about 3 miles 5 days a week. By the time a sneaker looks trashed on the outside, the inside support and cushioning are long gone.

4: Invest in "wicking" socks. Look for synthetic fabrics that wick moisture away, keeping your feet dry and making them less prone to blisters. Since some are thick and others are thin, wear your walking socks when you try shoes on because they can affect the fit. If you get the proper fit and fabric, you probably don't need to invest in specially marketed diabetic socks.

as you get older. Decreasing muscle mass also makes you weaker, and every-day tasks such as getting out of a chair and climbing the stairs become more difficult. As a result, you start to move less—further contributing to muscle loss and fat gain.

Strength training creates stronger muscles—the result you want, because stronger muscle mass makes our bodies look firmer, tighter, and more toned. Most importantly, though, regular strength training boosts your metabolism by about 7 percent, so you'll burn about 100 extra calories a day.

Strength training also increases your energy level, helps maintain bone density (guarding against osteoporosis and hence against fractures), improves sleep, boosts stamina, enhances balance, and smooths the appearance of lumpy cellulite. It also lowers your risk for diabetes. If you already have diabetes, it can help make blood sugar control easier—because denser muscle not only "sips" more blood sugar round the clock, it's also more sensitive to the hormone insulin, so it takes in that blood sugar more readily.

4 Reasons to Work Out to Music

1. You'll feel happier. A groundbreaking brain-imaging study from McGill University in Montreal showed for the first time that music activates the same reward or pleasure centers in the brain that respond to the good feelings associated with eating and—believe it or not—sex.[2]

2. You'll move faster. Australian researchers discovered that the faster the beat, the more vigorously you work out. Other research has shown that exercisers who listen to music have more endurance and thus exercise longer, burning more calories.

3. You'll get smarter. In the first study to look at the combined effects of music and exercise on mental performance, Charles Emery, the study's lead author and a professor of psychology at Ohio State University in Columbus, found that this duo increased scores on a verbal fluency test.[3]

4. You'll lose belly fat faster. Women who exercised to music lost as much as 8 pounds more than women who broke a sweat in silence.

BEFORE YOU BEGIN: STRENGTH-TRAINING BASICS

If you're not yet doing any strength training, now is the time to start! If you're currently lifting weights, try ramping it up a notch.

- THE TERMS: The word "rep" is short for repetition. For example, each time you lift and lower a dumbbell or roll your upper body off the floor and then lower it back down, it's considered one repetition.

- YOUR WEIGHTS: You will need two sets of dumbbells—light and heavy. We recommend that beginners choose 3- and 5-pound dumbbells; if you're already doing a strength-training program, try 5- and 8-pound dumbbells. But the right weight for you may be lighter or heavier than this.

- HOW TO TELL: If you can barely get through the last reps in an exercise, you need a lighter weight (try it out in the store before you buy!). If you can breeze through an exercise without fatigue, you may need a slightly heavier weight (or you could add a second set of reps).

- YOUR ROUTINE: In the Metabolism Boost, you'll begin with one set of 10 reps and progress to 15 reps during the 5-week plan. We recommend doing the routine on days 1, 3, and 5, but you can choose any 3 days—just leave a day of "rest" between workouts so that your muscles can repair themselves.

Lunge Press

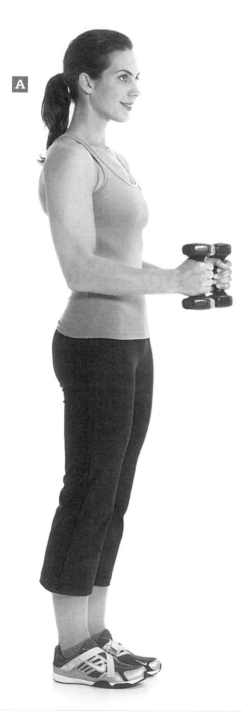

A

MAIN
MOVE

A. Stand with your feet together. Holding a dumbbell in each hand, bend arms to 90 degrees so dumbbells are in front of you, forearms parallel to the floor, palms facing each other.

B. Step right foot 2 to 3 feet behind you, landing on ball of foot. Bend knees, lowering your right knee toward the floor until the left thigh is parallel to the floor. Keep your left knee directly over your ankle. At the same time, press dumbbells behind you, straightening arms. Hold for a second, then press into left foot, standing back up, bringing feet together, and bending arms back to start position. Do one set, then repeat with the opposite leg.

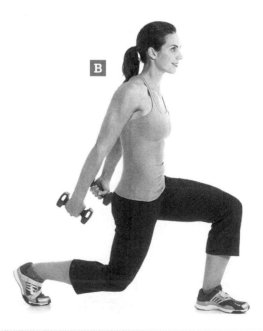

B

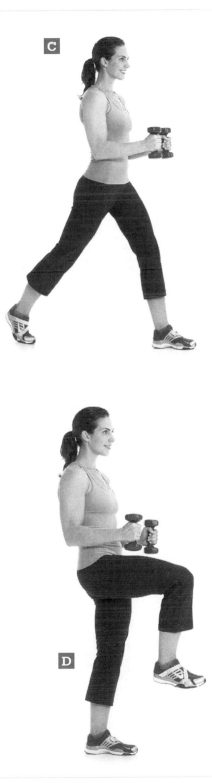

MAKE IT EASIER

. . . .

C. Do stationary lunges by starting with your left foot 2 to 3 feet in front of your right foot, right heel off floor. Maintain this position for one set, then switch legs and repeat.

MAKE IT HARDER

. . . .

D. As you stand back up from the lunge position, raise your right knee in front of you to hip height, leg bent 90 degrees. At the same time, bend your arms back to the start position. Hold for 1 second, balancing on left foot, then swing your right foot behind you and repeat. Complete one set, and then repeat with the opposite leg.

Squat Curl

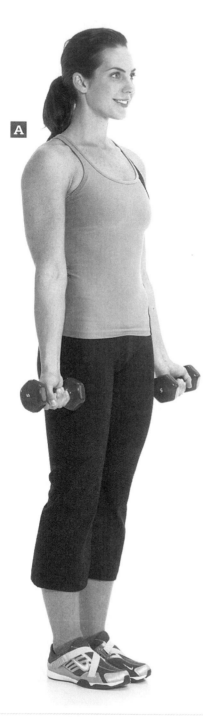

A. Stand with your feet together, holding a dumbbell in each hand, arms down at your sides, palms facing forward.

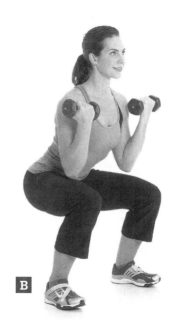

B. Step your right foot about 2 feet out to the side and bend knees and hips as if you were sitting back into a chair. Sit back as far as possible, keeping knees behind toes. At the same time, bend your elbows, curling dumbbells up toward shoulders. Don't move your upper arms or shoulders. As you stand back up, bring your feet together and lower dumbbells. Complete one set, and then repeat, stepping to side with left foot.

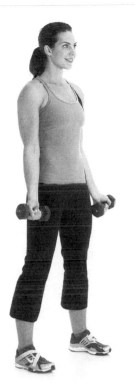

MAKE IT EASIER

C. Start with your feet about shoulder-width apart and maintain this position as you do the squats, without stepping to the side.

MAKE IT HARDER

D. As you stand back up from the squat position, raise your left knee, bringing it in front of you to hip height, leg bent 90 degrees. Hold for 1 second, balancing on your right foot, then swing your left foot out to the side and repeat. Complete one set, then repeat with the opposite leg.

Side Lunge & Raise

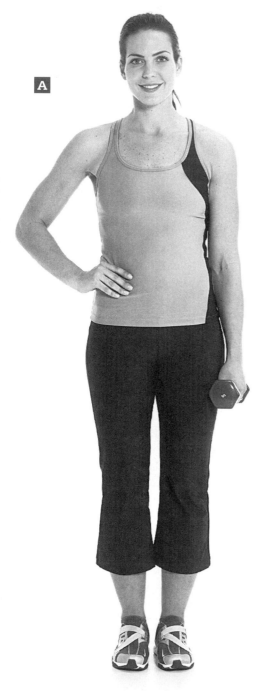

MAIN MOVE

A. Stand with your feet together and hold a dumbbell in your left hand with arm at side, palm facing in. Place your right hand on hip.

B. Step your right foot 2 to 3 feet out to the side and bend your right knee into a lunge, sitting back and bringing the dumbbell toward your right ankle. Keep your right knee behind toes. Press off your right foot and stand back up, bringing feet together. From this position, raise your left arm out to the left side until it's at shoulder height, and lift your right leg out to the opposite side, as high as possible (like photo at right). Hold for a second, then return to start position. Complete one set, then switch sides and repeat.

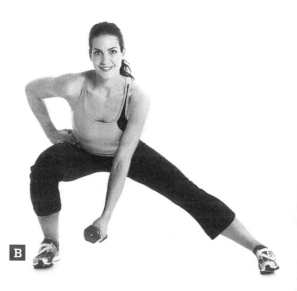

MAKE IT EASIER

C. Keep your foot on the floor as you raise your arm to shoulder height.

MAKE IT HARDER

D. From the lunge position, press off your right foot and stand back up, raising your left arm out to the left side until it's at shoulder height and lifting your right leg out to the opposite side, as high as possible, then immediately lower back into another lunge. Complete one set, then switch sides and repeat.

Pushup Row

MAIN MOVE

A. Holding a dumbbell in each hand, get down on your hands and knees. Walk your hands forward so your body forms a straight line from head to knees, and hands are directly beneath your shoulders and feet are in the air.

B. Bend your elbows out to the sides, lowering your chest almost to floor. Press into your hands, straightening arms back to start position. **C.** Then bend your right elbow back, pulling the dumbbell toward your chest, keeping your arm close to your body. Lower the dumbbell back to the floor, and repeat from the beginning, this time doing a row with your left arm. Continue alternating rows for a full set, doing an extra rep each time so you do an equal number of rows with each arm.

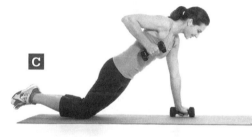

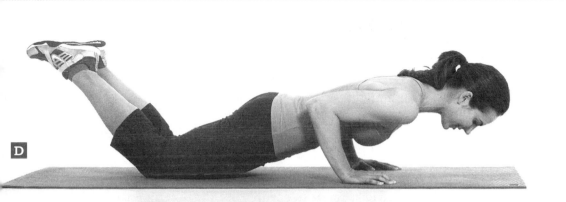

MAKE IT EASIER

D. Break up the moves. Do one set of pushups without dumbbells. Then get on your hands and knees and do a set of rows with each arm.

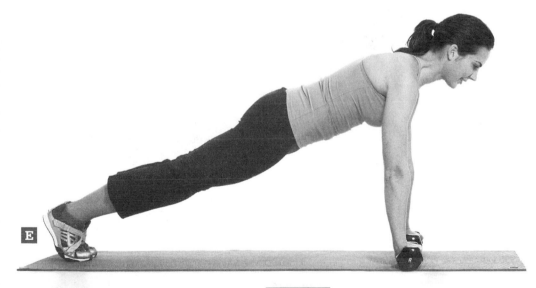

MAKE IT HARDER

E. Do full pushups, balancing on your hands and toes.

3 Days a Week: Tone Your Abs with the Belly Routine

THE THIRD COMPONENT OF the Flat Belly Workout focuses, of course, on your ab muscles. We've eliminated the crunches—a cause for celebration! Not only are they BO-RING, they never seemed to do much for any of us, and now there's scientific evidence that they're simply not effective.

Instead, we bring you five lab-tested moves that combine Pilates, traditional ab moves, and balance exercises to ensure that you're toning your midsection and core from every angle. All are guaranteed to deliver better results than ordinary crunches.

- The roll-up works the main belly muscle, the rectus abdominis, which runs from the bottom of your ribs down to your pelvis, and is *80 percent more effective* than a standard crunch.
- The bicycle move targets the main ab muscle more effectively while also working your obliques, the muscles that wrap around your torso. This generates 190 percent more activity than when you do a simple crunch, according to an American Council on Exercise study. (If you have time for just one move, this is the one!)
- The hover and arm and leg extension work both your abdominal and back muscles at the same time. Strong back muscles allow you to stand taller, improving posture—bonus—and helping your belly look flatter almost instantly.
- The pike zeros in on those lower abs. Since the rectus abdominis is one long, continuous muscle, you can't completely isolate your upper and lower abs. But this exercise allows you to maximize the amount of work that the muscle fibers in the lower portion of that muscle are doing, activating it more than regular crunches, while also stimulating the upper portion.

Bottom line? Not a crunch in the bunch. And now you know why.

Stretch Your Workout Benefits

The most important thing you can do before exercise is to warm up with gentle activity, such as walking for 5 minutes. The best time to stretch is post-workout, when your muscles are warm and pliable. Stretching then also helps promote recovery and will improve your posture so you stand taller, making your belly look flatter instantly.

These five stretches target the major muscle groups used in your workout. Gently ease in and out of the stretches, holding each for 10 seconds. Don't bounce. Do each stretch three to six times, taking deep breaths throughout.

Chest Stretch. Stand with your feet about shoulder-width apart and grasp your hands behind your back, fingers intertwined and palms facing each other. Keeping your chest lifted and shoulders down, squeeze your shoulder blades and gently lift your arms as high as comfortable. Don't arch your back. You should feel a stretch across your chest. Hold for 10 seconds and release.

Back Stretch. Stand with your feet about shoulder-width apart. Bending at the hips, lean forward and place your hands on your thighs just above the knees. Tuck your hips in, round your back, and drop your chin toward your chest so your back forms a C shape and you feel a stretch across your shoulders and down your back. Hold for 10 seconds and release.

Quad Stretch. Standing with feet together, bend your left leg behind you, bringing that foot toward your buttocks. (You can hold on to a chair or wall with your right hand for balance if needed.) Grasp your left foot with your left hand and tuck hips under so you feel a stretch in the front of your left thigh and hip. Hold for 10 seconds and release. Switch legs and repeat.

Calf Stretch. Stand with your right foot about 2 to 3 feet in front of your left, toes pointing forward. Place your hands on your right thigh and your right knee, keeping your left leg straight and pressing your left heel into the floor so you feel a stretch in your left calf. Hold for 10 seconds and release. Switch legs and repeat.

Hamstring Stretch. From the calf stretch position, step your back foot in 6 to 12 inches. Straighten your front leg, lifting your front toes off the floor, and bend your back leg and sit back, placing your hands on the opposite thigh. It is very important not to lock your front knee. You should feel a stretch down the back of the thigh of your straight leg. Hold for 10 seconds and release. Switch legs and repeat.

Bicycle

A. Lie faceup with knees above hips, calves parallel to the floor, and hands behind head.

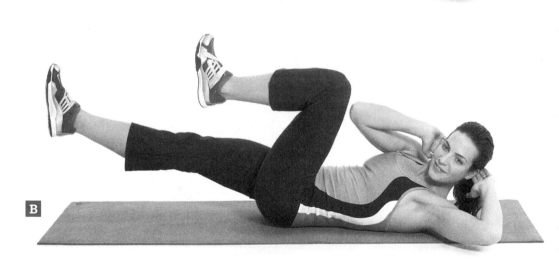

B. Contract your abs, raising your head and shoulders off the floor as you extend your right leg so it's about 10 inches off the floor. Twist to the left, bringing your right elbow and left knee toward each other. Don't pull on your neck; the work should come from your abs. Hold for a second, then switch sides, twisting to the right. That's one rep.

MAKE IT EASIER

C. Keep your feet flat on the floor with knees bent as you lift and twist your upper body.

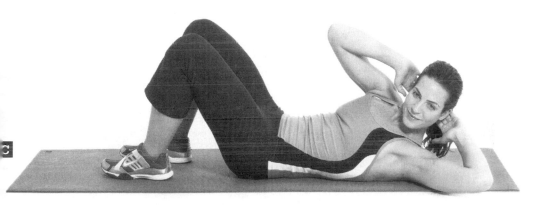

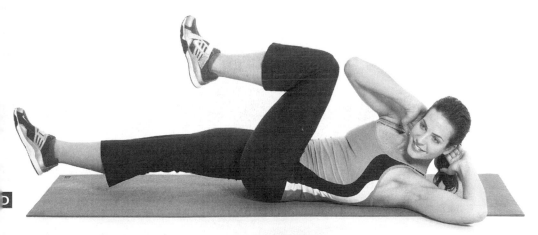

MAKE IT HARDER

D. Lower your extended leg farther so it's about 3 inches off the floor.

Hover

MAIN MOVE

A. Lie facedown with your upper body propped on your forearms and elbows directly beneath your shoulders. Toes are tucked.

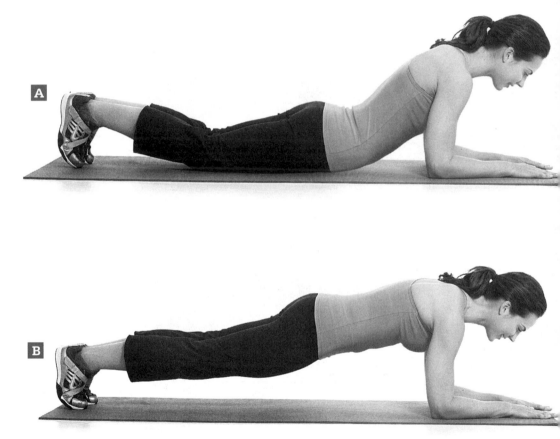

B. Contract your torso muscles, lifting your belly and legs off the floor so your body forms a straight line from head to heels. Keep your abs tight so your belly doesn't droop. Hold for 15 seconds (increase by 15 seconds each week so that by Week 4, you're holding for 1 minute). One rep is all you need to do.

C. Keep your knees on the floor and just lift your belly, balancing on your knees and forearms. Stay in this position.

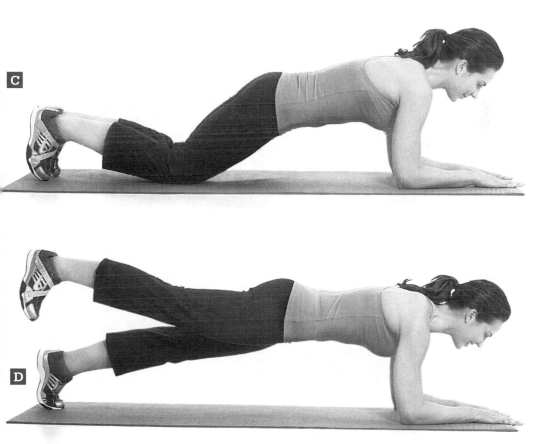

D. Raise your right foot off the floor and hold for half the time, then switch legs and hold for the remaining time.

Roll-Up

MAIN MOVE

A. Lie on your back with your arms extended overhead and legs bent, feet flat on the floor.

B. Inhale and raise your arms over your chest. Then exhale and roll your head toward your chest, lifting your head and shoulders off the floor. (Keep your arms next to your ears throughout the move.) Press your inner thighs together and your navel in toward your spine. Slowly peel off the floor until you're sitting up.

Then extend your legs so you're in a C shape—back rounded, head toward knees, and arms extended in front of you. Gradually reverse the movement, inhaling and squeezing your abs as you roll back down to the floor, one vertebra at a time.

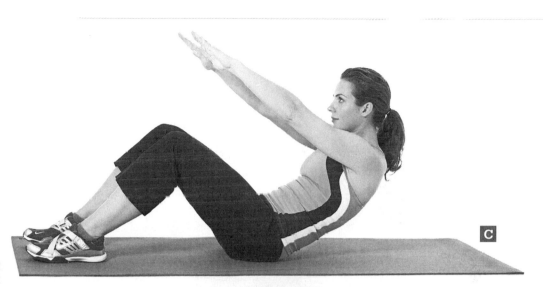

C. Sit upright on the floor with your knees bent, feet flat, and arms extended at shoulder height in front of you. As you exhale, roll back only about 45 degrees, one vertebra at a time, keeping your abs tight. Then roll back up.

D. Do the move with your legs extended the entire time.

Arm & Leg Extension

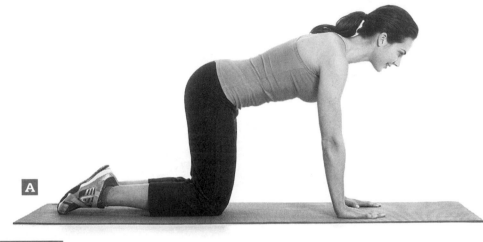

A. Kneel with your hands directly beneath your shoulders, and your knees directly beneath your hips.

B. Keeping your back straight and your head in line with your spine, simultaneously raise your left arm and right leg, extending them in line with your back so your fingers are pointing straight ahead and your toes are pointing behind you. Hold for a second, then lower. Perform one set, then switch arms and legs and repeat.

MAKE IT EASIER

C. Instead of lifting and lowering your arm and leg, hold them in line with your back for 15 seconds, then repeat on the opposite side. One rep on each side is enough. Increase the amount of time you hold the move until you can do it for a full minute.

C

MAKE IT HARDER

D. When your arm and leg are raised, contract your abs and draw your left elbow and right knee together beneath your torso, holding for a second. Extend and repeat. Perform one set, then switch arms and legs and repeat.

D

Ab Pike

A. Lie faceup with your arms at sides. Bend your legs so your feet are off the floor, thighs over hips.

A

B. As you pull your abs toward your spine, lift your hips off the floor, keeping your legs bent. Keep your hands and arms relaxed so you don't use them to help lift. Hold for a second, then slowly lower your hips to the floor and bend your legs.

B

C. Lie with your legs bent, feet flat on the floor. Contract your abs, pressing the small of your back into the floor, and curl your hips up, doing a pelvic tilt, without lifting your feet.

D. As you lift your hips, extend your legs, and then bend them as you lower.

READ A FLAT BELLY
SUCCESS
STORY

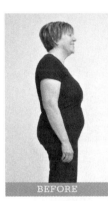

BEFORE

AFTER

Anne Harrington

AGE: 65

POUNDS LOST:

0

IN 35 DAYS

ALL-OVER INCHES LOST:

2

✳ BLOOD SUGAR: A1C STAYED STABLE AT

6.4

PERCENT

---

* The A1c is a test of long-term blood sugar control; levels under 7 percent are considered ideal for most people with diabetes.

"MY DAILY BLOOD SUGARS WERE ABSOLUTELY AMAZING!"
Anne, a retired technical writer, already keeps her blood sugar at healthy levels with diet and exercise. Her A1c level—an important check of long-term blood sugar control—held steady at a healthy 6.4 throughout the 5-week plan. That's stellar for someone with diabetes. But Anne was thrilled at the improvement in her daily blood sugar checks. "That was really, really inspiring," she says. "My numbers were down in the ranges people without diabetes would have. Two hours after a meal, they were around 89 to 96 mg/dL, because the meals were smaller than I had been eating."

Anne's weight remained stable on the 5-week plan, but she lost an inch from her waist, an inch from her hips, and her percentage of body fat fell by nearly 3 percent.

Spending a few minutes every day writing down her food choices helped Anne stay on track. "Writing down what I've eaten keeps me honest about portion control. A half-cup of pasta really has to be a half-cup. If I go back for seconds, I have to write it down. But for people with diabetes, tracking has a second benefit," she says. "It can help you discover hidden connections between foods you're eating and your blood sugar levels. At one point, I was having high blood sugars after meals and couldn't figure out why. But my certified diabetes educator noticed my blood sugar was always high after I ate brown rice. For me, rice is a food that raises my blood sugar! Everybody's high blood sugar foods are going to be different, but the way to find them is the same—keep a food diary, and test your blood sugar after meals."

Anne is also a big advocate of the benefits of two other essential components of the Flat Belly Diet Diabetes: exercise and stress reduction. "I take my dog Sadie—a 14-year-old mix of German shepherd, terrier, and boxer—on a half-hour walk most days. She goes slowly, so I do leg lifts and other exercises while she sniffs around. I also swim and use the weight machines at my local YMCA. I don't overdo it; it's more important to pace myself so I don't get hurt or feel too tired. I want to get out there and exercise again tomorrow!"

A daily meditation routine helps her tame tension—a move that lifts fatigue and helps protect against overeating. "I've learned that the brain needs to rest and to focus," she says. "If I get mentally tired, I eat. So I relax as preventive medicine."

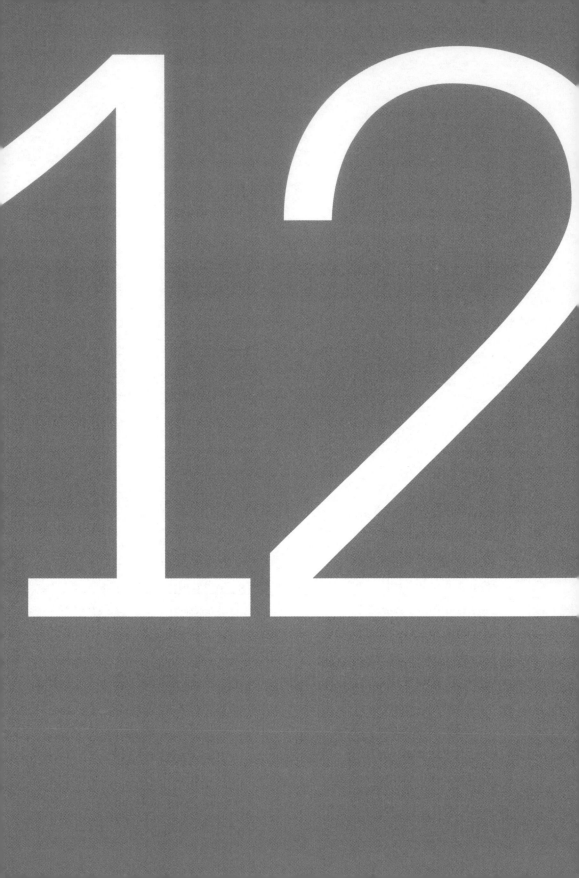

THE FLAT BELLY DIET
DIABETES
JOURNAL

MAKING A GRAND entrance at a party—in your most slimming pants or skirt—requires poise and confidence. Achieving your goals for your weight, for (say it with us) a flatter belly, and for better blood sugar control takes a *deeper* kind of confidence. It comes from mastering cause-and-effect connections—between mood and food; between food, exercise, and blood sugar; and between everyday life and whether you found time for exercise, stress reduction, and simply collecting your thoughts.

That's where the Flat Belly Diet Diabetes Journal comes in.

Behavioral scientists now understand how to uncover—and unravel—those mysterious connections. Therapy is one way, and it can be great if you can afford it and have the time and interest. Another, more practical way is to maintain a journal. Unlike a diary where you recount last night's dreams or confide your most intimate secrets, this journal is a tracking device that can quickly give you useful insights. It can help you recognize emotional connections you have with food, see links between what you've eaten and a later blood sugar reading, and notice patterns in your exercise habits.

In Phase 1, we gave you quick Mind Tricks to help you swiftly put the focus back on yourself and your goals when you came in contact with food. You can use these little strategies anytime, anywhere, to put the brakes on "mindless" and emotional eating. In Phase 2, you'll take it to the next level. You'll explore your relationship with food, attempt to dissect the whys and hows of your eating behavior, and try to pinpoint the psychological hot buttons that will help propel you to success. On every page, with just a few strokes of your pen, you'll jot down vital statistics that will help you make other key connections, too.

Every day we'll also ask you to reflect on what we call a Core Confidence. These exercises are all about your confidence and your attitude, both of which are at the core of your ability to succeed. There's no need to take all day to complete these exercises—15 minutes or less is all it takes.

Core Confidences are essential to forging a true and fruitful mind-belly connection. They will help you discover and understand your motivations, your barriers to success, and the wellsprings of ambition and ability that have driven you to achieve major life goals. It may sound strange, but the same qualities that helped you get that promotion or build a solid relationship with your spouse or raise a healthy, well-adjusted child are what will help you flatten your belly. Confidence, self-awareness, determination, love, acceptance, compassion, organization—if you have any of these qualities, the Core Confidence exercises will help you tap into and exploit them for your belly's benefit.

As you fill out these pages, remember to periodically look back and read what you've written in previous entries. That's how you'll spot behavior patterns and notice your progress. And remember, this is just for you, and all about being true to yourself. So:

- Forget spelling and punctuation.
- Write quickly to ward off your inner critic.
- Speak from your heart.

If you prefer keeping an electronic journal, we've got one for you! Go to www.prevention.com/healthtrackers, where you can customize a tracking system to keep tabs on your weight, blood sugar, waistline, meals, mood, and many other health and fitness goals.

The Rest of the Story

YOU'LL ALSO RECORD your hunger level before and after each meal, using the same scale (from 1 for ravenous to 10 for stuffed to the gills) that you used in Phase 1. There's room to log your exercise choices and times, as well as whether or not you made time for yourself—the all-important "me time" for relaxation.

And if you check your blood sugar daily with a glucose monitor, we've included space for those readings, too. Again, we recommend checking 2 hours after meals in addition to whatever checks your doctor has recommended. That way, you can see how various Flat Belly Diet Diabetes meals and foods affect your blood sugar.

Now, let's get writing!

■ **CORE CONFIDENCE:** Today you begin Phase 2! Take a moment to write down how you're feeling about the next 28 days, and what you expect of yourself in terms of healthy eating, physical activity, stress reduction, and, if applicable, blood sugar checks.

_____

_____

_____

■ FOOD LOG:

BREAKFAST			
What I Ate:		Thoughts:	
Time:	Location:	Hunger Before: 1 3 5 8 10	Hunger After: 1 3 5 8 10

LUNCH			
What I Ate:		Thoughts:	
Time:	Location:	Hunger Before: 1 3 5 8 10	Hunger After: 1 3 5 8 10

DINNER			
What I Ate:		Thoughts:	
Time:	Location:	Hunger Before: 1 3 5 8 10	Hunger After: 1 3 5 8 10

SNACK			
What I Ate:		Thoughts:	
Time:	Location:	Hunger Before: 1 3 5 8 10	Hunger After: 1 3 5 8 10

OPTIONAL 200-CALORIE SNACK			
What I Ate:		Thoughts:	
Time:	Location:	Hunger Before: 1 3 5 8 10	Hunger After: 1 3 5 8 10

■ EXERCISE LOG:

WALKING/CARDIO	METABOLISM/BELLY		PROGRESSIVE MUSCLE RELAXATION
Minutes:	# Reps:	Weight:	Thoughts:

■ DAILY BLOOD SUGAR LOG:

CHECK 1	CHECK 2	CHECK 3	CHECK 4	CHECK 5
Time:	Time:	Time:	Time:	Time:
Reading:	Reading:	Reading:	Reading:	Reading:

DAY 2

■ **CORE CONFIDENCE:** Wondering how to fit everything in? Spend a few minutes thinking about the little bits of "downtime" in your schedule—stretches of 5 to 30 minutes when you might take a short walk, do the Belly Routine, or simply relax. Write them all down, proving to yourself that you *do* have time!

_____

_____

■ **FOOD LOG:**

BREAKFAST			
What I Ate:		Thoughts:	
Time:	Location:	Hunger Before: 1 3 5 8 10	Hunger After: 1 3 5 8 10

LUNCH			
What I Ate:		Thoughts:	
Time:	Location:	Hunger Before: 1 3 5 8 10	Hunger After: 1 3 5 8 10

DINNER			
What I Ate:		Thoughts:	
Time:	Location:	Hunger Before: 1 3 5 8 10	Hunger After: 1 3 5 8 10

SNACK			
What I Ate:		Thoughts:	
Time:	Location:	Hunger Before: 1 3 5 8 10	Hunger After: 1 3 5 8 10

OPTIONAL 200-CALORIE SNACK			
What I Ate:		Thoughts:	
Time:	Location:	Hunger Before: 1 3 5 8 10	Hunger After: 1 3 5 8 10

■ **EXERCISE LOG:**

WALKING/CARDIO	METABOLISM/BELLY		PROGRESSIVE MUSCLE RELAXATION
Minutes:	# Reps:	Weight:	Thoughts:

■ **DAILY BLOOD SUGAR LOG:**

CHECK 1	CHECK 2	CHECK 3	CHECK 4	CHECK 5
Time:	Time:	Time:	Time:	Time:
Reading:	Reading:	Reading:	Reading:	Reading:

DAY 3

■ **CORE CONFIDENCE:** Write a note to your body. Detail three things you deeply appreciate about it. Then tell it three things you'll do today to nurture it (such as choosing healthy food or getting to bed earlier).

_____

_____

_____

■ **FOOD LOG:**

BREAKFAST		
What I Ate:	Thoughts:	
Time:	Location:	Hunger Before: 1 3 5 8 10	Hunger After: 1 3 5 8 10

LUNCH		
What I Ate:	Thoughts:	
Time:	Location:	Hunger Before: 1 3 5 8 10	Hunger After: 1 3 5 8 10

DINNER		
What I Ate:	Thoughts:	
Time:	Location:	Hunger Before: 1 3 5 8 10	Hunger After: 1 3 5 8 10

SNACK		
What I Ate:	Thoughts:	
Time:	Location:	Hunger Before: 1 3 5 8 10	Hunger After: 1 3 5 8 10

OPTIONAL 200-CALORIE SNACK		
What I Ate:	Thoughts:	
Time:	Location:	Hunger Before: 1 3 5 8 10	Hunger After: 1 3 5 8 10

■ **EXERCISE LOG:**

WALKING/CARDIO	METABOLISM/BELLY		PROGRESSIVE MUSCLE RELAXATION
Minutes:	# Reps:	Weight:	Thoughts:

■ **DAILY BLOOD SUGAR LOG:**

CHECK 1	CHECK 2	CHECK 3	CHECK 4	CHECK 5
Time:	Time:	Time:	Time:	Time:
Reading:	Reading:	Reading:	Reading:	Reading:

CORE CONFIDENCE: What are your overeating triggers? List them—common ones include eating out, parties, having a glass of wine or other alcoholic beverage (because it loosens inhibition), stress, and even celebrations. Write a brief escape plan for each situation.

FOOD LOG:

BREAKFAST			
What I Ate:		Thoughts:	
Time:	Location:	Hunger Before: 1 3 5 8 10	Hunger After: 1 3 5 8 10

LUNCH			
What I Ate:		Thoughts:	
Time:	Location:	Hunger Before: 1 3 5 8 10	Hunger After: 1 3 5 8 10

DINNER			
What I Ate:		Thoughts:	
Time:	Location:	Hunger Before: 1 3 5 8 10	Hunger After: 1 3 5 8 10

SNACK			
What I Ate:		Thoughts:	
Time:	Location:	Hunger Before: 1 3 5 8 10	Hunger After: 1 3 5 8 10

OPTIONAL 200-CALORIE SNACK			
What I Ate:		Thoughts:	
Time:	Location:	Hunger Before: 1 3 5 8 10	Hunger After: 1 3 5 8 10

EXERCISE LOG:

WALKING/CARDIO	METABOLISM/BELLY		PROGRESSIVE MUSCLE RELAXATION
Minutes:	# Reps:	Weight:	Thoughts:

DAILY BLOOD SUGAR LOG:

CHECK 1	CHECK 2	CHECK 3	CHECK 4	CHECK 5
Time:	Time:	Time:	Time:	Time:
Reading:	Reading:	Reading:	Reading:	Reading:

CORE CONFIDENCE: Forgiveness isn't just for others. If you're feeling guilty about or can't excuse yourself for your weight, your health concerns, or your past eating and exercise habits, it's time to clear the slate and start fresh. Write yourself a letter of forgiveness, then reread it.

FOOD LOG:

BREAKFAST			
What I Ate:		Thoughts:	
Time:	Location:	Hunger Before: 1 3 5 8 10	Hunger After: 1 3 5 8 10

LUNCH			
What I Ate:		Thoughts:	
Time:	Location:	Hunger Before: 1 3 5 8 10	Hunger After: 1 3 5 8 10

DINNER			
What I Ate:		Thoughts:	
Time:	Location:	Hunger Before: 1 3 5 8 10	Hunger After: 1 3 5 8 10

SNACK			
What I Ate:		Thoughts:	
Time:	Location:	Hunger Before: 1 3 5 8 10	Hunger After: 1 3 5 8 10

OPTIONAL 200-CALORIE SNACK			
What I Ate:		Thoughts:	
Time:	Location:	Hunger Before: 1 3 5 8 10	Hunger After: 1 3 5 8 10

EXERCISE LOG:

WALKING/CARDIO	METABOLISM/BELLY		PROGRESSIVE MUSCLE RELAXATION
Minutes:	# Reps:	Weight:	Thoughts:

DAILY BLOOD SUGAR LOG:

CHECK 1	CHECK 2	CHECK 3	CHECK 4	CHECK 5
Time:	Time:	Time:	Time:	Time:
Reading:	Reading:	Reading:	Reading:	Reading:

■ **CORE CONFIDENCE:** List at least five activities you've always wanted to try, but never quite got around to doing. Rank them in order of importance to you. Now, beside each one, list the very first step you'd have to take to make it happen. What can you do this week to bring #1 closer to reality?

■ FOOD LOG:

BREAKFAST			
What I Ate:		Thoughts:	
Time:	Location:	Hunger Before: 1 3 5 8 10	Hunger After: 1 3 5 8 10

LUNCH			
What I Ate:		Thoughts:	
Time:	Location:	Hunger Before: 1 3 5 8 10	Hunger After: 1 3 5 8 10

DINNER			
What I Ate:		Thoughts:	
Time:	Location:	Hunger Before: 1 3 5 8 10	Hunger After: 1 3 5 8 10

SNACK			
What I Ate:		Thoughts:	
Time:	Location:	Hunger Before: 1 3 5 8 10	Hunger After: 1 3 5 8 10

OPTIONAL 200-CALORIE SNACK			
What I Ate:		Thoughts:	
Time:	Location:	Hunger Before: 1 3 5 8 10	Hunger After: 1 3 5 8 10

■ EXERCISE LOG:

WALKING/CARDIO	METABOLISM/BELLY		PROGRESSIVE MUSCLE RELAXATION
Minutes:	# Reps:	Weight:	Thoughts:

■ DAILY BLOOD SUGAR LOG:

CHECK 1	CHECK 2	CHECK 3	CHECK 4	CHECK 5
Time:	Time:	Time:	Time:	Time:
Reading:	Reading:	Reading:	Reading:	Reading:

■ **CORE CONFIDENCE:** Fast rescue for emotional eating: Jot down a list of five instant indulgences you can substitute for food when cravings or emotions threaten to get the best of you. How about a 5-minute stroll, a cup of your favorite tea served in your favorite mug, or a neck or hand self-massage?

■ **FOOD LOG:**

BREAKFAST			
What I Ate:		Thoughts:	
Time:	Location:	Hunger Before: 1 3 5 8 10	Hunger After: 1 3 5 8 10

LUNCH			
What I Ate:		Thoughts:	
Time:	Location:	Hunger Before: 1 3 5 8 10	Hunger After: 1 3 5 8 10

DINNER			
What I Ate:		Thoughts:	
Time:	Location:	Hunger Before: 1 3 5 8 10	Hunger After: 1 3 5 8 10

SNACK			
What I Ate:		Thoughts:	
Time:	Location:	Hunger Before: 1 3 5 8 10	Hunger After: 1 3 5 8 10

OPTIONAL 200-CALORIE SNACK			
What I Ate:		Thoughts:	
Time:	Location:	Hunger Before: 1 3 5 8 10	Hunger After: 1 3 5 8 10

■ **EXERCISE LOG:**

WALKING/CARDIO	METABOLISM/BELLY		PROGRESSIVE MUSCLE RELAXATION
Minutes:	# Reps:	Weight:	Thoughts:

■ **DAILY BLOOD SUGAR LOG:**

CHECK 1	CHECK 2	CHECK 3	CHECK 4	CHECK 5
Time:	Time:	Time:	Time:	Time:
Reading:	Reading:	Reading:	Reading:	Reading:

DAY 8

■ **CORE CONFIDENCE:** Have you slipped up anytime over the past 2 weeks? List your slipup (maybe you never found time to exercise) on the left side of the page. On the right, list all the things you did right that day (hugged your child, completed a project). In the context of the "big picture" of your day, how big a deal was that slipup, really?

■ **FOOD LOG:**

BREAKFAST		
What I Ate:	Thoughts:	
Time:	Location:	Hunger Before: 1 3 5 8 10 · Hunger After: 1 3 5 8 10

LUNCH		
What I Ate:	Thoughts:	
Time:	Location:	Hunger Before: 1 3 5 8 10 · Hunger After: 1 3 5 8 10

DINNER		
What I Ate:	Thoughts:	
Time:	Location:	Hunger Before: 1 3 5 8 10 · Hunger After: 1 3 5 8 10

SNACK		
What I Ate:	Thoughts:	
Time:	Location:	Hunger Before: 1 3 5 8 10 · Hunger After: 1 3 5 8 10

OPTIONAL 200-CALORIE SNACK		
What I Ate:	Thoughts:	
Time:	Location:	Hunger Before: 1 3 5 8 10 · Hunger After: 1 3 5 8 10

■ **EXERCISE LOG:**

WALKING/CARDIO	METABOLISM/BELLY		PROGRESSIVE MUSCLE RELAXATION
Minutes:	# Reps:	Weight:	Thoughts:

■ **DAILY BLOOD SUGAR LOG:**

CHECK 1	CHECK 2	CHECK 3	CHECK 4	CHECK 5
Time:	Time:	Time:	Time:	Time:
Reading:	Reading:	Reading:	Reading:	Reading:

■ **CORE CONFIDENCE:** Describe a (non-diet) failure or setback from your recent past. What helped you persevere and get through it? How can you apply the lessons you learned to your experience on the Flat Belly Diet Diabetes?

_____

_____

_____

■ **FOOD LOG:**

BREAKFAST		
What I Ate:		Thoughts:
Time:	Location:	Hunger Before: 1 3 5 8 10 Hunger After: 1 3 5 8 10

LUNCH		
What I Ate:		Thoughts:
Time:	Location:	Hunger Before: 1 3 5 8 10 Hunger After: 1 3 5 8 10

DINNER		
What I Ate:		Thoughts:
Time:	Location:	Hunger Before: 1 3 5 8 10 Hunger After: 1 3 5 8 10

SNACK		
What I Ate:		Thoughts:
Time:	Location:	Hunger Before: 1 3 5 8 10 Hunger After: 1 3 5 8 10

OPTIONAL 200-CALORIE SNACK		
What I Ate:		Thoughts:
Time:	Location:	Hunger Before: 1 3 5 8 10 Hunger After: 1 3 5 8 10

■ **EXERCISE LOG:**

WALKING/CARDIO	METABOLISM/BELLY		PROGRESSIVE MUSCLE RELAXATION
Minutes:	# Reps:	Weight:	Thoughts:

■ **DAILY BLOOD SUGAR LOG:**

CHECK 1	CHECK 2	CHECK 3	CHECK 4	CHECK 5
Time:	Time:	Time:	Time:	Time:
Reading:	Reading:	Reading:	Reading:	Reading:

■ **CORE CONFIDENCE:** Think about the people you listed in Chapter 5 as being on "team me." Have you talked with them about your commitment to healthy eating, exercise, and stress reduction? Asked them for what you need? If so, what were the results? If not, what's holding you back? How can you enlist their support?

_____

_____

■ FOOD LOG:

BREAKFAST

What I Ate:		Thoughts:	
Time:	Location:	Hunger Before: 1 3 5 8 10	Hunger After: 1 3 5 8 10

LUNCH

What I Ate:		Thoughts:	
Time:	Location:	Hunger Before: 1 3 5 8 10	Hunger After: 1 3 5 8 10

DINNER

What I Ate:		Thoughts:	
Time:	Location:	Hunger Before: 1 3 5 8 10	Hunger After: 1 3 5 8 10

SNACK

What I Ate:		Thoughts:	
Time:	Location:	Hunger Before: 1 3 5 8 10	Hunger After: 1 3 5 8 10

OPTIONAL 200-CALORIE SNACK

What I Ate:		Thoughts:	
Time:	Location:	Hunger Before: 1 3 5 8 10	Hunger After: 1 3 5 8 10

■ EXERCISE LOG:

WALKING/CARDIO	METABOLISM/BELLY		PROGRESSIVE MUSCLE RELAXATION
Minutes:	# Reps:	Weight:	Thoughts:

■ DAILY BLOOD SUGAR LOG:

CHECK 1	CHECK 2	CHECK 3	CHECK 4	CHECK 5
Time:	Time:	Time:	Time:	Time:
Reading:	Reading:	Reading:	Reading:	Reading:

◼ **CORE CONFIDENCE:** Check in with your body. Is it feeling stronger, tighter, slimmer, more energized? Compare this to how you felt before you started the Flat Belly Diet Diabetes—chances are you've accomplished more than you realize!

_____

_____

_____

◼ **FOOD LOG:**

BREAKFAST			
What I Ate:		Thoughts:	
Time:	Location:	Hunger Before: 1 3 5 8 10	Hunger After: 1 3 5 8 10

LUNCH			
What I Ate:		Thoughts:	
Time:	Location:	Hunger Before: 1 3 5 8 10	Hunger After: 1 3 5 8 10

DINNER			
What I Ate:		Thoughts:	
Time:	Location:	Hunger Before: 1 3 5 8 10	Hunger After: 1 3 5 8 10

SNACK			
What I Ate:		Thoughts:	
Time:	Location:	Hunger Before: 1 3 5 8 10	Hunger After: 1 3 5 8 10

OPTIONAL 200-CALORIE SNACK			
What I Ate:		Thoughts:	
Time:	Location:	Hunger Before: 1 3 5 8 10	Hunger After: 1 3 5 8 10

◼ **EXERCISE LOG:**

WALKING/CARDIO	METABOLISM/BELLY		PROGRESSIVE MUSCLE RELAXATION
Minutes:	# Reps:	Weight:	Thoughts:

◼ **DAILY BLOOD SUGAR LOG:**

CHECK 1	CHECK 2	CHECK 3	CHECK 4	CHECK 5
Time:	Time:	Time:	Time:	Time:
Reading:	Reading:	Reading:	Reading:	Reading:

■ **CORE CONFIDENCE:** What are you grateful for? Make a list of all the things, the people, the circumstances in your life. Reread it before you go to bed and again when you wake up tomorrow morning.

_____

_____

_____

■ **FOOD LOG:**

BREAKFAST			
What I Ate:		Thoughts:	
Time:	Location:	Hunger Before: 1 3 5 8 10	Hunger After: 1 3 5 8 10

LUNCH			
What I Ate:		Thoughts:	
Time:	Location:	Hunger Before: 1 3 5 8 10	Hunger After: 1 3 5 8 10

DINNER			
What I Ate:		Thoughts:	
Time:	Location:	Hunger Before: 1 3 5 8 10	Hunger After: 1 3 5 8 10

SNACK			
What I Ate:		Thoughts:	
Time:	Location:	Hunger Before: 1 3 5 8 10	Hunger After: 1 3 5 8 10

OPTIONAL 200-CALORIE SNACK			
What I Ate:		Thoughts:	
Time:	Location:	Hunger Before: 1 3 5 8 10	Hunger After: 1 3 5 8 10

■ **EXERCISE LOG:**

WALKING/CARDIO	METABOLISM/BELLY		PROGRESSIVE MUSCLE RELAXATION
Minutes:	# Reps:	Weight:	Thoughts:

■ **DAILY BLOOD SUGAR LOG:**

CHECK 1	CHECK 2	CHECK 3	CHECK 4	CHECK 5
Time:	Time:	Time:	Time:	Time:
Reading:	Reading:	Reading:	Reading:	Reading:

■ **CORE CONFIDENCE:** Explore the links between mood and food in your life. Remember the last couple of times you craved a food when you were angry, sad, fearful, and happy. Write down the emotion, the food you craved, and what you actually ate. Look for patterns—sometimes, we feel the craving before we notice the emotion.

■ **FOOD LOG:**

BREAKFAST			
What I Ate:		Thoughts:	
Time:	Location:	Hunger Before: 1 3 5 8 10	Hunger After: 1 3 5 8 10

LUNCH			
What I Ate:		Thoughts:	
Time:	Location:	Hunger Before: 1 3 5 8 10	Hunger After: 1 3 5 8 10

DINNER			
What I Ate:		Thoughts:	
Time:	Location:	Hunger Before: 1 3 5 8 10	Hunger After: 1 3 5 8 10

SNACK			
What I Ate:		Thoughts:	
Time:	Location:	Hunger Before: 1 3 5 8 10	Hunger After: 1 3 5 8 10

OPTIONAL 200-CALORIE SNACK			
What I Ate:		Thoughts:	
Time:	Location:	Hunger Before: 1 3 5 8 10	Hunger After: 1 3 5 8 10

■ **EXERCISE LOG:**

WALKING/CARDIO	METABOLISM/BELLY		PROGRESSIVE MUSCLE RELAXATION
Minutes:	# Reps:	Weight:	Thoughts:

■ **DAILY BLOOD SUGAR LOG:**

CHECK 1	CHECK 2	CHECK 3	CHECK 4	CHECK 5
Time:	Time:	Time:	Time:	Time:
Reading:	Reading:	Reading:	Reading:	Reading:

■ **CORE CONFIDENCE:** You've completed the 3rd week of the Flat Belly Diet Diabetes! Think of a way to reward yourself that doesn't involve food (or skipping exercise). Will it be a movie, a new outfit (or pair of socks), a book or a CD . . . or something else?

■ FOOD LOG:

BREAKFAST			
What I Ate:		Thoughts:	
Time:	Location:	Hunger Before: 1 3 5 8 10	Hunger After: 1 3 5 8 10

LUNCH			
What I Ate:		Thoughts:	
Time:	Location:	Hunger Before: 1 3 5 8 10	Hunger After: 1 3 5 8 10

DINNER			
What I Ate:		Thoughts:	
Time:	Location:	Hunger Before: 1 3 5 8 10	Hunger After: 1 3 5 8 10

SNACK			
What I Ate:		Thoughts:	
Time:	Location:	Hunger Before: 1 3 5 8 10	Hunger After: 1 3 5 8 10

OPTIONAL 200-CALORIE SNACK			
What I Ate:		Thoughts:	
Time:	Location:	Hunger Before: 1 3 5 8 10	Hunger After: 1 3 5 8 10

■ EXERCISE LOG:

WALKING/CARDIO	METABOLISM/BELLY		PROGRESSIVE MUSCLE RELAXATION
Minutes:	# Reps:	Weight:	Thoughts:

■ DAILY BLOOD SUGAR LOG:

CHECK 1	CHECK 2	CHECK 3	CHECK 4	CHECK 5
Time:	Time:	Time:	Time:	Time:
Reading:	Reading:	Reading:	Reading:	Reading:

■ **CORE CONFIDENCE:** Two weeks to go on the plan. What aspects are going well, and which need more effort and attention? Identify two special challenges that you'd like to work on this week, and three areas where you're experiencing real success.

_____

_____

_____

■ FOOD LOG:

BREAKFAST			
What I Ate:		Thoughts:	
Time:	Location:	Hunger Before: 1 3 5 8 10	Hunger After: 1 3 5 8 10

LUNCH			
What I Ate:		Thoughts:	
Time:	Location:	Hunger Before: 1 3 5 8 10	Hunger After: 1 3 5 8 10

DINNER			
What I Ate:		Thoughts:	
Time:	Location:	Hunger Before: 1 3 5 8 10	Hunger After: 1 3 5 8 10

SNACK			
What I Ate:		Thoughts:	
Time:	Location:	Hunger Before: 1 3 5 8 10	Hunger After: 1 3 5 8 10

OPTIONAL 200-CALORIE SNACK			
What I Ate:		Thoughts:	
Time:	Location:	Hunger Before: 1 3 5 8 10	Hunger After: 1 3 5 8 10

■ EXERCISE LOG:

WALKING/CARDIO	METABOLISM/BELLY		PROGRESSIVE MUSCLE RELAXATION
Minutes:	# Reps:	Weight:	Thoughts:

■ DAILY BLOOD SUGAR LOG:

CHECK 1	CHECK 2	CHECK 3	CHECK 4	CHECK 5
Time:	Time:	Time:	Time:	Time:
Reading:	Reading:	Reading:	Reading:	Reading:

▨ **CORE CONFIDENCE:** Brush up on mindful eating today. Banish all distractions—TV, radio, books, computers, newspapers. Eat slowly. Put your fork down between bites and savor every mouthful. Write about the experience.

_____

_____

_____

▨ FOOD LOG:

BREAKFAST		
What I Ate:	Thoughts:	
Time:	Location:	Hunger Before: 1 3 5 8 10 Hunger After: 1 3 5 8 10

LUNCH		
What I Ate:	Thoughts:	
Time:	Location:	Hunger Before: 1 3 5 8 10 Hunger After: 1 3 5 8 10

DINNER		
What I Ate:	Thoughts:	
Time:	Location:	Hunger Before: 1 3 5 8 10 Hunger After: 1 3 5 8 10

SNACK		
What I Ate:	Thoughts:	
Time:	Location:	Hunger Before: 1 3 5 8 10 Hunger After: 1 3 5 8 10

OPTIONAL 200-CALORIE SNACK		
What I Ate:	Thoughts:	
Time:	Location:	Hunger Before: 1 3 5 8 10 Hunger After: 1 3 5 8 10

▨ EXERCISE LOG:

WALKING/CARDIO	METABOLISM/BELLY		PROGRESSIVE MUSCLE RELAXATION
Minutes:	# Reps:	Weight:	Thoughts:

▨ DAILY BLOOD SUGAR LOG:

CHECK 1	CHECK 2	CHECK 3	CHECK 4	CHECK 5
Time:	Time:	Time:	Time:	Time:
Reading:	Reading:	Reading:	Reading:	Reading:

DAY 17

CORE CONFIDENCE: List five personal strengths you possess in regard to your relationships, your job, your health, your interests. Now list how you can use them to help you make changes to become more of the person you wish to become.

_____

_____

_____

FOOD LOG:

BREAKFAST		
What I Ate:	Thoughts:	
Time:	Location:	Hunger Before: 1 3 5 8 10 Hunger After: 1 3 5 8 10

LUNCH		
What I Ate:	Thoughts:	
Time:	Location:	Hunger Before: 1 3 5 8 10 Hunger After: 1 3 5 8 10

DINNER		
What I Ate:	Thoughts:	
Time:	Location:	Hunger Before: 1 3 5 8 10 Hunger After: 1 3 5 8 10

SNACK		
What I Ate:	Thoughts:	
Time:	Location:	Hunger Before: 1 3 5 8 10 Hunger After: 1 3 5 8 10

OPTIONAL 200-CALORIE SNACK		
What I Ate:	Thoughts:	
Time:	Location:	Hunger Before: 1 3 5 8 10 Hunger After: 1 3 5 8 10

EXERCISE LOG:

WALKING/CARDIO	METABOLISM/BELLY		PROGRESSIVE MUSCLE RELAXATION
Minutes:	# Reps:	Weight:	Thoughts:

DAILY BLOOD SUGAR LOG:

CHECK 1	CHECK 2	CHECK 3	CHECK 4	CHECK 5
Time:	Time:	Time:	Time:	Time:
Reading:	Reading:	Reading:	Reading:	Reading:

■ **CORE CONFIDENCE:** Do a personal energy audit today. Compared with 3 weeks ago, how do you feel when you wake up in the morning, in midafternoon, when you exercise or have to do a physically demanding task, and in the evening? Do you have more stamina and oomph?

_____

■ **FOOD LOG:**

BREAKFAST	
What I Ate:	Thoughts:
Time:　　　　Location:	Hunger Before:　1　3　5　8　10　Hunger After:　1　3　5　8　10

LUNCH	
What I Ate:	Thoughts:
Time:　　　　Location:	Hunger Before:　1　3　5　8　10　Hunger After:　1　3　5　8　10

DINNER	
What I Ate:	Thoughts:
Time:　　　　Location:	Hunger Before:　1　3　5　8　10　Hunger After:　1　3　5　8　10

SNACK	
What I Ate:	Thoughts:
Time:　　　　Location:	Hunger Before:　1　3　5　8　10　Hunger After:　1　3　5　8　10

OPTIONAL 200-CALORIE SNACK	
What I Ate:	Thoughts:
Time:　　　　Location:	Hunger Before:　1　3　5　8　10　Hunger After:　1　3　5　8　10

■ **EXERCISE LOG:**

WALKING/CARDIO	METABOLISM/BELLY		PROGRESSIVE MUSCLE RELAXATION
Minutes:	# Reps:	Weight:	Thoughts:

■ **DAILY BLOOD SUGAR LOG:**

CHECK 1	CHECK 2	CHECK 3	CHECK 4	CHECK 5
Time:	Time:	Time:	Time:	Time:
Reading:	Reading:	Reading:	Reading:	Reading:

CORE CONFIDENCE: What does a lifetime of optimal health look like for you? Write three short lists—what being healthy will allow you to do this year, in the next 5 years, and later in life. Refer to this list in the future, whenever your motivation flags.

_____

_____

_____

FOOD LOG:

BREAKFAST		
What I Ate:		Thoughts:
Time:	Location:	Hunger Before: 1 3 5 8 10 Hunger After: 1 3 5 8 10

LUNCH		
What I Ate:		Thoughts:
Time:	Location:	Hunger Before: 1 3 5 8 10 Hunger After: 1 3 5 8 10

DINNER		
What I Ate:		Thoughts:
Time:	Location:	Hunger Before: 1 3 5 8 10 Hunger After: 1 3 5 8 10

SNACK		
What I Ate:		Thoughts:
Time:	Location:	Hunger Before: 1 3 5 8 10 Hunger After: 1 3 5 8 10

OPTIONAL 200-CALORIE SNACK		
What I Ate:		Thoughts:
Time:	Location:	Hunger Before: 1 3 5 8 10 Hunger After: 1 3 5 8 10

EXERCISE LOG:

WALKING/CARDIO	METABOLISM/BELLY		PROGRESSIVE MUSCLE RELAXATION
Minutes:	# Reps:	Weight:	Thoughts:

DAILY BLOOD SUGAR LOG:

CHECK 1	CHECK 2	CHECK 3	CHECK 4	CHECK 5
Time:	Time:	Time:	Time:	Time:
Reading:	Reading:	Reading:	Reading:	Reading:

■ **CORE CONFIDENCE:** If you could have just three foods for the rest of your life, what would they be? Write them down, then figure out how to incorporate them into your Flat Belly Diet Diabetes eating plan. (Remember, no food is off-limits!)

_____

_____

■ FOOD LOG:

BREAKFAST			
What I Ate:		Thoughts:	
Time:	Location:	Hunger Before: 1 3 5 8 10	Hunger After: 1 3 5 8 10

LUNCH			
What I Ate:		Thoughts:	
Time:	Location:	Hunger Before: 1 3 5 8 10	Hunger After: 1 3 5 8 10

DINNER			
What I Ate:		Thoughts:	
Time:	Location:	Hunger Before: 1 3 5 8 10	Hunger After: 1 3 5 8 10

SNACK			
What I Ate:		Thoughts:	
Time:	Location:	Hunger Before: 1 3 5 8 10	Hunger After: 1 3 5 8 10

OPTIONAL 200-CALORIE SNACK			
What I Ate:		Thoughts:	
Time:	Location:	Hunger Before: 1 3 5 8 10	Hunger After: 1 3 5 8 10

■ EXERCISE LOG:

WALKING/CARDIO	METABOLISM/BELLY		PROGRESSIVE MUSCLE RELAXATION
Minutes:	# Reps.	Weight:	Thoughts:

■ DAILY BLOOD SUGAR LOG:

CHECK 1	CHECK 2	CHECK 3	CHECK 4	CHECK 5
Time:	Time:	Time:	Time:	Time:
Reading:	Reading:	Reading:	Reading:	Reading:

■ **CORE CONFIDENCE:** Think of an individual you admire (it may be someone you know personally or someone you've only heard about). What makes him or her so special? If you could absorb two of his or her best qualities, what would they be and why?

_____

_____

■ **FOOD LOG:**

BREAKFAST		
What I Ate:	Thoughts:	
Time:	Location:	Hunger Before: 1 3 5 8 10 | Hunger After: 1 3 5 8 10

LUNCH		
What I Ate:	Thoughts:	
Time:	Location:	Hunger Before: 1 3 5 8 10 | Hunger After: 1 3 5 8 10

DINNER		
What I Ate:	Thoughts:	
Time:	Location:	Hunger Before: 1 3 5 8 10 | Hunger After: 1 3 5 8 10

SNACK		
What I Ate:	Thoughts:	
Time:	Location:	Hunger Before: 1 3 5 8 10 | Hunger After: 1 3 5 8 10

OPTIONAL 200-CALORIE SNACK		
What I Ate:	Thoughts:	
Time:	Location:	Hunger Before: 1 3 5 8 10 | Hunger After: 1 3 5 8 10

■ **EXERCISE LOG:**

WALKING/CARDIO	METABOLISM/BELLY		PROGRESSIVE MUSCLE RELAXATION
Minutes:	# Reps:	Weight:	Thoughts:

■ **DAILY BLOOD SUGAR LOG:**

CHECK 1	CHECK 2	CHECK 3	CHECK 4	CHECK 5
Time:	Time:	Time:	Time:	Time:
Reading:	Reading:	Reading:	Reading:	Reading:

▨ **CORE CONFIDENCE:** Which Flat Belly Diet Diabetes benefits matter most to you? Under columns labeled HIGH, MEDIUM, and LOW, list your motivators according to their priority in your life. For example, HIGH might include better blood sugar control, and MEDIUM might be walking up a hill without feeling tired.

▨ **FOOD LOG:**

BREAKFAST			
What I Ate:		Thoughts:	
Time:	Location:	Hunger Before: 1 3 5 8 10	Hunger After: 1 3 5 8 10

LUNCH			
What I Ate:		Thoughts:	
Time:	Location:	Hunger Before: 1 3 5 8 10	Hunger After: 1 3 5 8 10

DINNER			
What I Ate:		Thoughts:	
Time:	Location:	Hunger Before: 1 3 5 8 10	Hunger After: 1 3 5 8 10

SNACK			
What I Ate:		Thoughts:	
Time:	Location:	Hunger Before: 1 3 5 8 10	Hunger After: 1 3 5 8 10

OPTIONAL 200-CALORIE SNACK			
What I Ate:		Thoughts:	
Time:	Location:	Hunger Before: 1 3 5 8 10	Hunger After: 1 3 5 8 10

▨ **EXERCISE LOG:**

WALKING/CARDIO	METABOLISM/BELLY		PROGRESSIVE MUSCLE RELAXATION
Minutes:	# Reps:	Weight:	Thoughts:

▨ **DAILY BLOOD SUGAR LOG:**

CHECK 1	CHECK 2	CHECK 3	CHECK 4	CHECK 5
Time:	Time:	Time:	Time:	Time:
Reading:	Reading:	Reading:	Reading:	Reading:

■ **CORE CONFIDENCE:** Make a list of all the things and people you're angry with. Then write beside each name, in capital letters, the words I FORGIVE YOU.

_____

_____

_____

■ **FOOD LOG:**

BREAKFAST			
What I Ate:		Thoughts:	
Time:	Location:	Hunger Before: 1 3 5 8 10	Hunger After: 1 3 5 8 10

LUNCH			
What I Ate:		Thoughts:	
Time:	Location:	Hunger Before: 1 3 5 8 10	Hunger After: 1 3 5 8 10

DINNER			
What I Ate:		Thoughts:	
Time:	Location:	Hunger Before: 1 3 5 8 10	Hunger After: 1 3 5 8 10

SNACK			
What I Ate:		Thoughts:	
Time:	Location:	Hunger Before: 1 3 5 8 10	Hunger After: 1 3 5 8 10

OPTIONAL 200-CALORIE SNACK			
What I Ate:		Thoughts:	
Time:	Location:	Hunger Before: 1 3 5 8 10	Hunger After: 1 3 5 8 10

■ **EXERCISE LOG:**

WALKING/CARDIO	METABOLISM/BELLY		PROGRESSIVE MUSCLE RELAXATION
Minutes:	# Reps:	Weight:	Thoughts:

■ **DAILY BLOOD SUGAR LOG:**

CHECK 1	CHECK 2	CHECK 3	CHECK 4	CHECK 5
Time:	Time:	Time:	Time:	Time:
Reading:	Reading:	Reading:	Reading:	Reading:

DAY 24

■ **CORE CONFIDENCE:** How have you surprised yourself over the last 5 weeks? Maybe you discovered that you can eat four 400-calorie meals a day and not go back for seconds, tried new foods, or packed your lunch. Give yourself a pat on the back for each one!

_____

_____

■ **FOOD LOG:**

BREAKFAST				
What I Ate:		Thoughts:		
Time:	Location:	Hunger Before: 1 3 5 8 10	Hunger After: 1 3 5 8 10	

LUNCH				
What I Ate:		Thoughts:		
Time:	Location:	Hunger Before: 1 3 5 8 10	Hunger After: 1 3 5 8 10	

DINNER				
What I Ate:		Thoughts:		
Time:	Location:	Hunger Before: 1 3 5 8 10	Hunger After: 1 3 5 8 10	

SNACK				
What I Ate:		Thoughts:		
Time:	Location:	Hunger Before: 1 3 5 8 10	Hunger After: 1 3 5 8 10	

OPTIONAL 200-CALORIE SNACK				
What I Ate:		Thoughts:		
Time:	Location:	Hunger Before: 1 3 5 8 10	Hunger After: 1 3 5 8 10	

■ **EXERCISE LOG:**

WALKING/CARDIO	METABOLISM/BELLY		PROGRESSIVE MUSCLE RELAXATION
Minutes:	# Reps:	Weight:	Thoughts:

■ **DAILY BLOOD SUGAR LOG:**

CHECK 1	CHECK 2	CHECK 3	CHECK 4	CHECK 5
Time:	Time:	Time:	Time:	Time:
Reading:	Reading:	Reading:	Reading:	Reading:

■ **CORE CONFIDENCE:** Think about a recent situation that left you feeling stressed out. Did you react differently than you might have in the past, thanks to what you've learned on this plan? Do you still see areas that need improvement?

_____

_____

_____

■ **FOOD LOG:**

BREAKFAST		
What I Ate:		Thoughts:
Time:	Location:	Hunger Before: 1 3 5 8 10 Hunger After: 1 3 5 8 10

LUNCH		
What I Ate:		Thoughts:
Time:	Location:	Hunger Before: 1 3 5 8 10 Hunger After: 1 3 5 8 10

DINNER		
What I Ate:		Thoughts:
Time:	Location:	Hunger Before: 1 3 5 8 10 Hunger After: 1 3 5 8 10

SNACK		
What I Ate:		Thoughts:
Time:	Location:	Hunger Before: 1 3 5 8 10 Hunger After: 1 3 5 8 10

OPTIONAL 200-CALORIE SNACK		
What I Ate:		Thoughts:
Time:	Location:	Hunger Before: 1 3 5 8 10 Hunger After: 1 3 5 8 10

■ **EXERCISE LOG:**

WALKING/CARDIO	METABOLISM/BELLY		PROGRESSIVE MUSCLE RELAXATION
Minutes:	# Reps:	Weight:	Thoughts:

■ **DAILY BLOOD SUGAR LOG:**

CHECK 1	CHECK 2	CHECK 3	CHECK 4	CHECK 5
Time:	Time:	Time:	Time:	Time:
Reading:	Reading:	Reading:	Reading:	Reading:

DAY 26

CORE CONFIDENCE: Make today another mindful eating day—and focus on how good it feels to eat enjoyable food and to be comfortably full at the end of the meal. Focus on these good feelings and remind yourself that you deserve to feel this way! Write about how it feels.

FOOD LOG:

BREAKFAST			
What I Ate:		Thoughts:	
Time:	Location:	Hunger Before: 1 3 5 8 10	Hunger After: 1 3 5 8 10

LUNCH			
What I Ate:		Thoughts:	
Time:	Location:	Hunger Before: 1 3 5 8 10	Hunger After: 1 3 5 8 10

DINNER			
What I Ate:		Thoughts:	
Time:	Location:	Hunger Before: 1 3 5 8 10	Hunger After: 1 3 5 8 10

SNACK			
What I Ate:		Thoughts:	
Time:	Location:	Hunger Before: 1 3 5 8 10	Hunger After: 1 3 5 8 10

OPTIONAL 200-CALORIE SNACK			
What I Ate:		Thoughts:	
Time:	Location:	Hunger Before: 1 3 5 8 10	Hunger After: 1 3 5 8 10

EXERCISE LOG:

WALKING/CARDIO	METABOLISM/BELLY		PROGRESSIVE MUSCLE RELAXATION
Minutes:	# Reps:	Weight:	Thoughts:

DAILY BLOOD SUGAR LOG:

CHECK 1	CHECK 2	CHECK 3	CHECK 4	CHECK 5
Time:	Time:	Time:	Time:	Time:
Reading:	Reading:	Reading:	Reading:	Reading:

CORE CONFIDENCE: Tomorrow is your last "official" day on the Flat Belly Diet Diabetes. You've come a long way. Today, look back at all of your successes—large and small—and how you're feeling about them.

_____

_____

_____

FOOD LOG:

BREAKFAST		
What I Ate:		Thoughts:
Time:	Location:	Hunger Before: 1 3 5 8 10 Hunger After: 1 3 5 8 10

LUNCH		
What I Ate:		Thoughts:
Time:	Location:	Hunger Before: 1 3 5 8 10 Hunger After: 1 3 5 8 10

DINNER		
What I Ate:		Thoughts:
Time:	Location:	Hunger Before: 1 3 5 8 10 Hunger After: 1 3 5 8 10

SNACK		
What I Ate:		Thoughts:
Time:	Location:	Hunger Before: 1 3 5 8 10 Hunger After: 1 3 5 8 10

OPTIONAL 200-CALORIE SNACK		
What I Ate:		Thoughts:
Time:	Location:	Hunger Before: 1 3 5 8 10 Hunger After: 1 3 5 8 10

EXERCISE LOG:

WALKING/CARDIO	METABOLISM/BELLY		PROGRESSIVE MUSCLE RELAXATION
Minutes:	# Reps:	Weight:	Thoughts:

DAILY BLOOD SUGAR LOG:

CHECK 1	CHECK 2	CHECK 3	CHECK 4	CHECK 5
Time:	Time:	Time:	Time:	Time:
Reading:	Reading:	Reading:	Reading:	Reading:

DAY 28

■ **CORE CONFIDENCE:** You've reached the final day of our 35-day plan! Describe how it feels to have set and reached this goal. How happy are you with the results? How will you reward yourself? Write a pledge to yourself that you'll keep on taking care of your body and your health this way.

_____

_____

■ **FOOD LOG:**

BREAKFAST		
What I Ate:		Thoughts:
Time:	Location:	Hunger Before: 1 3 5 8 10	Hunger After: 1 3 5 8 10

LUNCH		
What I Ate:		Thoughts:
Time:	Location:	Hunger Before: 1 3 5 8 10	Hunger After: 1 3 5 8 10

DINNER		
What I Ate:		Thoughts:
Time:	Location:	Hunger Before: 1 3 5 8 10	Hunger After: 1 3 5 8 10

SNACK		
What I Ate:		Thoughts:
Time:	Location:	Hunger Before: 1 3 5 8 10	Hunger After: 1 3 5 8 10

OPTIONAL 200-CALORIE SNACK		
What I Ate:		Thoughts:
Time:	Location:	Hunger Before: 1 3 5 8 10	Hunger After: 1 3 5 8 10

■ **EXERCISE LOG:**

WALKING/CARDIO	METABOLISM/BELLY		PROGRESSIVE MUSCLE RELAXATION
Minutes:	# Reps:	Weight:	Thoughts:

■ **DAILY BLOOD SUGAR LOG:**

CHECK 1	CHECK 2	CHECK 3	CHECK 4	CHECK 5
Time:	Time:	Time:	Time:	Time:
Reading:	Reading:	Reading:	Reading:	Reading:

CONCLUSION

DAY 36
AND BEYOND

"KEEPING MY WEIGHT and my blood sugar at healthy levels is going to be a lifetime thing—and I'm ready for it," test panelist Donna Branson told us. "This is definitely going to be a permanent change. And no matter what I do, I know that having a MUFA at every meal will be a part of it!"

Donna was where you are now: She had recently finished our 5-week plan, seen some amazing results, and was looking to the future. She loved the progress she'd made—her blood sugar and cholesterol were better than they'd been in a long time, and she was fitting into clothing styles she hadn't worn in years. Best of all, she felt ready to move ahead. "I'm definitely making better choices," she said. "I've learned so much and seen what a difference it makes."

As you stand here on the threshold of "the rest of your life," let's take a look back at what you've achieved. You've finished the first 35 days of the Flat Belly Diet Diabetes. If you've followed the parameters of this plan (eating your MUFAs and other healthy foods at every meal, limiting calories to 1,600 a day, exercising regularly in a smart, efficient way, and coming to a deeper realization about how you think about food), then you've taken the first and most difficult step toward a healthier future. These are the steps that can lower your risk for developing diabetes. If you already have diabetes, they can make blood sugar control easier in the short term and lower your odds for serious, diabetes-related complications (such as vision loss, kidney function problems, and nerve damage). And you've most likely whittled away a few pounds of the deadliest fat you can have: belly fat.

What will you do tomorrow? When we asked our test panelists that question, every one responded that they would keep on using the tools, skills, and lessons learned on the Flat Belly Diet Diabetes. We hope you will, too—and not for a trimmer physique alone, but for a lifetime of optimal health.

With passion and eloquence, one of our test panelists described the real goals—and rewards—of a healthy lifestyle. Her words inspired us—and we

Don't Skip Meals!

It doesn't pay to try to dip below the 1,600-calories-a-day mark. If you drastically reduce the amount of food you eat for any extended period of time, your body's natural response is to slow things down to conserve fat. For those of us who aspire to flatter bellies, that "starvation response" is the last thing we need.

Why? Your body starts breaking down muscle tissue to use for fuel. Muscle is metabolically active tissue that requires a certain number of calories each day to maintain itself, whether or not it's in use. So the more muscle you have, the more calories you burn, 24/7. As your muscle mass drops, so does your body's need for calories to sustain it. You eventually need fewer and fewer calories just to maintain your new weight. It's far better to eat all of your allotted calories—and bolster muscle mass with our Metabolism Boost routine!

think they'll inspire you as you transition from Phase 2 to happily ever after: "I won't *diet*," Anne Harrington told us a few weeks after she finished Phase 2. "I've found that dieting to simply lose pounds and to try to turn my body into someone else's is counterproductive. My goal is all-around health. So I work hard to maintain my weight and I choose healthy, unprocessed foods so that my blood sugar, my blood pressure, and my cholesterol stay within a healthy range. I've lost a few pounds in the past few years, at a time of life when many women gain weight because of hormonal changes. The thing that really inspired me on the Flat Belly Diet Diabetes was seeing my blood sugar numbers—that's my real motivation. Keeping my blood sugar inside a healthy range will cut my chances for complications in the future. And for a person with diabetes, that's extremely important."

This chapter arms you to reap all of the benefits of the Flat Belly Diet Diabetes—from a longer, healthier life to, yes, a trimmer torso—for decades to come. Let's get started!

Eat and Exercise by the Rules

THE RULES FOR YOUR journey ahead are the ones you already know intimately:

- **RULE #1: STICK TO 400 CALORIES PER MEAL.**
- **RULE #2: NEVER GO MORE THAN 4 HOURS WITHOUT EATING.**
- **RULE #3: EAT A MUFA AT EVERY MEAL.**
- **RULE #4: EXERCISE MOST DAYS OF THE WEEK.**

RULE #1: STICK TO 400 CALORIES PER MEAL

WE'RE NOT GOING TO mince words: Keeping your weight down and your belly fat under control means continuing to "right size" your daily calories—by sticking to about 400 calories per meal, 1,600 per day. If you've added the extra 200-calorie snack, you can keep that up as well. Whether you've reached your goals—for weight, waist size, and/or blood sugar control—or are still in the process of getting there, maintaining the same daily calorie intake is crucial. The fact is, 1,600 calories is enough to keep up your energy, support your immune system, deliver the nutrients your whole body needs, and maintain your precious calorie-burning muscle (so you won't feel run-down, cranky, or hungry). Just as important, it's *not* enough calories to allow you to gain back your belly fat (and make you more vulnerable to all the attendant health risks).

We're not sentencing you to a lifetime of dull eating or downright deprivation, however. After 35 days on the Flat Belly Diet Diabetes, you've experienced the satisfaction and the range of high-taste, high-pleasure foods you can rustle up in a matter of minutes on this plan. As our test panelists discovered, the food is nothing short of fabulous. They served it to company, proudly put it on the table for their spouses and children, and got rave reviews when they brought it along to social events. One panelist's relatives loved the Chocolate-Zucchini Snack Cake so much that it became their most-requested favorite. And boredom? Forget about it. Without being prompted, they raved about the meals and snacks: One called the whole wheat tortilla roll-up with hummus, turkey, and pine nuts "as good as pizza" and a hearty snack of cheese and crackers "as good as filet mignon." And that snack cake? "As good as any dessert I've ever had," another said. One test panelist's family decided to cook the broiled cod, red potatoes, and snap pea dinner as a special Valentine's Day meal. Kudos poured in from panelists who cooked and from those whose busy lives left them with little to no kitchen time. Between the quick-fix meals, Snack Packs, and recipes, as well as a multitude of approved packaged and fast-food items, you have hundreds of choices, whether or not you have the time (or the inclination) to cook.

RULE #2: NEVER GO MORE THAN 4 HOURS WITHOUT EATING

THIS IS YOUR TRIED-AND-TRUE routine by now. You've established a rhythm, and your body has responded—by becoming accustomed to having three

DID YOU KNOW?

MUFA-rich 400-calorie meals at 4-hour intervals, as well as a healthy snack at whatever time of day suits you. The pattern helped our test panelists avoid hunger and maintain high levels of energy—in some cases, higher than they'd experienced for a while. Eating consistent, healthy quantities of healthy foods on a regular schedule, one panelist told us, also helped with blood sugar regulation. "You don't want to go a long time between meals when you have diabetes," he said. "You end up with roller-coaster blood sugar levels that leave you feeling kind of spacey and fuzzy. I truly believe that eating regularly like this, and eating reasonable portions, is teaching my body to become more sensitive to insulin. My body releases smaller amounts because the meals are smaller, and the exercise and weight loss make my cells more sensitive to it. That's healthier for my blood sugar."

RULE #3: EAT A MUFA AT EVERY MEAL

OVER THE PAST FEW weeks, you have come to know MUFAs well (and love them as dearly as we do, we're sure!), those little miracle workers in your belly that help you feel full, encourage the loss of visceral fat, and even help protect against blood sugar peaks and valleys. You've also discovered how easy—and tasty—it is to include small amounts of these healthy fats in your meals. Even if you can't work in a MUFA at every single meal you ever eat, you know that they are found mainly in vegetable oils, nuts, seeds, olives, and avocados (yes, and in the occasional piece of dark chocolate!). They are about as easy to come by as they are to love—test panelists found them on restaurant menus (as avocados and olive oil for dressing salads), in coffee shops (by having a small helping of nuts), and in convenience stores (again, many carry small bags of nuts). If you don't know the MUFA list by heart at this point, you can always flip to page 127.

RULE #4: EXERCISE MOST DAYS OF THE WEEK

WE'VE SHARED PLENTY OF convincing research showing that regular exercise is vital for controlling your blood sugar, lowering diabetes risk, losing pounds, and—of course—flattening your belly. We're confident that by now, 35 days after you first began this plan, you've experienced the pure pleasure and instant gratification of movement—it energizes, eases stress, even makes your skin glow and improves sleep. We hope you're also reaping deep, long-term benefits, too. Your baseline: a daily walk or other "cardio" exercise—swimming, biking (or using a pedaler if you have diabetes-related foot problems), or any other activity that gets your heart pumping. Keep up this healthy habit. It doesn't matter whether you fit short "bursts" of activity into your busy day or carve out a chunk of dedicated time for a walk or a workout. Fitting some physical activity into your schedule regularly is what counts. That's why our do-almost-anywhere, almost-anytime fitness program is flexible, so that you can keep it up no matter what else is swirling around in your life and on your calendar!

And keep up the Metabolism Boost and Belly Routine, too! There's no getting around the fact that we begin losing precious, calorie-burning, blood-sugarsipping muscle mass as we age—starting in our thirties! That means weight gain unless you take steps to preserve and rebuild muscle mass with strength-training (also called resistance-training) moves such as those in those two short, highly effective routines. If the moves become easy, add a second set of 10 repetitions for each exercise, with a short break (about a minute) in between as a breather. Once that's a cinch, add another short rest and another

The Flat Belly Diet Diabetes to Go: The Angst-Free Guide to Dining Out

Okay, you've got this gorgeous, flat belly, you're full of energy, and you feel absolutely wonderful. Now it's time to celebrate. Maybe it's your anniversary. Or your birthday. Or maybe you're just feeling happy. Dinner out? Why not?

It can be done—in fact, several of our test panelists tested our claim that you can enjoy a healthy meal out without blowing it. The result? Success! Paula Martin celebrated her 54th birthday with dinner at her favorite Chinese restaurant. "It was so delicious," she notes. "I had grilled tuna with no sauce, green tea soba noodles, and chicken lettuce wraps—reasonable portions and no dessert. It was the perfect amount of food, and I was back on the regular plan the next day. By the end of the program, I lost 35 pounds and several inches!"

Just remember, you are there to enjoy yourself, not binge. And if you stay with the plan—or even a slightly modified version—you will wake up feeling good, not guilty, tomorrow. Following these guidelines will help you stay on track:

- **Eat what you would normally eat throughout the day.** Skipping a meal to save calories for later just increases the chances that you will overeat at dinner. You can up your exercise—the added calorie burn will help offset a splurge like dessert.

- **If you can, find out what's on the menu** before you go (many are online now, and you can always call the restaurant to ask about healthy choices). In your mind, place your order before you leave the house, so you're not swayed by the sights, aromas, and waiter's descriptions!

- **Be the first at the table to order.** This will keep you from being tempted by others' choices.

- **Go for colors.** Fruits and vegetables have a rainbow of colors. High-fat, high-sugar, high-calorie stuff like cheese, cream sauce, and brownies come in shades of beige and brown.

- **Steer clear of anything that's breaded, crispy, creamy, or buttery.** Choose grilled, baked, steamed, or broiled foods instead, and select soups and sauces that are broth-based or tomato-based.

- **Hunt for the MUFAs.** Olive oil and/or a scattering of nuts on your salad, avocado in your sandwich, the olives on the salad bar—MUFAs may be hiding in plain sight all over the menu.

- **If you have diabetes: Watch the carbs.** If you normally eat a set amount of carbohydrates per meal, do so when eating out as well. This will help keep your blood sugar on an even keel.

- **Bring along our guide.** The *Flat Belly Diet Pocket Guide* includes recommendations for specific healthy, calorie-controlled, Flat Belly Diet–style meals at dozens of national fast-food and sit-down restaurant chains—plus strategies for eating well away from home whether you're facing the office vending machine or perusing the menu at your local Italian trattoria.

new results in the form of sleeker, more toned muscle and a new feeling of strength and stamina in everything else you do during the day!

Need a new "stretch" goal for fitness? How about walking farther and faster? If you're completely comfortable with our basic Fat Blast Walk and with the faster-paced intervals in our Calorie Torch Walk, consider adding an additional 5 minutes to your daily walks this week—raising your daily total to 40 minutes for beginners and 25 minutes for advanced walkers. Next week, add another 5 minutes. If you're feeling good, keep adding a few minutes each week until you're walking for 30 to 45 minutes.

A Flat Belly for Life: Your Mind-Set Matters

TIME AND AGAIN THROUGHOUT this book we've told you the Flat Belly Diet Diabetes is about attitude. Well, guess what—so is your healthy, flat-bellied future. We've supplied you with tools and tricks galore that, as you move forward beyond Day 35, are going to be no less important to nourishing and fortifying you than the Flat Belly Diet Diabetes meals and MUFAs. These tools and tricks have been as integral to your success as the foods you've eaten. You've used them to make major changes. And they'll be just as essential to

Off track? Hold the lecture.

Everyone has "off" days—when we eat a little too much, skip exercise, don't check blood sugar the way the doctor recommended, or make other unhealthy choices. The trigger could be stress, a special occasion, or vacation. The important thing to know is that, well, it happens to everyone. And what matters isn't the off day—it's what you do the next day. So don't punish yourself or let one off day throw you off track. Get back to healthy eating, physical activity, and regular blood sugar checks right away—no harm, no foul.

your ongoing health and well-being. Use these key practices and pointers as guides for the journey ahead:

KEEP JOURNALING

Tracking food, exercise, stress reduction—and blood sugar, if you have diabetes or if your doctor has recommended it—in a journal is probably the single most important thing you can do going forward to help you maintain your focus on your long-term health goals. Over and over again, our test panelists told us that journaling helped them stay on track with portion sizes, calories, and with eating every 4 hours. If you have diabetes, this written record can also help you spot the causes of blood sugar spikes and blood sugar lows that might otherwise seem mysterious and unfixable. Noting your emotions is just as powerful because it can help you spot patterns and situations that lead to unhealthy choices like overeating or even skipping meals or exercise. Your thoughts are the clues to all your destructive insecurities and all your inner power. Why on earth would you consider ignoring them? Just as no parent should be without a thermometer in the medicine cabinet, we firmly believe that no one committed to a healthy future should be without the means to record their thoughts, feelings, and actions.

STAY MINDFUL

Whenever you need a quick attitude adjustment from frantic to focused, call on the Mind Tricks from Chapter 5. They're fast—just minutes apiece—but extremely effective at jolting you out of a stress-fueled stupor and adjusting your emotional relationship to eating. They'll help you slow down, take your time, and savor your meals, so you won't be tempted to overindulge or eat too quickly.

MANAGE STRESS

The stress/belly fat and stress/blood sugar connections are emerging loud and clear from medical studies—and from the experiences of people who are battling both. Manage stress and you are one step closer to managing your belly fat forever. Writing in your journal can be a great stress reliever, but so can daily exercise and practicing a daily stress-reduction technique. We've given you a powerful, tension-melting tool called progressive muscle relaxation—a classic and proven stress tamer. Use it daily and it will become second nature, a strategy you can pull out of your bag of tricks whenever stress makes your muscles clench and your thoughts whirl. If you need more ideas to help get your stress under control, periodically revisit the stress-busting strategies in Chapter 5 and use them as a checklist.

GATHER A SUPPORT TEAM

One of the best ways to stay on track and stay motivated is to have a support team behind you. This is doubly important if you're coping with the daily challenges of living with diabetes. Support can help you avoid diabetes burnout, a common mental state that can be triggered if you feel overwhelmed, scared, or discouraged by your blood sugar readings or the demands of coping with diabetes when you'd rather be out loving the rest of your life! Regardless of how motivated you are, long-term success is always easier with help from others. Even one person will do—just someone to tell you you're doing great every once in a while. Having people in your life who understand and accept your dreams can make all the difference in the world. Your supporters don't have to be members of your family or even good friends, so long as they respect your goals. Support groups and online message boards are great ways to share experiences and emotional support with other people who know exactly what you're going through. Two that are highly recommended by Gillian and Dr. Edelman are the online discussion boards on the Web site of the Harvard Medical School–affiliated Joslin Diabetes Center at www.forums.joslin.org and the Web site of the Behavioral Diabetes Institute in San Diego, California, at www.behavioral diabetes.org. You can find an online "diabetes buddy" or mentor to provide support, information, and encouragement.

Track Your Blood Sugar

IF YOU DON'T HAVE diabetes, you may be wondering how often to have your blood sugar checked in the future to ensure that you're not developing it. On the basis of recommendations from the American Diabetes Association and the American College of Clinical Endocrinologists, talk to your doctor about these guidelines:

- **YOUR BLOOD SUGAR IS NORMAL NOW, BUT YOU'RE AT RISK FOR DIABETES:** Ask about an annual fasting blood sugar check. As a reminder, you're at risk if you have any of these factors: a waist measurement of 40 inches or more for men, 35 inches or more for women; overweight; physically inactive; age 45 or older; a family history of diabetes; a personal history of gestational diabetes (diabetes during pregnancy or if you've had a baby weighing 9 pounds or more); African American, Latino, Pacific Islander, or Native American descent; HDL cholesterol under 35; high blood levels of triglycerides, a type of fat molecule (normal is 150 mg/dl); or blood pressure levels of 130/85 or higher.

- **YOU HAVE SIGNS OF METABOLIC SYNDROME:** Ask about monitoring blood pressure, cholesterol, triglycerides, and blood sugar. You have metabolic syndrome if you have three of these: a waist measurement of 40 inches or more for men and 35 inches or more for women; triglyceride levels of 150 milligrams per deciliter (mg/dL) or above or taking medication for elevated triglyceride levels; HDL, or "good," cholesterol level below 40 mg/dL for men and below 50 mg/dL for women or taking medication for low HDL levels; blood pressure levels of 130/85 or above or taking medication for elevated blood pressure levels; fasting blood sugar levels of 100 mg/dL or above or taking medication for elevated blood glucose levels. Metabolic syndrome increases risk for diabetes and cardiovascular problems, so you and your doctor should take steps to reduce all of your risk factors. Typically, physicians retest blood pressure and cholesterol 3 to 6 months after you make healthy lifestyle changes to see if they're working. Ask your doctor how often you should be monitored.

- **YOU HAVE PREDIABETES:** Ask about more frequent office checks and home monitoring, too. Ask your doctor whether you should get a blood sugar meter for home blood sugar testing to uncover times of day when blood sugar is climbing toward the diabetic range. And make an appointment to have your blood sugar rechecked by your doctor in 6 months to a year.

- **YOU HAVE DIABETES:** Work with your doctor to establish a pattern of home blood sugar monitoring and get regular A1c checks. Depending on whether or not you use medications and on how tightly your blood sugar is controlled, you may need multiple daily checks or just a few tests per week. You also need two to four A1c tests a year. This measure of overall blood sugar level for the past 2 to 3 months shows how well your blood sugar was controlled around the clock, every day. High levels over

Outsmart Portion Distortion

Perhaps the most important tip for at-home and restaurant dining is to watch the size of your portions. It goes without saying that anything billed as "supersize" is something to be avoided, but beware dishes that don't advertise their generous proportions but still provide enough for two or three people. It always helps to have a visual reference to moderate your portions of different foods when you're dining out. For example:

One-half cup of cooked rice or pasta is considered one "serving." This is about the size of a mini fruit cup or half a baseball. If you're trying to limit your portion of rice or pasta to two servings, think two mini fruit cups or one baseball. Most Chinese restaurants provide far more than this amount of rice.

One standard-size slice of bread is considered one "serving" of bread. Compare rolls, buns, and other bread many years increase your odds for diabetes complications; in-control levels reduce risk. Home tests are available and can be convenient, but always share the results with your doctor and your diabetes care team so that changes can be made in your diabetes management plan if needed.

Over the years, you may find that your blood sugar levels begin to creep up—despite your best efforts. Your doctor may recommend that you begin using diabetes medications, add new ones, increase your doses, or even move to insulin. If that happens, take a deep breath and remember your top priority: good blood sugar control. Don't beat yourself up—and never, not for one second, doubt the benefits of healthy eating and exercise. These steps are proven to make your body more sensitive to insulin, the hormone that tells cells to let blood sugar in. They keep you healthy and lower your risk for diabetes-related complications. And they're absolutely worth continuing, even if you use blood-sugar-lowering medications.

products to this mental image and adjust your portion size accordingly: If the bun on your chicken sandwich or burger looks larger than two slices of bread, leave some bread on the plate.

Three ounces of cooked meat, the size of a deck of cards or a woman's palm, is considered one "serving." Most restaurants provide far more than this amount in an entrée. Savvy ways to cut back include ordering a half portion, having a sandwich instead of an entrée, or splitting a meal. You can also ask for a to-go box when your meal arrives and box up half of it before you even start eating.

One-fourth cup of shredded cheese is considered a single portion. That's about the size of a golf ball. According to the 2005 Dietary Guidelines, healthy adults need two to three servings of milk, yogurt, or cheese per day. If cheese is your weakness, think "golf ball" the next time you sprinkle cheese on your food.

Track Your Blood Pressure, Cholesterol, and Triglycerides

In Chapter 4, we also urged you to know these important numbers in addition to your blood sugar level—for two reasons. If you don't have diabetes, test results outside a normal healthy range—such as rising blood pressure or triglycerides or falling levels of "helpful" HDL cholesterol—can be indicators of rising diabetes risk. And if you have diabetes, prediabetes, or metabolic syndrome, you're also at high risk for heart disease and strokes, so keeping these important indicators of cardiovascular health within recommended ranges is vital.

When should you be rechecked? If any of your numbers were outside healthy ranges, ask your doctor about a retest in 3 to 6 months. It takes that long to see if healthy lifestyle changes (such as sticking with the Flat Belly Diet Diabetes) have made a difference. Your doctor or health-care practitioner should keep checking until a healthy lifestyle, or medication if necessary, brings these numbers in line. How often should you be retested after that? Your doc will probably check your blood pressure at every visit—and at the very least, once a year. Experts recommend cholesterol and triglyceride checks every 3 years between the ages of 20 and 39, every 2 years in your forties, and annually starting at age 50. If you have diabetes, Dr. Edelman recommends getting these checked every year.

In Closing

I'd like to close by reminding you of a crucial question I asked you earlier in this book: Who are you doing this for? There is still only one acceptable answer to that question. That answer is "for me." If you weren't quite sure of that back then, I hope that with the Core Confidences you've explored, you have the tools to arrive at that answer now.

This plan was created to help you see that focusing on yourself isn't an exercise in selfishness. In today's day and age, we are all overly committed to other people, whether it's the attention we lavish on our children and spouse, or the time we spend at our jobs, or the effort we put into building our communities. But none of those commitments is worth anything if you aren't first and foremost committed to yourself. The Flat Belly Diet Diabetes isn't a vanity ploy. It is a blood sugar–friendly weight-loss plan, formulated to meet the special needs of people with or at risk for diabetes. And it's based on the most credible—and safe—science that targets the most dangerous type of fat you carry on your body, the fat that threatens your very existence. If you want to live longer and healthier, keeping that fat is simply not an option.

This plan is less about achieving an ideal body than it is about creating a healthier life. If you remember nothing about the Flat Belly Diet but the fact that a healthy diet featuring a MUFA at every meal could help rescue your blood sugar and save your life, then I've done my job. And you've done yours.

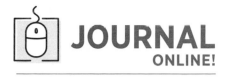

JOURNAL
ONLINE!

Log on to **www.prevention.com/ healthtrackers** for free access to *Prevention* magazine's comprehensive set of personal health-tracking tools. Perfect for keeping tabs on everything from meals and weight to blood sugar and cholesterol levels to your moods, energy level, and stress!

endnotes

Chapter 1

1. American Diabetes Association, "Total Prevalence of Diabetes & Pre-diabetes," http://www.diabetes.org/diabetes-statistics/prevalence.jsp.

2. S. Klein, D. B. Allison, S. B. Heymsfield, D. E. Kelley, R. L. Leibel, C. Nonas, and R. Kahn, "Waist Circumference and Cardiometabolic Risk: A Consensus Statement from Shaping America's Health: Association for Weight Management and Obesity Prevention; NAASO, The Obesity Society; the American Society for Nutrition; and the American Diabetes Association," *American Journal of Clinical Nutrition* 85, no. 5 (May 2007): 1197–202.

3. "Self-Reported Prediabetes and Risk-Reduction Activities—United States, 2006," *CDC: Morbidity and Mortality Weekly Report*, 57, no. 44 (November 7, 2008): 1203–5.

4. Centers for Disease Control and Prevention and the Agency for Healthcare Research and Quality, "Frequently Asked Questions: Prediabetes," 2008, http://www.cdc.gov/DIABETES/faq/prediabetes.htm.

5. I. Janssen, P. T. Katzmarzyk, and R. Ross, "Body Mass Index, Waist Circumference, and Health Risk: Evidence in Support of Current National Institutes of Health Guidelines," Archives of Internal Medicine 162, no. 18 (October 14, 2002): 2074–9.

6. American Diabetes Association, "Frequently Asked Questions about Women and Diabetes," http://www.diabetes.org/type-1-diabetes/women-diabetes-faqs.jsp.

7. Scott M. Grundy, James I. Cleeman, Stephen R. Daniels, Karen A. Donato, Robert H. Eckel, Barry A. Franklin, and David J. Gordon, et al., "Diagnosis and Management of the Metabolic Syndrome: An American Heart Association/National Heart, Lung, and Blood Institute Scientific Statement," Circulation 112 (2005): 2735–52.

8. Mark Stolar, "Metabolic Syndrome: Controversial but Useful," Cleveland Clinic Journal of Medicine 74, no. 3 (March 2007): 199–202, 205–8.

9. National Diabetes Education Program, "Type 2 Diabetes Risk After Gestational Diabetes," April 2006, http://www.ndep.nih.gov/resources/ResourceDetail.aspx?ResId=322.

10. B. E. Klein, R. Klein, S. E. Moss, and K. J. Cruickshanks, "Parental History of Diabetes in a Population-Based Study," *Diabetes Care* 19, no. 8 (1996): 827–30.

11. American Association of Clinical Endocrinologists, "Facts About Diabetes," http://www.aace.com/meetings/consensus/dcc/dc-facts.php.

12. K. M. V. Narayan, James P. Boyle, Theodore J. Thompson, Edward W. Gregg, and David F. Williamson, "Effect of BMI on Lifetime Risk for Diabetes in the U.S.," *Diabetes Care* 30 (2007): 1562–6.

13. Jamal S. Rana, Tricia Y. Li, JoAnn E. Manson, and Frank B. Hu, "Adiposity Compared With Physical Inactivity and Risk of Type 2 Diabetes in Women," *Diabetes Care* 30 (2007): 53–8.

Chapter 2

1. K. H. Liu, Y. L. Chan, W. B. Chan, W. L. Kong, M. O. Kong, and J. C. N. Chan, "Sonographic Measurement of Mesenteric Fat Thickness Is a Good Correlate with Cardiovascular Risk Factors: Comparison with Subcutaneous and Preperitoneal Fat Thickness, Magnetic Resonance Imaging and Anthropometric Indexes," *International Journal of Obesity* 27 (2003): 1267–73.

2. K. H. Liu, Y. L. Chan, W. B. Chan, J. C. N. Chan, and C. W. N. Chiu, "Mesenteric Fat Thickness Is an Independent Determinant of Metabolic Syndrome and Identifies Subjects With Increased Carotid Intima-Media Thickness," *Diabetes Care* 29, no. 2 (February 2006): 379–84.

3. Y. Cao, C. Hu, X. Meng, D. Wang, and J. Zhang, "Expression of TNF-α protein in Omental and Subcutaneous Adipose Tissue in Obesity," *Diabetes Research and Clinical Practice* 79, no. 2 (2008): 214–19.

4. Luigi Fontana, J. Christopher Eagon, Maria E. Trujillo, Philipp E. Scherer, and Samuel Klein, "Visceral Fat Adipokine Secretion Is Associated With Systemic Inflammation in Obese Humans," *Diabetes* 56, no. 4 (2007): 1010–13.

5. C. M. Steppan, S. T. Bailey, S. Bhat, E. J. Brown, R. R. Banerjee, C. M. Wright, H. R. Patel, R. S. Ahima, and M. A. Lazar, "The Hormone Resistin Links Obesity to Diabetes," *Nature* 409, no. 6818 (January 18, 2001): 307–12.

6. Chamukuttan Snehalatha, Bheekamchand Mukesh, Mary Simon, Vijay Viswanathan, Steven M. Haffner, and Ambady Ramachandran, "Plasma Adiponectin Is an Independent Predictor of Type 2 Diabetes in Asian Indians," *Diabetes Care* 26 (2003): 3226–29.

7. Sanjeev R. Mehta, E. Louise Thomas, Jimmy D. Bell, Desmond G. Johnston, and Simon D. Taylor-Robinson, "Non-Invasive Means of Measuring Hepatic Fat Content," *World Journal of Gastroenterology* 14, no. 22 (June 14, 2008): 3476–83.

8. N. O. Litbarg, K. P. Gudehithlu, P. Sethupathi, J. A. Arruda, G. Dunea, and A. K. Singh, "Activated Omentum Becomes Rich in Factors That Promote Healing and Tissue Regeneration," *Cell and Tissue Research* 328, no. 3 (June 2007): 487–97. Epub February 14, 2007.

9. T. Tran, Y. Yamamoto, S. Gesta, and C. Kahn, "Beneficial Effects of Subcutaneous Fat Transplantation on Metabolism," *Cell Metabolism* 7, no. 5 (May 2008): 410–20.

10. A Thörne, F. Lönnqvist, J. Apelman, G. Hellers, and P. Arner, "A Pilot Study of Long-term Effects of a Novel Obesity Treatment: Omentectomy in Connection with Adjustable Gastric Banding," *International Journal of Obesity* 26 (2002): 193–9.

11. "Thin People May Be Obese on the Inside," *Medical Research News* (May 14, 2007) Report on a study funded by the Medical Research Council under the direction of Dr. Jimmy Bell, professor of molecular imaging at Imperial College, London. http://www.news-medical.net/news/2007/05/14/25076.aspx

12. National Diabetes Information Clearinghouse, National Institute of Diabetes and Digestive and Kidney Diseases, National Institutes of Health, "What Diabetes Is," http://diabetes.niddk.nih.gov/DM/pubs/type1and2/what.htm.

13. I. Janssen, P. T. Katzmarzyk, and R. Ross, "Body Mass Index, Waist Circumference, and Health Risk: Evidence in Support of Current National Institutes of Health Guidelines," *Archives of Internal Medicine* 162 (October 14, 2002): 2074–9.

14. Amalia Gastaldelli, Yoshinori Miyazaki, Maura Pettiti, Masafumi Matsuda, Srihanth Mahankali, Eleonora Santini, Ralph A. DeFronzo, and Ele Ferrannini, "Metabolic Effects

of Visceral Fat Accumulation in Type 2 Diabetes," *Journal of Clinical Endocrinology & Metabolism* 87, no. 11 (November 2002): 5098–103.

15. Rena R. Wing, Randi Koeske, Leonard H. Epstein, Mary Patricia Nowalk, William Gooding, and Dorothy Becker, "Long-Term Effects of Modest Weight Loss in Type II Diabetic Patients," *Archives of Internal Medicine* 147, no. 10 (1987): 1749–53.

16. National Diabetes Information Clearinghouse, National Institute of Diabetes and Digestive and Kidney Diseases, National Institutes of Health, "What I Need to Know about Gestational Diabetes," April 2006, http://diabetes.niddk.nih.gov/dm/pubs/gestational/index.htm.

17. Scott M. Grundy, James I. Cleeman, Stephen R. Daniels, Karen A. Donato, Robert H. Eckel, Barry A. Franklin, and David J. Gordon, et al., "Diagnosis and Management of the Metabolic Syndrome: An American Heart Association/National Heart, Lung, and Blood Institute Scientific Statement," *Circulation* 112 (2005): 2735–52.

18. Beverly Balkau, Pascaline Picard, Sylviane Vol, Leopold Fezeu, and Eveline Eschwège, for the DESIR Study Group, "Consequences of Change in Waist Circumference on Cardiometabolic Risk Factors Over 9 Years: Data from an Epidemiological Study on the Insulin Resistance Syndrome (DESIR)," *Diabetes Care* 30, no. 7 (July 2007): 1901–3. Epub April 27, 2007.

19. National Center for Chronic Disease Prevention and Health Promotion, US Centers for Disease Control and Prevention and the Agency for Healthcare Research and Quality, "Frequently Asked Questions: Prediabetes," 2008, http://www.cdc.gov/DIABETES/faq/prediabetes.htm.

20. Elizabeth L. M. Barr, Paul Z. Zimmet, Timothy A. Welborn, Damien Jolley, Dianna J. Magliano, David W. Dunstan, and Adrian J. Cameron, et al., "Risk of Cardiovascular and All-Cause Mortality in Individuals With Diabetes Mellitus, Impaired Fasting Glucose, and Impaired Glucose Tolerance: The Australian Diabetes, Obesity, and Lifestyle Study," *Circulation* 116 (2007): 151–7.

21. S. M. Haffner, M. P. Stern, H. P. Hazuda, B. D. Mitchell, and J. K. Patterson, "Cardiovascular Risk Factors in Confirmed Prediabetic Individuals: Does the Clock for Coronary Heart Disease Start Ticking before the Onset of Clinical Diabetes?" *Journal of the American Medical Association* 263, no. 21 (June 6, 1990): 2893–8.

22. C. Zhang, K. M. Rexrode, R. M. van Dam, T. Y. Li, and F. B. Hu, "Abdominal Obesity and the Risk of All-Cause, Cardiovascular, and Cancer Mortality: Sixteen Years of Follow-Up in U.S. Women," *Circulation* 117, no. 13 (April 1, 2008): 1624–6.

23. I. Janssen, P. Katzmarzyk, R. Ross, "Body Mass Index, Waist Circumference, and Health Risk: Evidence in Support of Current National Institute of Health Guidelines," *Archives of Internal Medicine* 162, no. 18 (October 2002): 2074–79.

24. Susan Sam, Steven Haffner, Michael H. Davidson, Ralph B. D'Agostino Sr., Steven Feinstein, George Kondos, Alfonso Perez, and Theodore Mazzone, "Relationship of Abdominal Visceral and Subcutaneous Adipose Tissue with Lipoprotein Particle Number and Size in Type 2 Diabetes," *Diabetes* 57, no. 8 (2008): 2022–7.

25. D. V. Schapira, R. A. Clark, P. A. Wolff, A. R. Jarrett, N. B. Kumar, and N. M. Aziz, "Visceral Obesity and Breast Cancer Risk," *Cancer* 74, no. 2 (July 15, 1994): 632–9.

26. P. von Hafe, F. Pina, A. Pérez, M. Tavares, and H. Barros, "Visceral Fat Accumulation as a Risk Factor for Prostate Cancer," *Obesity Research* 12, no. 12 (December 2004): 1930–5.

27. Tobias Pischon, P. H. Lahmann, C. Friedenreich, T. Norat, A. Tjønnland, J. Halkjaer, and K. Overvad, et al., "Body Size and Risk of Colon and Rectal Cancer in the European Prospective Investigation into Cancer and Nutrition," *Journal of the National Cancer Institute* 98, no. 13 (July 5, 2006): 920–31.

28. R. A. Whitmer, D. R. Gustafson, E. Barrett-Connor, M. N. Haan, E. P. Gunderson, and K. Yaffe, "Central Obesity and Increased Risk of Dementia More Than Three Decades Later," *Neurology* 71, no. 14 (September 30, 2008): 1057–64.

29. E. J. Mayer-Davis, R. D'Agostino Jr., A. J. Karter, S. M. Haffner, M. J. Rewers, M. Saad, and R. N. Bergman, "Intensity and Amount of Physical Activity in Relation to Insulin Sensitivity: The Insulin Resistance Atherosclerosis Study," *Journal of the American Medical Association* 279, no. 9 (March 4, 1998): 669–74.

30. Frank B. Hu, Tricia Y. Li, Graham A. Colditz, Walter C. Willett, and JoAnn E. Manson, "Television Watching and Other Sedentary Behaviors in Relation to Risk of Obesity and Type 2 Diabetes Mellitus in Women," *Journal of the American Medical Association* 289 (2003): 1785–91.

31. E. Epel, R. Lapidus, B. McEwen, and K. Brownell, "Stress May Add Bite to Appetite in Women: A Laboratory Study of Stress-Induced Cortisol and Eating Behavior," *Psychoneuroendocrinology* 26, no. 1 (January 2001): 37–49.

32. F. F. Ribeiro-Filho, A. N. Faria, S. Azjen, M. T. Zanella, and S. R. Ferreira, "Methods of Estimation of Visceral Fat: Advantages of Ultrasonography," *Obesity Research* 11, no. 12 (December 2003): 1488–94.

33. National Institute of Diabetes and Digestive and Kidney Diseases, National Institutes of Health, US Department of Health and Human Services, "Weight and Waist Measurement: Tools for Adults," NIH Publication No. 04–5283, November 2008, http://www.win.niddk.nih.gov/publications/PDFs/Weightandwaist.pdf.

34. H. Schunkert, S. Moebus, J. Hanisch, P. Bramlage, E. Steinhagen-Thiessen, H. Hauner, J. Weil, J. Wasem, and K. H. Jöckel, "The Correlation between Waist Circumference and ESC Cardiovascular Risk Score: Data from the German Metabolic and Cardiovascular Risk Project (GEMCAS)," *Clinical Research in Cardiology* 97, no. 11 (November 2008): 827–35.

35. Michael E. J. Lean and Thang S. Han, "Fat and Visceral Fat: Time for Cardiologists to Act Against Obesity," *British Journal of Cardiology* 12, no. 4 (July/August 2005): 249–53.

36. A. Misra, N. K. Vikram, R. Gupta, R. M. Pandey, J. S. Wasir, and V. P. Gupta, "Waist Circumference Cutoff Points and Action Levels for Asian Indians for Identification of Abdominal Obesity," *International Journal of Obesity* 30, no. 1 (2006): 106–11.

37. J. G. Fan and Y. D. Pent, "Metabolic Syndrome and Non-Alcoholic Fatty Liver Disease: Asian Definitions and Asian Studies," *Hepatobiliary and Pancreatic Diseases International* 6, no. 6 (December 2007): 572–8.

38. Samuel Klein, "The Case of Visceral Fat: Argument for the Defense," *Journal of Clinical Investigation* 113, no. 11 (June 1, 2004): 1530–2.

39. J. C. Lovejoy, C. M. Champagne, L. de Jonge, H. Xie, and S. R. Smith, "Increased Visceral Fat and Decreased Energy Expenditure during the Menopausal Transition," *International Journal of Obesity* 32 (2008): 949–58.

40. J. A. Kanaley, I. Giannopoulou, G. Tillapaugh-Fay, J. S. Nappi, and L. L. Ploutz-Snyder, "Racial Differences in Subcutaneous and Visceral Fat Distribution in Postmenopausal Black and White Women," *Metabolism* 52, no. 2 (February 2003): 186–91.

41. T. S. Han, E. Gates, E. Truscott, and M. E. Lean, "Clothing Size as an Indicator of Adiposity, Ischaemic Heart Disease and Cardiovascular Risks," *Journal of Human Nutrition and Dietetics* 18, no. 6 (December 2005): 423–30.

42. A.Pascot, J. Després, I. Lemieux, N. Alméras, J. Bergeron, A. Nadeau, D. Prud'homme et al, "Deterioration of the Metabolic Risk Profile in Women: Respective Contributions of Impaired Glucose Tolerance and Visceral Fat Accumulation," *Diabetes Care* 24, no. 5 (May 2001): 902–908.

43. Wilfred Y. Fujimoto, Kathleen A. Jablonski, George A. Bray, Andrea Kriska, Elizabeth Barrett-Connor, Steven Haffner, and Robert Hanson, et al., for the Diabetes Prevention Program Research Group, "Body Size and Shape Changes and the Risk of Diabetes in the Diabetes Prevention Program," *Diabetes* 56, no. 6 (June 2007): 1680–5.

44. M. Brochu, A. Tchernof, A. N. Turner, P. A. Ades, and E. T. Poehlman, "Is There a Threshold of Visceral Fat Loss That Improves the Metabolic Profile in Obese Postmenopausal Women?" *Metabolism* 52, no. 5 (May 2003): 599–604.

45. T. P. Markovic, L. V. Campbell, S. Balasubramanian, A. B. Jenkins, A. C. Fleury, L. A. Simons, and D. J. Chisholm, "Beneficial Effect on Average Lipid Levels from Energy Restriction and Fat Loss in Obese Individuals with or without Type 2 Diabetes," *Diabetes Care* 21, no. 5 (1988): 695–700.

46. André Tchernof, Amy Nolan, Cynthia K. Sites, Philip A. Ades, and Eric T. Poehlman, "Weight Loss Reduces C-Reactive Protein Levels in Obese Postmenopausal Women," *Circulation* 105 (2002): 564.

47. The Diabetes Prevention Program Research Group, "Intensive Lifestyle Intervention or Metformin on Inflammation and Coagulation in Participants with Impaired Glucose Tolerance," *Diabetes* 54, no. 5 (May 2005): 1566–72.

Chapter 3

1. Meals Matter, "Portion Distortion: Serving Sizes Are Growing," http://www.mealsmatter.org/EatingForHealth/Topics/article.aspx?articleId=53.

2. Centers for Disease Control and Prevention, "Obesity among Adults in the United States—No Statistically Significant Change Since 2003–2004. Data Brief Number 1," November 2007.

3. American Diabetes Association, "Prevalence of Diabetes Rose 5% Annually Since 1990," 2007, http://www.diabetes.org/diabetesnewsarticle.jsp?storyId=15351710&filename=20070623/ADA20070623118262585664IEDIT.xml.

4. Centers for Disease Control and Prevention, "State-Specific Incidence of Diabetes Among Adults—Participating States, 1995–1997 and 2005–2007," *Morbidity and Mortality Weekly Report* 57, no. 3 (October 31, 2008): 1169–73.

5. B. V. Howard, J. E. Manson, M. L. Stefanick, S. A. Beresford, G. Frank, B. Jones, and R. J. Rodabough, et al., "Low-Fat Dietary Pattern and Weight Change Over 7 Years: The Women's Health Initiative Dietary Modification Trial," *Journal of the American Medical Association* 295 (February 2006): 39–49.

6. Finding Your Way to a Healthier You: Based on the *Dietary Guidelines for Americans*, US Department of Health and Human Services, US Department of Agriculture, 2005, http://www.cnpp.usda.gov/Publications/DietaryGuidelines/2005/2005DGConsumerBrochure.pdf.

7. D. Grassi, G. Desideri, S. Necozione, C. Lippi, R. Casale, G. Properzi, and J. B. Blumberg, "Blood Pressure Is Reduced and Insulin Sensitivity Increased in Glucose-Intolerant, Hypertensive Subjects after 15 Days of Consuming High-Polyphenol Dark Chocolate," *The Journal of Nutrition* 138, no. 9 (September 2008): 1671–6.

8. Z. Faridi, V. Y. Njike, S. Dutta, A. Ali, and D. L. Katz, "Acute Dark Chocolate and Cocoa Ingestion and Endothelial Function: A Randomized Controlled Crossover Trial," *American Journal of Clinical Nutrition* 88, no. 1 (July 2008): 58–63.

9. University of Michigan, "Healing Foods Pyramid: Dark Chocolate," http://www.med.umich.edu/UMIM/food-pyramid/dark_chocolate.htm.

10. R. D. Mattes, P. M. Kris-Etherton, and G. D. Foster, "Impact of Peanuts and Tree Nuts on Body Weight and Healthy Weight Loss in Adults," *The Journal of Nutrition* 138, no. 9 (September 2008): 1741S–45S.

11. K. McManus, L. Antinoro, and F. Sacks, "A Randomized Controlled Trial of a Moderate-Fat, Low-Energy Diet Compared with a Low-Fat, Low-Energy Diet for Weight Loss in Overweight Adults," *International Journal of Obesity* 25, no. 10 (October 2001): 1503–11.

12. C. L. Pelkman, V. K. Fishell, D. H. Maddox, T. A. Pearson, D. T. Mauger, and P. M. Kris-Etherton, "Effects of Moderate-Fat (from Monounsaturated Fat) and Low-Fat Weight-Loss Diets on the Serum Lipid Profile in Overweight and Obese Men and Women," *American Journal of Clinical Nutrition* 79, no. 2 (February 2004): 204–12.

13. K. Z. Walker, K. O'Dea, L. Johnson, A. J. Sinclair, L. S. Piers, G. C. Nicholson, and J. G. Muir, "Body Fat Distribution and Non-Insulin-Dependent Diabetes: Comparison of a Fiber-Rich, High-Carbohydrate, Low-Fat (23%) Diet and a 35% Fat Diet High in Monounsaturated Fat," *American Journal of Clinical Nutrition* 63, no. 2 (February 1996): 254–60.

14. J. A. Paniagua, A. Gallego de la Sacristana, I. Romero, A. Vidal-Puig, J. M. Latre, E. Sanchez, and P. Perez-Martinez, et al., "Monounsaturated Fat-Rich Diet Prevents Central Body Fat Distribution and Decreases Postprandial Adiponectin Expression Induced by a Carbohydrate-Rich Diet in Insulin-Resistant Subjects," *Diabetes Care* 30, no. 7 (July 2007): 1717–23.

15. S. Lemieux, D. Prud'homme, A. Nadeau, A. Tremblay, C. Bouchard, and J. P. Després, "Seven-Year Changes in Body Fat and Visceral Adipose Tissue in Women: Association with Indexes of Plasma Glucose-Insulin Homeostasis," *Diabetes Care* 19, no. 9 (September 1996): 983–91.

16. B. Vessby, M. Unsitupa, K. Hermansen, G. Riccardi, A. A. Rivellese, L. C. Tapsell, and C. Nälsén, et al., "Dietary Saturated Fat for Monounsaturated Fat Impairs Insulin Sensitivity in Healthy Men and Women," *Diabetologia* 44, no. 3 (March 2001): 312–9.

17. P. M. Kris-Etherton, F. B. Hu, E. Ros, and J. Sabaté, "The Role of Tree Nuts and Peanuts in the Prevention of Coronary Heart Disease: Multiple Potential Mechanisms," *Journal of Nutrition* 138, no. 9 (September 2008): 1746S–51S.

18. J. A. Paniagua, A. G. de la Sacristana, E. Sánchez, I. Romero, A. Vidal-Puig, F. J. Berral, and A. Escribano, et al., "A MUFA-Rich Diet Improves Postprandial Glucose, Lipid and GLP-1 Responses in Insulin-Resistant Subjects," *Journal of the American College of Nutrition* 26, no. 5 (October 2007): 434–44.

19. Richard D. Mattes, Penny M. Kris-Etherton, and Gary D. Foster, "Impact of Peanuts and Tree Nuts on Body Weight and Healthy Weight Loss in Adults," Journal of Nutrition 138 (2008): 1741S–5S.

20. J. Salas-Salvadó, J. Fernández-Ballart, E. Ros, M. A. Martínez-González, M. Fitó, R. Estruch, D. Corella, and M. Fiol, et al., "Effect of a Mediterranean Diet Supplemented with Nuts on Metabolic Syndrome Status: One-Year Results of the PREDIMED Randomized Trial," *Archives of Internal Medicine* 168, no. 22 (December 2008): 2449–58.

21. I. Shai, D. Schwarzfuchs, Y. Henkin, D. R. Shahar, S. Witkow, I. Greenberg, and R. Golan, et al., "Weight Loss with a Low-Carbohydrate, Mediterranean, or Low-Fat Diet," *New England Journal of Medicine* 359, no. 3 (July 17, 2008): 229–41.

22. A. S. Rocca, J. LaGreca, J. Kalitsky, and P. L. Brubaker, "Monounsaturated Fatty Acid Diets Improve Glycemic Tolerance through Increased Secretion of Glucagon-Like Peptide-1," *Endocrinology* 142, no. 3 (March 2001): 1148–55.

23. A. C. Tierney and H. M. Roche, "The Potential Role of Olive Oil-Derived MUFA in Insulin Sensitivity," *Molecular Nutrition and Food Research* 51, no. 10 (October 2007): 1235–48.

24. M. D. Ashen and R. Blumental, "Low HDL Cholesterol Levels," *New England Journal of Medicine* 353, no. 12 (September 22, 2005). 1252–60.

25. I. Bondia-Pons, H. Schröder, M. I. Covas, A. I. Castellote, J. Kaikkonen, H. E. Poulsen, and A. V. Gaddi, et al., "Moderate Consumption of Olive Oil by Healthy European Men Reduces Systolic Blood Pressure in Non-Mediterranean Participants," *Journal of Nutrition* 137, no. 1 (January 2007): 84–7.

26. S. Terés, G. Barceló-Coblijn, M. Benet, R. Alvarez, R. Bressani, J. E. Halver, and P. V. Escribá, "Oleic Acid Content Is Responsible for the Reduction in Blood Pressure Induced by Olive Oil," *Proceedings of the National Academy of Sciences of the United States of America* 105, no. 37 (September 16, 2008): 13811–6.

27. K. Esposito, R. Marfella, M. Ciotola, C. Di Palo, F. Giugliano, G. Giugliano, and M. D'Armiento, et al., "Effect of a Mediterranean-Style Diet on Endothelial Dysfunction and Markers of Vascular Inflammation in the Metabolic Syndrome: A Randomized Trial," *Journal of the American Medical Association* 292, no. 12 (September 22, 2004): 1440–6.

28. H. Ueshima, J. Stamler, P. Elliott, Q. Chan, I. J. Brown, M. R. Carnethon, and M. L. Daviglus, et al., "Food Omega-3 Fatty Acid Intake of Individuals (Total, Linolenic Acid, Long-Chain) and Their Blood Pressure. INTERMAP Study," *Hypertension* 50, no. 2 (August 2007): 313–9.

29. E. B. Rimm, W. C. Willett, F. B. Hu, L. Sampson, G. A. Colditz, J. E. Manson, C. Hennekens, and M. J. Stampfer, "Folate and Vitamin B_6 from Diet and Supplementation in Relation to Risk of Coronary Heart Disease among Women," *Journal of the American Medical Association* 279, no. 5 (February 1998): 359–64.

30. N. Z. Unlu, T. Bohn, S. K. Clinton, and S. J. Schwartz, "Carotenoid Absorption from Salad and Salsa by Humans Is Enhanced by the Addition of Avocado or Avocado Oil," *Journal of Nutrition* 135, no. 3 (March 2005): 431–6.

31. D. Taubert, R. Roesen, C. Lehmann, N. Jung, and E. Schömig, "Effects of Low Habitual Cocoa Intake on Blood Pressure and Bioactive Nitric Oxide: A Randomized Controlled Trial," *Journal of the American Medical Association* 298, no. 1 (July 2007): 49–60.

32. T. T. Fung, K. M. Rexrode, C. S. Mantzoros, J. E. Manson, W. C. Willett, and F. B. Hu, "Mediterranean Diet and Incidence of and Mortality from Coronary Heart Disease and Stroke in Women," *Circulation* 118, no. 8 (March 2009): 1093–100.

33. A. Esmaillzadeh, M. Kimiagar, Y. Mehrabi, L. Azadbakht, F. B. Hu, and W. C. Willett, "Fruit and Vegetable Intakes, C-Reactive Protein, and the Metabolic Syndrome," *American Journal of Clinical Nutrition* 84, no. 6 (December 2006): 1489–97.

34. World Cancer Research Fund, American Institute for Cancer Research, "Food, Nutrition, Physical Activity, and the Prevention of Cancer: A Global Perspective," 2007, http://www.dietandcancerreport.org/.

35. F. J. He, C. A. Nowson, and G. A. MacGregor, "Fruit and Vegetable Consumption and Stroke: Meta-Analysis of Cohort Studies," *Lancet* 367, no. 9507 (2006): 320–6.

36. H. C. Hung, K. J. Joshipura, R. Jiang, F. B. Hu, D. Hunter, S. A. Smith-Warner, and G.A. Colditz, "Fruit and Vegetable Intake and Risk of Major Chronic Disease," *Journal of the National Cancer Institute* 96, no. 21 (November 2004): 1577–84.

37. J. S. de Munter, F. B. Hu, D. Spiegelman, M. Franz, and R. M. van Dam, "Whole Grain, Bran, and Germ Intake and Risk of Type 2 Diabetes: A Prospective Cohort Study and Systematic Review," *PLoS Medicine* 4, no. 8 (August 2007): e261.

38. D. R. Jacobs Jr., L. F. Andersen, and R. Blomhoff, "Whole-Grain Consumption Is Associated with a Reduced Risk of Noncardiovascular, Noncancer Death Attributed to Inflammatory Diseases in the Iowa Women's Health Study," *American Journal of Clinical Nutrition* 85, no. 6 (June 2007): 1606–14.

39. M. C. Gannon, F. Q. Nuttall, A. Saeed, K. Jordan, and H. Hoover, "An Increase in Dietary Protein Improves the Blood Glucose Response in Persons with Type 2 Diabetes," *American Journal of Clinical Nutrition* 78, no. 4 (October 2003): 734–41.

40. P. L. Lutsey, L. M. Steffen, and J. Stevens, "Dietary Intake and the Development of the Metabolic Syndrome: The Atherosclerosis Risk in Communities Study," *Circulation* 117, no. 6 (February 2008): 754–61.

41. D. K. Layman and J. I. Baum, "Dietary Protein Impact on Glycemic Control during Weight Loss," *Journal of Nutrition* 134, no. 4 (April 2004): 968S–73S.

42. US Environmental Protection Agency, "Mercury Levels in Commercial Fish and Shellfish," May 7, 2009, http://www.cfsan.fda.gov/~frf/sea-mehg.html.

43. W. S. Harris, D. Mozaffarian, E. Rimm, P. Kris-Etherton, L. L. Rudel, L. J. Appel, and M. M. Engler, "Omega-6 Fatty Acids and Risk for Cardiovascular Disease: A Science Advisory from the American Heart Association Nutrition Subcommittee of the Council on Nutrition, Physical Activity, and Metabolism; Council on Cardiovascular Nursing; and Council on Epidemiology and Prevention," *Circulation* 119, no. 6 (February 2009): 902–7.

Chapter 4

1. American College of Endocrinology, "Consensus Statement on Guidelines for Glycemic Control," *Endocrine Practice* 8, supplement 1 (January/February 2002): 5–11.

2. T. D. Wiggin, K. A. Sullivan, R. Pop-Busui, A. Amato, A. A. Sima, and E. L. Feldman, "Elevated Triglycerides Correlate with Progression of Diabetic Neuropathy," *Diabetes* 58, no. 7 (July 2009): 1634–40.

3. S. M. Grundy, J. I. Cleeman, S. R. Daniels, K. A. Donato, R. H. Eckel, B. A. Franklin, and D. J. Gordon, et al., "Diagnosis and Management of the Metabolic Syndrome: An American Heart Association/National Heart, Lung, and Blood Institute Scientific Statement," *Circulation* 112, no. 17 (October 25, 2005): 2735–52.

4. M. Stolar, "Metabolic Syndrome: Controversial but Useful," *Cleveland Clinic Journal of Medicine* 74, no. 3 (March 2007): 205–8.

5. S. G. Wannamethee, A. G. Shaper, L. Lennon, and R. W. Morris, "Metabolic syndrome vs. Framingham risk score for prediction of coronary heart disease, stroke, and type 2 diabetes mellitus," *Archives of Internal Medicine* 165, no. 22 (December 2005): 2644–50.

6. M. P. Stern, K. Williams, C. González-Villalpando, K. J. Hunt, and S. M. Haffner, "Does the Metabolic Syndrome Improve Identification of Individuals at Risk of Type 2 Diabetes and/or Cardiovascular Disease?" *Diabetes Care* 27, no. 11. (November 2004): 2676–81.

7. S. M. Grundy, "A Changing Paradigm for Prevention of Cardiovascular Disease: Emergence of the Metabolic Syndrome as a Multiplex Risk Factor," *European Heart Journal* 10, Suppl B (2008): B16–23.

8. American Diabetes Association, "Prevalence of Diabetes in the United States 2009," http://www.diabetes.org/diabetes-statistics/prevalence.jsp.

9. National Diabetes Information Clearinghouse, National Institute of Diabetes and Digestive and Kidney Diseases, National Institutes of Health, "Am I At Risk For Type 2 Diabetes?" 2008, http://diabetes.niddk.nih.gov/dm/pubs/riskfortype2/index.htm.

10. E. S. Ford, W. H. Giles, and W. H. Dietz, "Prevalence of the Metabolic Syndrome among U.S. Adults: Findings from the Third National Health and Examination Survey," *Journal of the American Medical Association* 287, no. 3 (January 2002): 356–9.

11. Yong-Woo Park, Shankuan Zhu, Latha Palaniappan, Stanley Heshka, Mercedes R. Carnethon, and Steven B. Heymsfield, "The Metabolic Syndrome: Prevalence and Associated Risk Factor Findings in the US Population From the Third National Health and Nutrition Examination Survey, 1988–1994," *Archives of Internal Medicine* 163 (2003): 427–36.

12. M. M. Engelgau, L. S. Geiss, J. B. Saaddine, J. P. Boyle, S. M. Benjamin, E. W. Gregg, and E. F. Tierney, et al., "The Evolving Diabetes Burden in the United States," *Annals of Internal Medicine* 140, no. 11 (June 2004): 945–50.

13. R. H. Cobin, J. A. Davidson, O. P. Ganda, A. J. Garber, R. Hellman, P. S. Jellinger, and C. S. Levetan, et al., for the Consensus Statement Writing Committee, "American College of Endocrinology Consensus Statement on Guidelines for Glycemic Control," *Endocrine Practice* 8, no. S1 (January/February 2002): 6–9.

14. Centers for Disease Control and Prevention, "Self-Reported Prediabetes and Risk-Reduction Activities—United States, 2006," *Morbidity and Mortality Weekly Report* 57, no. 44 (November 7, 2008): 1203–5.

15. Centers for Disease Control and Prevention, "Prevalence of Self-Reported Cardiovascular Disease among Persons Aged >35 Years with Diabetes—United States, 1997-2005," *Morbidity and Mortality Weekly Report* 56, no. 43 (November 2, 2007): 1133–7.

16. American Association of Clinical Endocrinologists, "State of Diabetes Complications in America: Washington, D.C., May 18, 2005," http://www.stateofdiabetes.com.

17. E. S. Ford, W. H. Giles, and W. H. Dietz, "Prevalence of the Metabolic Syndrome among U.S. Adults: Findings from the Third National Health and Examination Survey," *Journal of the American Medical Association* 287, no. 3 (January 2002): 356–9.

18. Yong-Woo Park, Shankuan Zhu, Latha Palaniappan, Stanley Heshka, Mercedes R. Carnethon, and Steven B. Heymsfield, "The Metabolic Syndrome: Prevalence and Associated Risk Factor Findings in the US Population From the Third National Health and Nutrition Examination Survey, 1988–1994," *Archives of Internal Medicine* 163 (2003): 427–36.

19. L. B. Tankó, Y. Z. Bagger, G. Qin, P. Alexandersen, P. J. Larsen, and C. Christiansen, "Enlarged Waist Combined with Elevated Triglycerides Is a Strong Predictor of Accelerated Atherogenesis and Related Cardiovascular Mortality in Postmenopausal Women," *Circulation* 111, no. 15 (April 2005): 1883–90.

20. Centers for Disease Control and Prevention and the Agency for Healthcare Research and Quality, "Frequently Asked Questions: Prediabetes," July 8, 2008, http://www.cdc.gov/DIABETES/faq/prediabetes.htm.

21. W. C. Knowler, E. Barrett-Connor, S. E. Fowler, R. F. Hamman, J. M. Lachin, E. A. Walker, and D. M. Nathan, for the Diabetes Prevention Program Research Group, "Reduction in the Incidence of Type 2 Diabetes with Lifestyle Intervention or Metformin," *New England Journal of Medicine* 346, no. 6 (February 2002): 393–403.

Chapter 5

1. R. S. Surwit, M. A. van Tilburg, N. Zucker, C. C. McCaskill, P. Parekh, M. N. Feinglos, and C. L. Edwards, et al., "Stress Management Improves Long-Term Glycemic Control in Type 2 Diabetes," *Diabetes Care* 25, no. 1 (January 2002): 30–4.

2. K. E. Innes, C. Bourguignon, and A. G. Taylor, "Risk Indices Associated with the Insulin Resistance Syndrome, Cardiovascular Disease, and Possible Protection with Yoga: A Systematic Review," *Journal of the American Board of Family Practice* 18, no. 6 (November–December 2005): 491–519.

3. E. Newman, D. B. O'Connor, and M. Conner, "Daily Hassles and Eating Behaviour: The Role of Cortisol Reactivity Status," *Psychoneuroendocrinology* 32, no. 2 (February 2007): 125–32.

4. G. Oliver, J. Wardle, and E. L. Gibson, "Stress and Food Choice: A Laboratory Study," *Psychosomatic Medicine* 62, no. 6 (November–December 2000): 853–65.

5. G. Hawley, C. Horwath, A. Gray, A. Bradshaw, L. Katzer, J. Joyce, and S. O'Brien, "Sustainability of Health and Lifestyle Improvements Following a Non-Dieting Randomised Trial in Overweight Women," *Preventive Medicine* 47, no. 6 (December 2008): 593–9.

6. N. Grant, M. Hamer, and A. Steptoe, "Social Isolation and Stress-Related Cardiovascular, Lipid, and Cortisol Responses," *Annals of Behavioral Medicine* 37, no. 1 (February 2009): 29–37.

7. N. I. Eisenberger, M. D. Lieberman, and K. D. Williams, "Does Rejection Hurt? An fMRI Study of Social Exclusion," *Science* 302, no. 5643 (October 2003): 290–2.

8. L. E. Carlson, M. Speca, P. Faris, and K. D. Patel, "One Year Pre-Post Intervention Follow-Up of Psychological, Immune, Endocrine and Blood Pressure Outcomes of Mindfulness-Based Stress Reduction (MBSR) in Breast and Prostate Cancer Outpatients," *Brain, Behavior, and Immunity* 21, no. 8 (November 2007): 1038–49.

9. S. L. Shapiro, J. A. Astin, S. R. Bishop, and M. Cordova, "Mindfulness-Based Stress Reduction for Health Care Professionals: Results from a Randomized Trial," *International Journal of Stress Management* 12, no. 2 (2005): 164–76.

10. E. Epel, S. Jimenez, K. Brownell, L. Stroud, C. Stoney, and R. Niaura, "Are Stress Eaters at Risk for the Metabolic Syndrome?" *Annals of the New York Academy of Science* 1032 (December 2004): 208–10.

11. T. Okura, Y. Nakata, D. J. Lee, K. Ohkawara, and K. Tanaka, "Effects of Aerobic Exercise and Obesity Phenotype on Abdominal Fat Reduction in Response to Weight Loss," *International Journal of Obesity* 29, no. 10 (October 2005): 1259–66.

12. E. J. Mayer-Davis, R. D'Agostino, A. J. Karter, S. M. Haffner, M. J. Rewers, M. Saad, and R. N. Bergman, "Intensity and Amount of Physical Activity in Relation to Insulin Sensitivity: The Insulin Resistance Atherosclerosis Study," *Journal of the American Medical Association* 279, no. 9 (March 1998): 669–74.

13. F. Hu, T. Y. Li, G. A. Colditz, W. C. Willett, and J. E. Manson, "Television Watching and Other Sedentary Behaviors in Relation to Risk of Obesity and Type 2 Diabetes Mellitus in Women," *Journal of the American Medical Association* 289, no. 14 (April 2003): 1785–91.

14. C. Castaneda, J. E. Layne, L. Munoz-Orians, P. L. Gordon, J. Walsmith, M. Foldvari, and R. Roubenoff, "A Randomized Controlled Trial of Resistance Exercise Training to Improve Glycemic Control in Older Adults with Type 2 Diabetes," *Diabetes Care* 25, no. 12 (December 2002): 2335–41.

15. R. Sigal, G. P. Kenny, N. G. Boulé, G. A. Wells, D. Prud'homme, M. Fortier, and R. D. Reid, "Effects of Aerobic Training, Resistance Training, or Both on Glycemic Control in Type 2 Diabetes: A Randomized Trial," *Annals of Internal Medicine* 147, no. 6 (September 2007): 357–69.

16. M. G. Flynn, B. K. McFarlin, and M. M. Markofski, "State of the Art Reviews: The Anti-Inflammatory Actions of Exercise Training," *American Journal of Lifestyle Medicine* 1, no. 3 (2007): 220–35.

17. Mayo Clinic, "Depression and Anxiety: Exercise Eases Symptoms," October 23, 2007, http://www.mayoclinic.com/health/depression-and-exercise/MH00043.

18. P. Hassmen, N. Koivula, and A. Uutela, "Physical Exercise and Psychological Well-Being: A Population Study in Finland," *Preventive Medicine* 30, no. 1 (January 2000): 17–25.

19. J. E. Gangwisch, S. B. Heymsfield, B. Boden-Albala, R. M. Buijs, F. Kreier, T. G. Pickering, and A. G. Rundle, "Sleep Duration as a Risk Factor for Diabetes Incidence in a Large U.S. Sample," *Sleep* 30, no. 12 (December 2007): 1667–73.

20. K. Knutson, A. M. Ryden, B. A. Mander, and E. K. Van Cauter, "Role of Sleep Duration and Quality in the Risk and Severity of Type 2 Diabetes Mellitus," *Archives of Internal Medicine* 166, no. 16 (September 2006): 1768–74.

21. K. Spiegel, E. Tasali, P. Penev, and E. Van Cauter, "Brief Communication: Sleep Curtailment in Healthy Young Men Is Associated with Decreased Leptin Levels, Elevated Ghrelin Levels, and Increased Hunger and Appetite," *Annals of Internal Medicine* 141, no. 11 (December 7, 2004): 846-50.

22. A. V. Nedeltcheva, L. Kessler, J. Imperial, and P. D. Penev, "Exposure to Recurrent Sleep Restriction in the Setting of High Caloric Intake and Physical Inactivity Results in Increased Insulin Resistance and Reduced Glucose Tolerance," *The Journal of Clinical Endocrinology and Metabolism*, published online ahead of print June 30, 2009.

23. D. Einhorn, D. A. Stewart, M. K. Erman, N. Gordon, A. Philis-Tsimikas, and E. Casal, "Prevalence of Sleep Apnea in a Population of Adults with Type 2 Diabetes Mellitus," *Endocrine Practice* 13, no. 4 (July–August 2007): 355–62.

24. Rosalind Cartwright, "Sleeping Together: A Pilot Study of the Effects of Shared Sleeping on Adherence to CPAP Treatment in Obstructive Sleep Apnea," *The Journal of Clinical Sleep Medicine* 4, no. 2 (April 15, 2008): 123–7.

25. H. Landolt, J. V. Rétey, K. Tönz, J. M. Gottselig, R. Khatami, I. Buckelmüller, and P. Achermann, "Caffeine Attenuates Waking and Sleep Electroencephalographic Markers of Sleep Homeostasis in Humans," *Neuropsychopharmacology* 29, no. 10 (July 2004): 1933–39.

26. J. Chawla and A. Suleman, "Neurologic Effects of Caffeine" (November 26, 2008), http://emedicine.medscape.com/article/1182710-overview

27. M. J. Shirlow and C. D. Mathers, "A Study of Caffeine Consumption and Symptoms: Indigestion, Palpitations, Tremor, Headache and Insomnia," *International Journal of Epidemiology* 14, no. 2 (June 1985): 239–48.

Chapter 6

1. J. F. Hollis, C. M. Gullion, V. J. Stevens, P. J. Brantley, L. J. Appel, J. D. Ard, and C. M. Champagne, "Weight Loss during the Intensive Intervention Phase of the Weight-Loss Maintenance Trial," *American Journal of Preventive Medicine* 35, no. 2 (August 2008): 118–26.

Chapter 7

1. J. W. Pennebaker, J. K. Kiecolt-Glaser, and R. Glaser, "Disclosure of Traumas and Immune Function: Health Implications for Psychotherapy," *Journal of Consulting and Clinical Psychology* 56, no. 2 (April 1988): 239–45.
2. J. F. Hollis, C. M. Gullion, V. J. Stevens, P. J. Brantley, L. J. Appel, J. D. Ard, and C. M. Champagne, "Weight Loss during the Intensive Intervention Phase of the Weight-Loss Maintenance Trial," *American Journal of Preventive Medicine* 35, no. 2 (August 2008): 118–26.

Chapter 8

1. US Department of Agriculture, "Dietary Guidelines for Americans, 2005," updated July 9, 2008, http://www.health.gov/DIETARYGUIDELINES/dga2005/document/html/chapter2.htm.

Chapter 9

1. B. Wansink and P. Chandon, "Meal Size, Not Body Size, Explains Errors in Estimating the Calorie Content of Meals," *Archives of Internal Medicine* 145, no. 5 (September 5, 2006): 326–32.

Chapter 11

1. American Council on Exercise, "New Study Puts the Crunch on Ineffective Ab Exercises," http://www.acefitness.org/getfit/studies/bestworstabexercises.pdf.
2. A. J. Blood and R. J. Zatorre, "Intensely Pleasurable Responses to Music Correlate with Activity in Brain Regions Implicated in Reward and Emotion," *Proceedings of the National Academy of Sciences* 98, no. 20 (September 25, 2001): 11818–23.
3. C. F. Emery, E. T. Hsiao, S. M. Hill, and D. J. Fried, "Short-Term Effects of Exercise and Music on Cognitive Performance Among Participants in a Cardiac Rehabilitation Program," *Heart and Lung: The Journal of Acute and Critical Care* 32, no. 6 (November/December 2003): 368–73.

index

Underscored page references indicate sidebars and tables.
Boldface references indicate photographs.

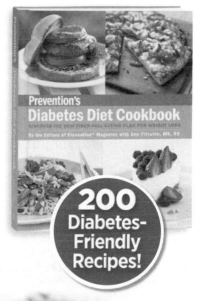

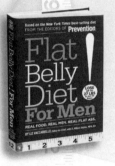
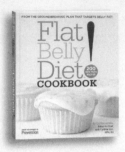
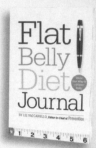
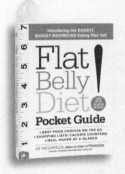
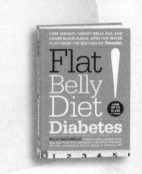
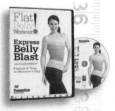
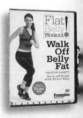